Nursing

Ethics

and

Law

Nursing Ethics and Law

JACQULYN K. HALL, R.N., J.D.

W. B. SAUNDERS COMPANY

A Division of Harcourt Brace & Company

Philadelphia London Toronto Montreal Sydney Tokyo

W. B. SAUNDERS COMPANY
A Division of Harcourt Brace & Company
The Curtis Center
Independence Square West
Philadelphia, PA 19106

This publication is designed to provide accurate and authoritative information in regard to the subject matter covered. In publishing this book neither the author nor the publisher is engaged in rendering legal, accounting or other professional service. If legal advice or other expert assistance is required, the services of a competent professional should be sought.

Library of Congress Cataloging-in-Publication Data

Hall, Jacqulyn Kay.
  Nursing ethics and law / Jacqulyn Kay Hall.
    p.   cm.
  ISBN 0-7216-4991-2
  1. Nursing ethics. 2. Nursing—Law and legislation—United States. I. Title.
  [DNLM: 1. Ethics, Nursing. 2. Legislation, Nursing—United States. WY 85 H177n 1996]
  RT85.H24   1996
  174'.2—dc20
  DNLM/DLC
                                                95-42001

Cover photograph: R. Krubner/H. Armstrong Roberts

NURSING ETHICS AND LAW   ISBN 0-7216-4991-2

Printed in the United States of America

Last digit is the print number: 9 8 7 6 5 4 3 2 1

To Hal

"And, when he shall die, cut him out in little stars,
and he shall make the face of heaven so fine that
all the world will be in love with night,
and pay no worship to the garish sun."
—SHAKESPEARE, *Romeo and Juliet*

PREFACE

This unique book is the essence I have distilled from years of learning and practice in nursing and law, experiences in sailing the Caribbean and Atlantic, and from living and studying history and philosophy in Europe—all the while observing nursing and America close up and from a distance. This is a labor of love, written for nurses who care for patients and who will care some day for me, to dispel their fear. They can lay down at last the tomes of ethics and law and get on with the work of nursing, certain in the knowledge that doing good nursing is right and legal.

CONTENTS

ONE

Values in Ethics and Law • 1
INTRODUCTION • ETHICS • LAW

Introduction—*2* • Ethics → Law—*3* • Organization of the Book—*7* • Limits to Ethics and Law—*10*

Ethics—*13* • Values Underlying Illness Care Law—*14* • History: A Brief Overview—*15* • Professional Ethics—*18* • Codes of Ethics—*26* • Preambles of the Codes—*29* • Competence—*30* • Values in Conflict?—*37* • Interests and Emotions—*38* • Philosophy and Religion—*40* • The Ideal and the Real: Two Views of the World—*42*

Law—Based on Ethics, but Not the Highest Ethic—*49* • Theory of Morality Development—*52* • Feminist Morality—*56* • Ethics Committees—*58* • Ethicists and Decision Making—*60* • Law—*67* • Philosophies of Law—*68* • History of Law: A Brief Overview—*69* • Rights—Limits on Government Power—*74* • Divisions of Law: Criminal and Civil Law—*79* • Statutes—*82* • Regulations and Rules—*88* • Case Law—*93*

TWO

Ethics and Law of
Doing Good (Beneficence) • 105
MALPRACTICE

Beneficence (Doing Good): The Value As Basis for the Law—*106* • Pater/Maternalism—*107* • Malpractice: Laws Enforcing the Ethic—*108* • Four Essentials of Malpractice—*110* • Defenses in Malpractice Law—*119* • Malpractice Insurance—*123* • General Tort Law—*126* • Vicarious Liability—*126* • Strict Liability (Assumption of Risk, Product Liability)—*129* • Immunities—*132* • Joint and Several Liability—*134* • Statutes of Limitation—*136* • Tort Reform—*139* • Avoiding Lawsuits—*146* • Managing Lawsuits—*149* • Documentation—*151*

THREE

Ethics and Law of
Doing No Harm (Non-maleficence) • 161
INTENTIONAL TORTS • LICENSURE

Non-maleficence: The Value As Basis for the Law—*162* • Laws Enforcing the Value, Doing No Harm—*164* • Intentional Torts—*164* • Quasi-intentional Torts—Injury to Economics and Dignity—*173* • Statutes Prohibiting Maltreatment—*178* • Anti-dumping—*182* • Non-maleficence in Research—*185* • Licensure—*192* • Education—*207*

FOUR

Ethics and Law of
Freedom (Autonomy) • 219
CONSENT • ADVANCE DIRECTIVES • TRANSPLANTS
HIV/AIDS • TB • AUTONOMY FOR THE NURSE • FUTILITY

Autonomy—The Value and Consequences—*220* • Law Enforcing the Value, Freedom, for the Patient—*222* • Consent—*222* • Kinds of Consent—*225* • Specific Consents—*233* • Advance Directives—*240* • Living Wills—*244* • Durable (Springing) Power of Attorney—*249* • Transplants—*263* • HIV/AIDS Autonomy Issues—*270* • Autonomy for the Nurse—*279*

FIVE

Ethics and Law of
Fairness (Justice) • 299
JUSTICE • SOCIAL JUSTICE
ECONOMICS • LABOR LAW

Fairness (Justice)—*300* • Theories of Fairness—*303* • Economics of Illness Care Law—*307* • Labor Ethics and Law—*317* • Fair Labor Standards Act—*320* • Drug Testing—*321* • Americans with Disabilities Act—*322* • Civil Rights—*324* • National Labor Relations Act—*328* • Anti-trust Law (The Sherman Act)—*330* • Family and Medical Leave Act of 1993—*332* • Occupational Safety and Health Act (OSHA)—*333* • Worker Compensation—*333*

SIX

Ethics and Law of
Being True (Fidelity) • 337
KEEPING PROMISES (CONTRACTS)
KEEPING SECRETS • TELLING TRUTH

Discussion of the Value, Being True: The Ethics—*338* • Keeping Promises: Loyalty—*339* • Keeping Secrets: Confidentiality—*339* • Ethics

Code for Fidelity—*339* • Keeping Promises: The Law Enforcing the Ethic—*341* • Contracts—*341* • Covenants Not to Compete—*345* • Employment "At Will"—*346* • Loyalty to the Managed Care Patient—*350* • Law Enforcing Confidentiality—*355* • Telling Truth (Veracity)—*358* • Whistle-Blowing—*360*

<u>SEVEN</u>

Ethics and Law of Life • 367

A TIME TO BE BORN • A TIME TO DIE

General Discussion of the Value, Life—*368*

A Time to Be Born—*370* • Artificial Insemination—*371* • In Vitro Fertilization—*373* • Surrogate Motherhood—Adoption—*376* • Contraception and Technology—*379* • Abortion—*383* • Neonates—*405*

A Time to Die—*411* • Who Dies? The Old, the Sick—*413* • Life Expectancy, Averages, Risk Probability—*417*

Why Do People Die? • Cost of Care—*423* • Quality of Life—*426* • Competency/Capacity—*430*

How Do People Die?—*434* • CPR/DNR—*434* • Withdrawing Vs. Withholding—to Treat or Limit Treatment—*439* • Dehydration—*443* • Cases: The "Right" to Die—*452*

What Is Death? What Is Dying?—461 • PVS—*462* • Brain Death and Higher Brain Death—*466*

When Do People Die—and Who Chooses?—*467* • The Nazis and Euthanasia—*468* • Assisted Suicide—*472* • Euthanasia—*473* • Analysis by Degree of Intent—*475* • Self-killing—*477* • Official Positions on Suicide, Assisted Suicide, and Euthanasia—*479* • The Holland Experience—*481* • Pain Control—*482*

Index • 493

ONE

Values in
Ethics and Law

TOPICS COVERED

Introduction

Ethics is the basis of law

Organization of the book

Limits to ethics and law

Ethics

History of ethics in illness care

Professional ethics

Codes of ethics

Interests and emotions

Philosophy and religion

Two views of the world: Idealism and Realism

Law is based on ethics, but it is not the highest ethic

Theory of morality development
    FEMINIST MORALITY

Ethics committees

Ethicists and the decision-making process

Law

Philosophy and history of law

Ethics vs. law

Lobbying

Rights—limits on government power

Divisions of law: criminal and civil law
STATUTE • REGULATIONS AND RULES • CASE LAW

INTRODUCTION

Good nursing practice is ethical and legal.

The shared values (ethics) of a people are the basis of their law.

Law is a *minimum* standard of morality.

The ethics incorporated into good nursing practice are more important than knowledge of the law; practicing ethically saves the effort of trying to know all the laws.

Nurses who follow specific legal mandates that violate good nursing practice and ethical principles could be legal but not right (and eventually, not even legal).

Good practice reflects ethical behavior that results in action that is legal— this is a theory of law.

A legal duty does not exist without a higher ethical duty, but there may exist an ethical duty without a lower legal duty.

The minimum behavior required by law is not the same as the maximum of ethical behavior.

GOOD NURSING PRACTICE IS GOOD ETHICS IS GOOD LAW. With this statement as guide, good nurses can practice with confidence, knowing their practice is ethical and legal. They do not need complicated legal advice for every situation. Good practice → good ethics → good law is taught and demonstrated throughout this book. Good practice is ethical; it is axiomatic that mere technical competence is not professional practice.

Nurses consider themselves professionals, and they are assumed to have certain values. If taught and indeed held, such values ensure that one who practices good nursing also practices good ethics.

PROFESSIONAL NURSING VALUES

Doing good (caring) for the patient (*beneficence*).

Doing no harm to the patient (*non-maleficence*).

Being fair to the patient (*justice*).

Preserving the freedom of the patient (and nurse) (*autonomy*).

Being true: Keeping promises to the patient (*loyalty*); telling the truth to the patient (*veracity*); and keeping secrets of the patient (*confidentiality*).

Treasuring the life of the patient (*life*).

Students enter nursing school with some values incorporated into their personal ethic. Their professional education should formalize and systematize those values, becoming the basis of their professional ethic. Then, as nurses practice good ("professional") nursing, they should adhere to those values appropriately.

Some authorities identify slightly different values; for example, calling them "moral principles"—beneficence, non-maleficence, respect for persons (instead of autonomy), and justice—but life is not always mentioned as a specific value.

Ethics → Law

Ideally, the shared values (ethics) of a people are the basis of law. In an ideal world, law would be the same as a minimum ethic; law would be the basic ethic that all agree upon, written and enforced. Certain behavior would be considered the minimum ethic, so essential that everyone would be held to that behavior. People would write law to *enforce* such ethical behavior.

Some behavior would be considered right without its having to be written as law (that is, not mandated). That behavior would be beyond the minimum standard of law. If nurses adhere to the professional ethics outlined in this book, their behavior would be at a minimum lawful, and probably also beyond the minimum standard of law. *Nursing Ethics and Law* won't prescribe to nurses the right "answer" to a problem; instead, this book will assure the nurses who search for answers that an answer that is consistent with good nursing and its values—will be lawful too.

Law Is Not the Same As Ethics

Law is not completely coincident with ethics or morality; it is a *minimum* morality. The danger in confusing or equating law with ethics is that minimum "good" behavior—the law—is taken to be the same as the ideal behavior.

Some believe the law should enforce the highest ethic. That is the position of people who believe, for example, that abortion is murder. But if the law is equivalent to the ethic, then the law becomes the highest ethic and there is no difference between the ethic and the law.

In a free society, the law will not (should not?) reflect that highest standard of behavior. If law and ethics are equated, the lower standard of behavior may come to be seen as ethical. Using the example of abortion in the United States: Instead of abortion being seen, as it is now, as legal but unethical to some, abortion might be seen as legal *and* ethical.

The ideal of law being the minimum ethic of *all* the people is attained some of the time, but most of the time it is not. Laws are not always considered the agreed-upon, minimal ethic of all the people. In a democracy, the laws are the enforced minimum ethic only of those values shared by the *majority* of the people; the minority may share a minimum ethic not enforced by the minimum of law. The immediate example in the United States is abortion law, discussed in Chapter Seven.

An act can be legal—consistent with the written expressions of laws of the society. It can be moral (ethical)—what feels right or wrong. And it can be practical—what actually happens.

Throughout this book, ideal (ethical) and real (legal) premises are demonstrated in various ways. For each area of nursing values, the desired ideal ethical behavior is described along with the minimum legal behavior resulting from the ideal of the ethic. The ethic incorporated into good nursing practice is always more important for the nurse to know and follow than the specific law.

Nurses cannot learn all the laws, even if it were desirable to do so. Even if they could be learned, they would be out of date immediately. Indeed, as this book is being read, American lawmakers are enacting thousands of *new* regulations, statutes, and case law in 50 state capitals and courthouses across the United States, and in Washington, D.C.

Ethical Behavior Is Efficient

Ethical behavior saves the nurse the valuable time and effort that would be needed trying to learn law. Following correct nursing practice and professional ethics will keep the nurse in compliance with the law 99 percent of the time; the one percent of the instances when law does not follow the ethic, the law will not be enforced. In the unlikely event that it is attempted, the nurse has an excellent defense if charged with noncompliance of law. In addition to keeping the nurse "safe" legally, ethical behavior allows for sleeping with a clear conscience.

The farther lawmakers stray from enforcing a minimum ethic, the harder it is to predict the law only by knowing what is good practice (ethical). That a law required recording medications in three places would be hard to predict. But it is not hard to predict that giving a poison is prohibited by law (because it is not good nursing practice; it's unethical). The good news: If the legality of an act is not obvious, then guessing wrong will have little consequence. (If law requires recording in three places, recording in only one carries little or no punishment; but giving the poison can be predicted to carry penalty.)

The reverse is not true: Nurses who follow specific legal mandates, although violating good nursing practice and ethical principle, could be legal but not right. They may even be risking violation of the law, if and when it is changed to reflect underlying ethical norms.

"LEGAL" BUT NOT ETHICAL AND EVENTUALLY NOT LEGAL

Example: German nurses were censured at the Nuremberg trials for administering barbiturates to mentally retarded children, who slept for days, contracted pneumonia and died of it. Legal at the time? Yes. Doctor's orders? Yes, directly or by innuendo. Good nursing practice? No. Ethical? No. And, in the end not even held legal.[1]

The concepts of law and ethics are inseparable. Being a nurse in society incorporates certain ethical principles. An adherence to good nursing practice produces certain ethical actions and almost always results in behavior that is legal, too. When that rule fails, the consequences are usually inconsequential.

This book is written for practicing staff nurses and student nurses. Additionally, for graduate students, specialists, and nurse managers, it will serve as a quick reference. The approach is elementary, but the concept is sophisticated. The idea that good practice reflects ethical behavior that results in legal action is a theory of law—different from Rawls's *Theory of Justice*[2] (discussed in Chapter Five, Ethics and Law of Fairness)—but of equal validity.

Behavior (CAN) leads to ethics (SHOULD) leads to law (MUST).

Practice → Ethics → Law

Ethical Behavior Is Practical

The nurse's actual practice (the *ability* to care for the patient's needs) leads to the ethic (the *ethical duty* to care for the patient's needs). That ethic is then reflected in law (the *legal duty* to care for the patient's needs). If the nurse in practice can give the patient sufficient food and water to maintain life (if the patient can be fed without causing more harm than good), then the nurse has an ethical duty to feed the patient. A legal duty enforces that ethic.

If for some reason the nurse is unable to give food and water (for instance, the patient is competent and refuses nourishment), then the nurse is unable to feed as a practical matter (the root of the word *practical* is "practice"). If that's the case, there's no ethical duty—and no ethical duty, then no legal duty. A legal duty will never exist without there first being a higher ethical duty, but the reverse is *not* true: An ethical duty may exist without a lower legal duty.

As an example, the nurse has the actual (practical) power to kill a person with a lethal injection. If the nurse works for the prison system, there may exist a legal power to kill in some situation (execution); but the nurse may feel an ethical duty *not* to kill. No law may forbid the act (execution), but there may be an ethical principle beyond and different from the minimal ethic of the law.

The same ethic may hold for participating in abortions, or for dehydrating to death a patient who is not dying. If assisted suicide or euthanasia (killing the patient) becomes legal, nurses must confront whether the legality will be sufficient for their assisting in preparing the syringe for the physician, or for pushing the lethal bolus. If the law says nurses *may* do so, they must confront whether they *will* kill a patient who requests death. The minimum behavior allowed by the law, then, will not be the same as the maximum of ethical behavior.

Note that when the law makes it impossible for nurses to do a specific practice, then the ethic doesn't require them to do so. (For example, nurses in Great Britain seldom do dialysis on patients over 55; people don't come in as patients because the system won't pay.) In those cases, the minimum ethic of the whole people as reflected in law may be different from the minority ethic of the nurse, but the nurse has no ethical and thus no legal duty to do the impossible.

In situations in which law is equated with the ethics of practice and also sets actual practice standards, law takes command and leads, instead of ethics and good practice (at least, law leads those who don't question it). "It's legal so it's ethical" is the lowest level of ethical reasoning, if one accepts a hierarchy of stages of reasoning (discussed under Kohlberg's theory, under Theory of Moral Development, later in this chapter).

In general, however, "good" nursing leads to nursing ethics, and those ethical values in turn are the base of nursing law.

The book's premise: A nurse needs to know few details of law (or even formal ethics) if she practices good nursing.

ORGANIZATION OF THE BOOK

This brief overview of the book may give the reader some idea as to *where* to look for *what*.

First chapter: Ethics and law—theories and sources.

Second chapter: Ethics and law of the value, Doing Good (Beneficence)—malpractice law

Third chapter: Ethics and law of the value, Doing No Harm (Non-maleficence)—intentional torts and licensure law.

Fourth chapter: Ethics and law of the value, Freedom (Autonomy)—law of consent, advance directives, and nurse autonomy.

Fifth chapter: Ethics and law of the value, Fairness (Justice)—due process, antidiscrimination law, and social justice.

Sixth chapter: Ethics and law of the value, Being True (Fidelity: loyalty, confidentiality, veracity)—contract law and whistle-blowing.

Seventh chapter: Ethics and law of the value, Life—ethical and legal aspects of life surrounding birth and death.

The Contents, plus use of the Index, allows the nurse to find the topic sought quickly. The goal is to help the nurse find the information needed immediately, without reading the entire book. Endnotes reveal sources so that nurses on their own can find more information if they need it; in addition, the name and citation of important legal cases are given. It has been the work of the author, however, to study the source material, distill it, and pass it on so the reader can use it. The reader should not have to consult the original sources to understand the law and ethics of nursing.

The theories and sources of nursing ethics and law are addressed in the balance of Chapter One. The section on ethics defines ethics (custom), discusses the role and content of some professional codes of ethics, discusses professionalism, and notes that ethics entails conflict and personal feelings.

Ethics is described in relation to philosophy and religion, and the philosophies that nurses will usually encounter in ethical discussions are identified, described, and categorized as either "real" or "ideal." Ethics is differentiated from law, and theories of moral development are covered.

A feminist morality is introduced, and ethics committees are described. A new process is outlined to help nurses make decisions about ethical problems.

In the section on law, ethics is identified as the source of law, and ethics and law are differentiated. Rights under the law are differentiated from entitlements, and law is separated into different categories, for ease of study and explanation.

Law is identified by its effect on the nurse (whether it is criminal or civil) and is divided by sources, starting with statutes (and constitutions made in the same way), then regulations and accompanying administrative law rules, and lastly case law (more complex). The section on sources of law includes information that nurses can use if they are interested in politics, but its main purpose is to inform the nurse where the law originates. At this point, it is only fair to let the reader know the author's philosophy of law, expressed by one of the great thinkers about law and ethics, John Stuart Mill:

> That the only purpose for which power can be rightfully exercised over any member of a civilised community, against his will, is to prevent harm to others. His own good, either physical or moral, is not a sufficient warrant. He cannot rightfully be compelled to do or forbear because it will be better for him to do so, because it will make him happier . . . [or] in the opinions of others, to do so would be wise, or even right. These are good reasons for remonstrating with him, reasoning with him, or persuading him, or entreating him, but not for compelling him, or visiting him with any evil in case he do otherwise.[3]

After Chapter One, the next six chapters elaborate on the common values of nursing practice: The ethics and law of each value.

Values

Nursing ethics is based on values. Each value found in nursing ethics results in some laws of nursing practice that enforce the minimum ethic. These laws, related to the nursing ethics value they spring from, are identified specifically. The description of nursing ethics and resulting law covers virtually all of the usual nurse's practice.

The foundation of law is ethics. In this book's approach, the ethics are separated into values. For each value identified, the minimum—the law that flows from that value—is discussed.

No fewer than ten "virtues" were identified by William Bennett as desirable to teach young people: self-discipline, responsibility, courage (the value: Freedom); compassion (the value: Doing Good); friendship, loyalty, faith, honesty (the value: Being True); perseverance, work.[4] Neither these, nor those discussed throughout this book, are exhaustive of *all* values held by people, but the following are used often in nursing and suffice for this book. Each value is the topic of a chapter that explains the ethics and resulting law of that value.

Value: Doing Good (Beneficence) Beneficence, discussed in Chapter Two, is what nurses call caring. Note that the general public is not mandated to do good; their only duty is not to harm others. Only if one undertakes a duty to care, as nurses do, is the person mandated to follow through and actually benefit the other person. (Doing good for the patient is also discussed in Chapter Seven under concepts such as benefits versus burden, and ordinary versus extraordinary care.)

Tort law, specifically malpractice (professional negligence), is the biggest area of law based on the value of Doing Good. The essentials needed to establish negligence and defenses, documentation, standards of care, and other areas of tort law are discussed there.

Value: Doing No Harm (Non-maleficence) Tort law and some other statutory law reflect the mandate that all people have (not just nurses), *not* to harm others. The law, discussed in Chapter Three, includes the intentional torts. Battery, assault, false imprisonment, intentional infliction of emotional distress, are explored; and defenses to those acts are given, for example under consent (also discussed in Chapter Four) and assumption of risk.

Also listed under Doing No Harm are those called quasi-intentional torts that sometimes affect nurses; now called "economic dignity interests," these are the traditional torts of defamation (slander and libel), invasion of privacy, and some others, together with the defenses to those lawsuits.

Other statutes prohibit nurses and others from maltreating people (children, dependents, old people), and they also require some people (specifically nurses) to report abuse they know about. (This topic is also discussed in Chapter Six under keeping patients' secrets and telling the truth, both *to* and *about* patients.)

Licensure statutes and related statutory protection are also addressed in Chapter Three. This kind of law is a mandate to care for (not to harm) the patient. The ethics and law of education for nurses are enforced through licensure law.

Value: Freedom (Autonomy) Consent law enforces the minimum of the value in illness care and is discussed in Chapter Four. Related laws are the advance directives (durable power of attorney and living will). Laws related to AIDS are also addressed under this value as a consequence of a freely chosen lifestyle. Transplant law and ethics are grouped here also as an issue of free choice.

The freedom (autonomy) of the nurse is a concomitant value, expressed in autonomous practice and its legal consequences. The giving of "futile" care is discussed under this value as a determination made by the autonomous caregiver.

Value: Fairness (Justice) The value of fairness under the law, discussed in Chapter Five, is important, not merely because it's "good" to be fair. Without fairness in law there is no peace within a country. The assumption that law should be just is so basic that it doesn't stir much ethical controversy.

Chapter Five also contains discussion of the similar term *social justice*, an attempt to use the force of law to implement the value Doing Good. The discussions of law belonging to justice include rights, limits on the power of lawmakers to control our lives (rights to liberty, life, property; due process, and equal protection). Disputed rights (rights to privacy, to die, to refuse treatment, to abortion, to life) are also discussed in Chapter One, under Rights—Limits on Government Power.

Social justice, as noted, represents a value completely different from justice, an attempt to mandate doing good. Since mandating social justice would affect and change the economics of nursing, some instruction on the basis of economics affecting illness care is given. Labor laws (especially antidiscrimination laws) are also discussed in Chapter Five.

Value: Being True (Fidelity) The value of keeping promises (loyalty), one subject of Chapter Six, is enforced in contract law, employment law, and whistle-blowing (also related to telling the truth). The value of telling the truth is reflected in requiring the "informed" in consent and protecting the patient's friend when the patient won't (and may conflict with keeping promises to, and the secrets of, the patient). Keeping secrets of patients is required by case and statute law, but note the conflicts with the value of Doing No Harm (the reporting). Also note its conflict with the value of telling the truth (encouraging whistle-blowing with laws that protect the public or other individuals).

Value: Life The value, Life, is discussed at length in Chapter Seven, which is divided chronologically into two sections (A Time to Be Born and A Time to Die) for ease of study. One division contains the issues surrounding the beginning of human life, and the other contains issues confronted near the end of human life. The chronological division is convenient and logical, grouping issues with common themes. Several of the issues in each division have common values and law, and these are cross-referenced.

A Time to Be Born discusses the ethics and law of artificial insemination, in vitro fertilization, surrogate motherhood, abortion, and neonates.

A Time to Die discusses the ethics of dying, as well as the assumptions and myths of society that surround this action. The law and ethics discussed include:

Who dies (attitudes and statistics about old people).

What is death (brain death, persistent vegetative state [PVS]).

Why they die (quality of life considerations).

How they die (dehydrated, no cardiopulmonary resuscitation [CPR]).

When they die (suicide, euthanasia, assisted suicide).

The preceding, brief overview of the book may give the reader some help as to where to look for what.

Limits to Ethics and Law

The values that are held by all peoples underlie the theory of natural law (natural rights), for example, not killing, stealing, lying, hurting other people.

Unintended consequences of actions (or laws) can never be known with certainty, but they can be estimated with knowledge of personal and others' experiences.

Humans can arrange their lives in any way they want—nearly. There are some limits on behavior toward other humans, often not known in advance but apparent only when the limits have been exceeded and trouble results. These limits have been called religion, natural law (natural rights), or moral imperatives. Whatever the label, there are limits that are constant in all human societies or civilizations—in most societies, it is in some measure wrong to kill, to steal, to lie, or to hurt other people. The bioethical issues and law discussed in this book all come back to these "shalt nots" and how they are applied to nursing.

Consequences of Actions

People act rationally to achieve intended consequences; they can usually see what the intended consequences will be. Problems come with the *unintended* consequences of actions, which can never be known with certainty. The unintended consequences of actions, however, can be *estimated* with knowledge of personal and others' experiences—a good reason to study the history of law and ethics. How others act can be seen, and the unintended consequences of their actions can be analyzed. The unintended consequences of proposed actions can also be anticipated to some extent, when people use experience that others have already had (as is done when one does a literature search on a topic, or when a committee hears testimony about a proposed law).[5]

RESOURCES

Many of the references and resources in this book are from medical and nursing journals, from articles discussing the same issues as the bioethics and law journals. The advantage to the nurse of using these journals is that they may be found in the agency or hospital library if it's large enough; if not, the local branch librarian may be able to collaborate with a medical or nursing school library in the state to get the article.

The book is limited to the subject of ethics and law; the focus is on issues most important in the United States (and in countries with a similar Western cultural foundation). It will also be helpful to nurses in countries that use theories of medical and nursing care like those prevalent in the United States. The discussions should be helpful to all readers, since ethical principles cut across cultural lines. There is much to be learned from other cultures, other religions, other countries, but limits on time and space mean the nurse is left to explore those according to personal interest.

The goal of this book is to give the nurse information about the subjects of ethics and law as they pertain to nursing practice. It will succeed if it convinces the nurse that what is already known (good nursing practice) is also ethical and legal practice. The mission of the book is to help nurses stop worrying about "the ethics" and "the law" and concentrate on what they do best, on what needs doing—nursing.

Following are some of the better known centers of ethics study that can provide more information:

Institute of Society, Ethics and the Life Sciences, The Hastings Center, 255 Elm Road Briarcliff Manor, NY 10510-9974 (established 1969).

Midwest Bioethics Center, 410 Archibald Suite 200, Kansas City, MO 64111.

National Reference Center for Bioethics Literature (established 1971), Kennedy Institute of Ethics, Georgetown University, Washington, DC 20057. 1-800-MED-ETHX   1-202-687-3885   FAX: 1-202-687-6770.

A bibliographic **BIOETHICS** database, produced by the National Reference Center, is available online through the National Library of Medicine's MEDLARS system. The Reference Center has also produced and made available: Scope Notes, on several specific bioethical issues (for example, Maternal-Fetal Conflict), and *The International Directory of Bioethics Organizations*, listing one or more bioethics organizations, in 25 states in the United States and 25 countries.

Other major resources are the following books:

American College of Physicians, "Ethics Manual," *Annals of Internal Medicine*, 1984; 101:129–137, and 101:263–274. Available from Annals of Internal Medicine, Subscriber Service Division, American College of Physicians, 4200 Pine Street, Philadelphia, PA 19104.

Anderson, G.R., and Glesnes-Anderson, V.A., *Health Care Ethics*, Rockville, MD: Aspen, 1987.

Beauchamp, T.L., and Walters, L. (Eds.), *Contemporary Issues in Bioethics*, Belmont, CA: Wadsworth, 1989.

Cassell, E.J., *The Place of the Humanities in Medicine*, Hastings-on-Hudson, NY: The Hastings Center, 1984.

Guidelines on the Termination of Life-Sustaining Treatment and the Care of the Dying, Hastings-on-Hudson, NY: The Hastings Center, 1984. (Note newer address above.)

Halverson, W.H., *A Concise Introduction to Philosophy*, New York: Random House, 1981.

Halverson, W.H., *Concise Readings in Philosophy*, New York: Random House, 1981.

Hayek, F.A., *New Studies in Philosophy, Politics, Economics and the History of Ideas*, Chicago: University of Chicago Press, 1985.

Monagle, J.F., and Thomasma, D.C., *Medical Ethics*, Rockville, MD: Aspen, 1988.

Ross, J.W., *Handbook for Ethics Committees*, Chicago: American Hospital Association, 1994.

Waymack, M.H., and Taler, G.A., *Medical Ethics and the Elderly*, Chicago: Pluribus Press, 1988.

Additional resources are located in the Endnotes of each chapter.

ETHICS

∇

"The louder he spoke of his honor, the faster we counted our spoons."
—**RALPH W. EMERSON**

$\triangle$

Why Study Ethics?

Nurses need to study ethics in order to care *fully* for their patients.

At minimum, nurses should study ethics as part of the "liberal arts," like philosophy, literature, art, history. Nurses study liberal arts as well as nursing for good reasons.

GOOD REASON TO STUDY ETHICS

Edmund Pellegrino, an influential writer on the humanities in medicine, gives nurses a reason:

The liberal arts are attitudes of mind, not disciplines or bodies of knowledge. They have since classical times been those intellectual skills needed to be a free man—not only in the political sense, but more critically in the sense of being free of the tyranny of other men's thinking and opinions, free to make up one's own mind and take one's own position. The liberal arts comprise those skills most commonly associated with being human—the capability to think clearly and critically, to read and understand language, to write and speak clearly, *to make moral judgments*, to recognize the beautiful, and to possess a sense of the continuity between man's present and inherited past. [EMPHASIS ADDED].[6]

Since nurses care for sick people, they may face more difficult and immediate ethics conflicts than people in other jobs. The people cared for are less able to fend for themselves. When they need nurses, people are in a weaker position, and they have less information at hand than when they need other, nonnursing services.

Every medical and nursing school in the United States teaches ethics and law in one form or another. Graduates and nursing students should have the opportunity for a systematic exposure to ethics and law, equivalent to at least one semester, say the experts.[7] Indeed, a separate course in nursing school on ethics and law would seem to be in order, especially when one realizes that even associate degree correspondence schools for respiratory therapists offer separate courses on ethics.[8]

When the word *bioethics* is used, it refers to ethics applied to biology. Bioethics is not a subject different from ethics, however; the principles of ethics can apply in every field, as in nursing ethics and medical ethics. This book is about ethics and law applied to nursing, so the word *bioethics* will not be needed. Ethics, like the terms *law, philosophy, sociology, religion, history*, and *science*, is not a physical thing; it's a construct. Constructs (ideas and concepts) exist only in the minds of people, and they are only what people make of them—what people decide the concepts are.

VALUES UNDERLYING ILLNESS CARE LAW

> Humans are born with some instinctive values and develop them with the experience of living.

This book will elaborate on the six most-mentioned values in ethics and the laws that enforce those values. That is not to say that there are only six values, but these are the most prevalent values in the ethics and law of American nurses. As listed earlier, they include doing good, doing no harm, freedom, fairness, being true (encompassing keeping promises, keeping secrets, and telling truth), and life. As much as possible, the values that underlie the law of patient care will be described in Anglo-Saxon terms since they are usually more direct and positive. Inherent in all the values is the primary self-interest of human beings, discussed under each value. Other writers may describe fewer, or more, values; the value, Life, is left out of some current writing on ethics for nurses.

Ethical principles and law arise from each value described. Understanding the values first, makes ethics and the law that arise from them logical and understandable, in the correct order of the creation of the law. People first hold a value, then they write laws to reflect those values.

Where values come from (economic need or social pressures, from the construction of the human brain, from the unconscious millennia of human experience, or from God) is beyond the scope of this book. The six values chosen here are observed to be the major values in illness care at this time; all the law written about nurses enforces some minimum part of one of these.

If nurses recognize the basic values humans hold important, they will know in general terms the law that results from those values. When nurses understand the value, and realize that humans make laws that follow that value, they can predict the law governing any area of human activity (especially nursing). If they're ethical, they'll be legal.

Licensure law is a good example: Nurses know that humans value doing good for people, and not harming people. With that knowledge nurses can predict that as a part of nursing law, licensure law will have developed to *enforce* the values of Doing Good and Doing No Harm. The nurse can predict that in general terms the licensure law *prescribes* good behavior on the part of the nurse, and *proscribes* bad behavior by the nurse.

The details of the laws change, and it's important that nurses stay as informed as possible about the specific laws in their state pertaining to their practice. But it is more important to know the ethics underlying the laws and adhere to those ethics.

In some writing other values are mentioned. The president of the American Medical Association wrote that medical schools should add "business management, socioeconomics, and politics to the curriculum, along with [new] *ethics of limited resources*." [BRACKETS AND EMPHASIS ADDED].[9]

All people have some innate values, including some that may be instinctive, modified by what is learned early, and what is learned as the individual grows and ages; those teachings are dependent on the kind of world or society lived in.

That humans have instinctive values may not be surprising; humans have at minimum the values of their living cohabitants of Earth. Observing animal behavior reveals "values" such as care and protection of the young, mating for life, loyalty, cooperation with the pack, protection of territory, will to survive, a drive toward freedom of movement, and possibly "acceptance" of death when inevitable. Chimpanzees and gorillas even exhibit what some call healing behavior, from "cure" (removing splinters, draining abscesses) to "care" (healing gestures, touch).[10]

Beyond the probability that people are born with "ethical instincts," humans learn more about what is the "right" thing to do from their life experiences. With more experience they can see the intended consequences and some of the unintended consequences of their acts. In fact, experience may be more valuable in teaching nurses about right behavior than a course in ethics.

HISTORY: A BRIEF OVERVIEW

The history of ethics reveals that the issues are constant; only the particular application of the principles changes.

The concepts of ethics and law to prevent and punish harming patients, and to resolve conflicts between patient and practitioner, are not new. Two thousand years before Christ, Egyptians who had been injured by physicians could obtain compensation for their losses. That ancient government set up a schedule of payments to compensate patients injured by physicians—a cross between malpractice insurance and workers' compensation—issues still present and discussed in Chapter Two, Doing Good.

Recent ethics history is instructive: Not long ago people worried about who would receive kidney dialysis. When the taxpayers began to pay for everyone who needed dialysis, the ethical problem diminished. If the taxpayers cease paying for dialysis for everyone, the problem will return.

Another ethical issue that has come back (or never went away) is the definition of death. Brain death statutes have replaced the older "cessation of pulse and respiration" of the common law, in order to allow for removal of donated organs from a live body. The ethical issue returns in the form of a proposed new legal definition of death: higher brain death, the patient declared dead because the brain is only partially functioning.

It might seem that euthanasia is a new ethical issue for nurses, since the advent of Intensive Care Units (ICUs) and expensive care. But a 1939 Gallup Poll found that 46 percent of Americans favored killing "incurables" (at the time there were no ICUs and the cost of care was cheap). Over and over again each generation has to re-solve similar problems of living and dying—*deja vu*.[11]

Looking at history, one can see that conflict about doing the right thing with sick people has been going on since records have been kept (and doubtless before recorded history, if one can speculate from the behavior of aboriginal people of the present). Records exist of early peoples who feared newborn children who looked different from the tribe, or children born twins; some people killed such babies at birth. The degree of "difference" of individual babies must have been debated; certainly the mother of the baby must have had something to say. The Greek philosopher Plato recommended that children born handicapped or inferior in some way be left to die. Is that so far from the modern situation in which the fear of bearing a Down's syndrome baby motivates abortion of the fetus?

Contrasted with the above is other evidence from American prehistory. Archeological studies support the thesis that aboriginal peoples in what is now the United States held to the value, Life: Skeletal remains have been found of a child born with spina bifida, the spinal cord exposed. (These children are difficult to care for even now with high technology.) The remains show that the child lived to be a teenager and did not die of obvious trauma, which to archeologists indicates the aboriginals' high degree of care for a "different" child.

Nursing Ethics History

Nursing ethics is as old as the action of nursing itself; the ethics of modern nursing began with the advent of modern nursing (dating since the mid-1800s).

Space constraints prevent a thorough discussion of nursing ethics history here, but note that in the *Encyclopedia of Bioethics* (an internationally known standard bioethics reference text, developed with support of the Kennedy Institute of Ethics) nursing ethics including its history covers only nine pages out of 1,813.[12]

One of the earliest documents, a combination of nursing ethics and standards of care, was written in India in 1000 B.C. by Charaka, who said that people who care for the sick should be

> . . . of good behavior, distinguished for purity; possessed of cleverness and skill; imbued with kindness; skilled in every service a patient may require; competent to cook food; skilled in bathing and washing the patient; rubbing and massaging the limbs; lifting and assisting him to walk about; well skilled in the art of making beds; ready, patient and skillful on waiting upon one who is ailing and never unwilling to do anything that is ordered.[13]

The early Christian deaconesses of the fourth and fifth centuries A.D. were the models for the late nineteenth-century deaconesses at Kaiserwerth who taught nursing to Florence Nightingale. (She also learned nursing from the physician-established Sisters of St. John's House in London.) The original deaconesses had as their goals in the first 500 years A.D.:

to feed the hungry

to give water to the thirsty

to clothe the naked

to visit the imprisoned

to shelter the homeless

to care for the sick

to bury the dead.[14]

The term "professional" originally distinguished a nurse who was paid, as opposed to an "amateur" or unpaid nurse. The Anglican nursing orders (sisterhoods, religious women) were helped to create modern nursing by physicians like Robert Bentley Todd who, in the early 1800s, grew dissatisfied with the lack of good nursing help in London teaching hospitals. Dr. Todd created a training institution that educated professional nurses, the Sisters of Saint John's House, affiliated with King's College Hospital, whose model in turn was that of English teacher reform (to professionalize school teachers).[15]

The Sisters' eventual decline was said to be a defeat for autonomous nursing, while the ascendancy of the Nightingale school of nursing began producing an alternative, a cheaper, more tractable nurse—a nurse "morally trained," meaning, at that time, that she was trustworthy and reliable. The Nightingale nurse was respectable, but less independent, and not instructed in the basic principles of what she was doing; thus she was restrained from exercising professional judgment.[16]

Nurses in the United States were concerned with ethics from the first, as exemplified by Isabel Hampton Robb's *Nursing Ethics for Hospital and Private Use*, written in 1903. And, later, ethics courses were prevalent in nursing curricula in the 1930s and 1940s (for examples, see Densford and Millard's *Ethics for Modern Nurses*, cited in note 11). Then, after deletion from the nursing curricula for a couple of decades, ethics courses came back.

The International Council of Nurses established a nursing ethics committee in 1933, but did not issue a code of conduct until 1953. This code was revised in 1965 at the insistence of Canadian student nurses that "nursing's subservience to medicine" be removed.

Economics and politics have, in the past as now, been included in nursing ethics teaching and studies. One heading in Densford's 1946 *Ethics for Modern Nurses* is Political and Economic Ethics, in which the author concluded that nurses have a role to play in the arena of economics and politics: ". . . the nurse . . . has a larger responsibility [than just as a nurse] for using far-sighted intelligence" to work for political and economic goals.[17]

Largely omitted from the history of nursing ethics has been information on the behavior of nurses in Germany during the National Socialist era, the 1930s thru the end of World War II.[18] Books have been written about how German doctors and their professional organizations collaborated with the Nazis during the Holocaust, but until very recently the mention of "killing" done by nurses with the complicity of their nurse associations was absent. Some documentation of the independent and cooperative role of the German and Axis nurses in euthanizing their patients is now available.[19]

PROFESSIONAL ETHICS

Almost all professions have a written code of ethics that distinguishes them from other occupations.

Organized nursing (ANA and its state affiliates, other general and specialty nurse associations) have great influence on the ethics and the law of nursing.

Lengthening and standardization of education is seen as the route to professionalism for most illness care occupations.

The altruism of the professional is the act of putting one's professional interest above other self-interests.

The ideas of "profession" and "ethics" are related and both should be understood by nurses. The idea of "profession" is a concept, a construct, with definition and meaning often subject to individual interpretation.

The traditional professions of law, medicine, clergy, military, were first formalized in England as something for the younger sons to do; the oldest son inherited the farm, under a system of primogeniture, so the younger boys needed an honorable occupation.

It is asserted that historically there are three qualities exhibited by a profession: organization of the practitioners, learning by the practitioners, and a spirit of public service on the part of the practitioners, as individuals and as a group. Earning a livelihood is secondary in that interpretation—or perhaps underlies all of it.[20] The provision of enough necessities of life to survive is the basic self-interest of all people, including professionals.

People who work in occupations that don't fit the traditional or sociologist's definitions (such as nurses) seek to mold their occupations to those definitions. Being a member of a profession is valued; people labeled as professional are seen as more educated, thoughtful, wise, wealthy, trustworthy, or powerful than the average person. But, it might be asked: Which came first, the profession or the attributes? Did certain professions have *status*, thus entitling its members be defined "professional"?

In the history of illness care, the obvious professional role model was medicine. The reverse was not true: Doctors did not view nursing as their role model.[21]

Professionals Are Organized

The Codes of Ethics of the American Medical Association (AMA) and the American Nurses Association (ANA), discussed below, have added sections suggesting that, to be ethical, the practitioner must work for improvements in the profession and in the community. One way to do that is to work through the association(s) of nurses.

CONTACTING THE STATE NURSE ASSOCIATION

Many books on nurse ethics or law (few are about ethics *and* law, as is this one) list the state nurses association addresses and telephone numbers (including Licensed Practical Nurses [LPNs]). Such a list is only useful for the one nurses association of the nurse's state (one rarely needs other than one's own SNA's number). Such lists are outdated as soon as printed for some states. Nurses who want to contact the SNA should call the information operator in the state's capital or larger cities and ask for the nurse's association of the state.

The membership of the ANA is about 200,000, less than ten percent of the nurses in the country; yet it is still the largest nurse organization representing nurses in general. Many other nurse organizations exist that represent nurses in generalist and specialty areas. Together and in council, they represent nurses at the state and national level.

The ANA plays a large role in the ethics and the law of nursing. ANA members actually write its Code of Ethics and provide interpretive statements on ethical problems through a division called the Center for Ethics and Human Rights (600 Maryland Avenue SW, Suite 100 West, Washington, DC 20024-2571).

State nurses' associations (and other national nurse organizations) are heavily involved in writing, passing and/or defeating legislation that affects nurses. Nurse practice acts in all the states have been written almost single-handedly by ANA affiliates. The ethical standards and laws that affect every nurse are influenced by who belongs to the ANA, who runs the organization, and who makes the positions that the ANA advocates. The positions of the association often become the statement of ethics and the law for all nurses.

ANA leaders respond to members in two very different categories: One category is Masters-degreed educators with six years or more of post–high school education (many of whom belong to ANA because they want to change/improve nursing). The other group is Associate-degreed nurses with two years of training (many of whom belong to the ANA because they are under collective bargaining contracts and represented by their state nurses' associations).

Although the ANA union movement was hampered in the past by an insistence that the professional association not represent any other category of worker in bargaining units—only RNs[22]—ANA and its state affiliates have become the bargaining agent for some nurses. Even in an attenuated form, union activity alienated some nurses, who left the organization because of it.

From the union influence of the staff nurses in collective bargaining, and from the usually more liberal views of the academics in nursing who were the largest influence among the elected officials, ANA became more politically active and more polarized. Nurses who had been a moderating influence left the organization, leaving power to those who remained, many of whose views were in favor of government solutions to social problems. The remaining members of ANA are thus somewhat different from the nurses who are not members.

The organization for the first time endorsed a candidate for U.S. President in 1992 (Bill Clinton). ANA leaders pursued the goal of nursing as a profession, independent and different from medicine. To that end, they have pursued more education requirements for entry into the occupation.

Professionals Are Educated

Doctors are seen to have a long education relative to nurses. But British doctors get six years of education beyond high school (this is true also in some medical schools in the United States); that is the same amount of education time spent getting a Master's degree in nursing. Doctors didn't begin to have a "long" education until about the turn of the twentieth century (changes commenced even before a report was issued stating there were a lot of quacks calling themselves doctors). Medicine gradually lengthened and set further standards of education for its practitioners.

This lengthening and standardization of education is still seen as the route to professionalism for most illness care occupations. Independent or solo practitioner job structures are preferred for the same reason—independence from, leading to equality with, the doctor (although increasing numbers of doctors work as employees and not entrepreneurs).

All the occupations seek to work in teams, making themselves independent of, equal to, and as professional as doctors. Workers in illness care seek autonomy in their practice, just as the physician has (is thought to have, or had). Doctors increasingly have lost freedom, in the form of people looking over their shoulders in managed care, quality review, payment review, peer review committees, and state medical boards—not to mention the ultimate review, malpractice suits.

A "review" within a profession is not a new idea. In the late 1300s the medical guild (union) of Florence required that "bad cases" be reviewed by a committee of the guild. This was voluntary peer review, an extension of the control of the law, much like review committees today function to control practice without the formality of law.

People in occupations that want to be "professionals" seek to increase the *thinking* part of their jobs and to decrease the portion of their time they spend doing physical things (although even some doctors' jobs are now composed of physical skills, such as catheterizations). The physical procedures done by doctors have been more highly valued than cognition, or thinking activity, and paid more under Medicare and insurance reimbursement.

Despite the wish to professionalize and differentiate the two jobs, can nursing and medicine be separated? The education and technology of caring for people is a continuum from unpaid, amateur nursing care done by mothers/fathers, sisters/brothers, and daughters/sons. Florence Nightingale wrote "Notes for Nurses," not for professional nurses but for those mothers and daughters whom she knew would be nurses at some time in their lives. The continuum continues from volunteers to people who are *paid* to care (professionals) and taught to do more complex procedures for patients, based on some knowledge of science. Still further along the continuum are the artificial distinctions of *nursing aide* to *nurse* to *doctor*: LPN to RN–ADN to BSN; to "advanced practice nurse," who has a Master's degree and is a clinical specialist; to the complex work of some doctors. All are engaged in some form of care.

CARE CONTINUUM—by complexity and scientific knowledge required, *not* by intensity or quality or importance of care. (The continuum showing quality and importance of care might well run from right to left!)

| | | Care by doctors |
| Care by family | Care by nurses | and nurse specialists |

> ___↑_____↑_____↑_____ >

Professionals Are Altruistic

In defining professionals, most sociologists mention as among the most important characteristics, the professional's putting the patient or client first (before self-interest). That is a poor description of the way it works. The practitioner's first self-interest is being a good practitioner/professional and that precedes *other* self-interests such as eating, going home early, or making a lot of money.

Being defined as "professional" has not kept lawyers and physicians from making a lot of money. But, on the other hand, merely being described as a "profession" will not make the occupation one that earns a lot of money. Teachers, clergy, military people, all are called professionals, but they do not make a lot of money.

More education does not cause an occupation to make a lot of money—the market does that. The market tells the person, based on what the person is paid in money, that people value what the person *does*. One doesn't have to agree that they're right (one may not believe that doctors should be more valued than nurses), but the patients and the payors do, as a whole. Otherwise, in the fairly unrestricted market that still exists in the United States, nurses would be paid more. People pay more money, through the market, for professional baseball and basketball players than they pay for professional doctors—they don't pay the players for their education.

The alternative to the market system is one like Plato's Republic, where all activity is controlled and values are set by the state. The former Soviet Union was an experiment in line with that philosophy, an attractive ideal, but it didn't/doesn't work because so few people *are* "the state." Rewards in such a system are not just for merit or according to need (only "state" people in the USSR drove the nice cars and shopped at the special stores and had good medical care when they were ill). Determining prices by the market, although it may seem unfair, is the only system that works consistently, and a system that "works" must at least allow the people to feed themselves—which the utopian systems do not.

Professional Employee Conflicts

> Nurses may experience legal and ethical conflicts as professionals who are also employed.

The conflicts nurses experience often arise in the context of being *employed* professionals. As downsizing of the illness industry increases and "managed care" limits care to decrease cost, the ethical (and even legal) conflicts for nurse employees increase. Nurses are usually employees, not independent practitioners, both in the United States and abroad. And, although some physicians are entrepreneurs (sole proprietors), or partners, or own part of their corporation, the trend is for physicians also to be employees. (Whether the nurse is technically an employee or independent contractor—and why that matters—is discussed further in Chapter Six.) In this section on professional ethical conflicts, an "employee" can mean an independent contractor or a person in a partnership or a corporation. Only the entrepreneur is apparently independent.

> Even self-employed people (doctors, nurse practitioners, therapists) have somewhat of an employee relationship with the organization that pays the bill—in effect, the third-party payor directs much of their work.

Even among self-employed people (doctors, nurse practitioners, therapists), the relationship of the practitioner to the payor—the insurance company, or the government, or managed care organization that pays the bill—looks increasingly like the traditional employee–employer relationship. And the payor, now seldom the patient, is usually the government or insurer or HMO.

In earlier days in nursing the nurse saw herself, and was seen, as an employee, a contractor, a servant—*of the patient*. With payment of the bill by either private or government insurers, the practitioner is not directly responsible to the patient, but to the (sometimes anonymous) third-party payor (3PP) (*eventually* the patient or taxpayer); the unseen 3PP in effect directs much of the work.

The Patient-3PP-Practitioner Relationship

In any work setting, there is some conflict between the interests of the employer and those of the employee. The usual differences are pay for work, hours of work, and conditions of work. Nurses and their employers may differ also about professional ethics and standards of practice.

The conflict about ethics is not unique to illness care. Engineers have a professional standard, perhaps different from their employer's, to build good and safe buildings and cars. Lawyers who work as employees have a standard of professional responsibility, not just to their employer, but also to their clients.

Nurses have yet an additional source of potential ethical conflict: the doctor. Although the doctor is not always an employee nor the nurse's employer, the nurse has traditionally been expected to take orders.[23] This "two masters" problem existed for nurses even when the patient and not the hospital was the actual employer, and it continued when having the hospital and the doctor as boss. Today the third "boss," the 3PP, has something to say about what the nurse does, to whom, and how.

The Professional Employee and Agency Policy

Because they set standards for practice, agency policies have ethical (and legal) implications for the professional.

Employers have policies or standards on a number of ethical and legal issues. For example, the employer probably has policies on living wills and other advance directives; policies on no-code orders; on reporting child abuse, elder abuse, and all other reportable conditions like gunshot wounds; policies to follow an organ donation; required pre-op pregnancy checks, ICU selection, determination of death, and code blue policies; and more, no doubt.

Any and all of these policies have ethical and legal implications for the professional. Some of them were probably made with the help of the ethics committee at the institution, and some with the help of the legal counsel. Discussion of their specifics is impossible here, but nurses should be aware of them and know their content generally. After reading this book the nurse should be able to analyze the values expressed in the policy; in addition, the nurse should be able to identify the interests of the people likely to be affected in a given situation.

Employer policies are not law, but they can be used as standards of practice in lawsuits or licensure actions, to measure the nurse's performance. The policies may not even be ethical by the nurse's personal or professional standards. When conflict arises (for example, if the nurse believes a policy is not ethical), the nurse may face the decision of whether to follow policy and keep the job or, as a professional, adhere to what is seen as the right, ethical, behavior. The nurse can work to change the policies seen as unethical according to professional standards (for instance, a policy that prescribes CPR for all patients found unresponsive, regardless of the patient's prior condition and wishes, or the nurse's professional judgment about whether CPR can succeed).

Nurses will experience professional conflict when they find unsafe practices in the workplace. These can include short staffing, floating out of specialty areas,[24] long hours, use of unprepared help, and patients' rights violations; or even poor physical plant, maintenance, and equipment.

Nurses may work with their peers to set up committees for broad problem areas, using the existing workplace and professional grievance systems. As a last resort (or if serious enough, mandated as a first action), nurses may work with the appropriate licensing board (hospital, doctor, or nurse board) to solve the problem.[25]

At least one state mandates that each agency employing licensed people must have a committee to monitor and enforce the appropriate licensure law. The Texas nursing law requires each agency employing ten nurses have such a committee for nursing practice to examine just such issues.

Professionals: Not Necessarily More Ethical

People called "professional" have duties different from other people, but do not necessarily have a higher ethic or moral sense. Professionals do put their self-interest in care higher than their other self-interests.

One difference between the professional's ethic and nonprofessional's ethic: The professional's obligations are formalized into a code of ethics.

Nurses do have an ethical interest (and a legal mandate too) in doing good for their patient (other workers may not have that ethical and legal duty). At times, nurses prioritize their own interest in doing good, instead of some other of their interests. That prioritizing of professional interests does good for their patients. The professional who cares for people is valuable to the society; professionals can be relied on to act in their own *professional* interest (which usually coincides with the patient's interest).

Some people get pleasure from helping other people. Such people are attracted to occupations that require interest in helping people. Others, however, sometimes find that the training or practice they experience in helping occupations convinces them that they chose the wrong job—they discover they would be happier doing jobs without such values as Doing Good for patients. People self-select themselves into nursing, or out of it, depending on how highly they value their own interest in doing good for other people.

But people classed as professionals do not necessarily have a higher ethic or moral sense than other people. (Other occupations also have self-interests that are "higher"—and definitely beyond immediate gratification.) The factory worker also has some concern for, and obligation to, the fellow human to make products that are as safe as possible. Some mechanics have a written code of ethics. The ethical and legal obligation not to harm other people pre-existed the concept of the professions. Humans all feel some obligation (duty) toward each other as people—at least enough not to harm them.

The professional assumption. If the interest of the client/patient/customer (stated as coincident with the professional interest of the nurse) conflicts with another self-interest of the professional, the professional will put the other self-interest second—the professional is putting a work (professional) interest first. The professional still acts out of self-interest, which benefits the patient, too.

PROFESSIONAL:

SELF-INTEREST IN DOING GOOD = PATIENT'S INTEREST

Both professional and patient benefit; the patient's need for care is met. The professional's need to be a good practitioner or help others (whatever the self-interest in doing the job) is met.

Professionals do not put others' interests ahead of their own; they prioritize their own interests so that their work interest (the interest in doing a good job) comes first most of the time. Usually the work interest in doing good comes first *more* of the time for professionals than nonprofessionals—that is what is implied by "professional." Any other implication, that professionals are better or kinder or more ethical than others, is difficult to prove.

This ethical standard is more pronounced in illness care. The people the nurse serves could be injured or die as a result of the nurse's act, or failure to act. But mechanics, too, have such responsibility. One hopes the mechanic too is a "professional" and puts the public's safety (the professional interest in doing a good brake job) ahead of another interest (such as leaving work early).

CODES OF ETHICS

The difference between the professional and nonprofessional's ethic: In professional occupations, obligations are formalized, somewhat agreed upon, written down, and taught. That's what is in this book. Professions usually have a written moral/ethical code of behavior. (This is not to imply that nonprofessionals have a lower standard of behavior; nonprofessional occupations often do have ethics, but they may not be standardized, formalized, or written [or written about, as here].) The code of behavior/ethics is a series of statements about what behavior or ideals are expected of a person in that occupation.

Some writers distinguish between codes of ethics (ideals) and codes of conduct (behavior). But the ideals of people can only be observed from what they do (indeed, their conduct). The two concepts are the same: Behavior is evidence of what the nurse believes. If the individual were to behave badly, her "ideal," whatever it was, obviously didn't help. If actions of people are right, ethics and law are not concerned that some evil thought motivated them.

Codes of ethics/conduct differ in detail, but they have some values in common: They put Doing Good and Freedom (Beneficence and Autonomy) in behalf of the patient first. They discuss Being True (Loyalty) to their occupations, and to their improvement of their profession.

Through promises to maintain competence, codes promote the value of Doing No Harm (Non-maleficence), in behalf of the patient. They promise Keeping Secrets (Confidentiality) and Being True (Loyalty, Advocacy) for the patient. They may hint at Doing Good in the form of social justice. Underlying all, as always, is the value of Life (promoting always the life of the patient).

Following the comment, the several values are exemplified and discussed in the context of portions of ethical codes.

Comment: In the 1960s the code of ethics for pathologists reflected the values most important to that specialty. The code was a long list of courtesies and protections for other pathologists. A variety of promises were made not to invade another's economic turf, much like covenants not to compete in employment contracts. The value strongest was Being True to the members of the specialty, and underlying that, the Money self-interest. After prosecution by the Federal Trade Commission on antitrust grounds, the College of Pathologists agreed not to enforce that code; they now adhere to the American Medical Association Code.[26] This incident is an example of an ethical code that was *un*enforced by the law, because it was an "ethic" not higher but seemingly lower than the minimum ethic of law. (Portions of the AMA Code appear below, beginning under Preambles of the Codes.)

Who Writes Codes of Ethics?

The professional association of the particular occupation writes its code of ethics. The most politically active people in the occupation—not necessarily the most ethical—may write the code. Even if "experts" in ethics help write the code, it could not reflect what every member of the group thinks is ethical behavior. The code is necessarily a compromise between what most of the group *thinks* are the most important ethical *attitudes* of members (code of ethics), or *behaviors* of members (code of conduct).

A code of ethics by definition is not law: If it mandates behavior, it is a written law instead of an ethical guide to action in situations commonly encountered.

If a code mandated behavior, it would then be written law and practitioners would be forced to follow it. The code is thus a guide, suggestions for action in situations that practitioners often encounter.

But violating the code, behaving differently from what the code recommends, doesn't always mean that the practitioner has behaved unethically.

To behave differently from the code of ethics means that the practitioner believes that a current situation calls for different action. In this situation the nurse believes her action to be either ethical, or the only possible choice for her in the situation.

Duncanis and Golin's *Interdisciplinary Health Care Team* reviewed 20 professional health care codes of ethics and said all the codes discussed five major concerns: professional competence (Doing Good for the patient), loyalty both to profession and to client (Fidelity, Being True), legal responsibilities and responsibility to society (both Being True and Doing Good to the greater society). The ANA Nursing Code was said to be the only one with concern for the individual and that individual's "uniqueness."[27]

> "As professionals, the nurses have a code which maintains that their primary ethical obligation is to the patient."[28]

Medical oaths (similar to codes of ethics) have been examined to see what ethical principles they contained. To researchers, few oaths clearly demonstrated respect for patient autonomy. Nor did the researchers note the principle of Telling Truth. But one-half to three-fourths of the oaths reflected the values of Doing No Harm, Doing Good, Fairness, and Keeping Secrets. The researchers believe that the oaths have not "kept pace" with the changing doctor-patient relationship since they appear to devalue patient freedom while retaining some paternalism.[29]

Codes of ethics for nurses were not always advocated by all: Densford, writing in the 1940s, said that the doctors have a code, but

> . . . nurses have never "frozen" their moral rules into a code subscribed to by all nursing organizations. The nursing profession has been wise in so doing, for thus its ethics is likely to be more responsive to new conditions, or in other words, more adaptable. A written code usually includes concessions to dogmatic, well organized, highly vocal minorities, and the more liberal [original use of the word] members of the nursing profession ought to keep clear of such commitments. Once a code is adopted, it is very difficult to get it changed, because of inertia if nothing else. [EMPHASIS ADDED].[30]

One might question how "adaptable" nursing codes should be.

Historical evolution of specific nurse codes can be found in the literature.[31] As noted above, some distinguish an ethical code of conduct (actions prescribed or prohibited) from a code of ethics (beliefs stated). And note that the codes change as nurses' relationship to society changes. And, further, that codes change as the society's wishes change—which is where a line may have to be drawn, especially if the society endorses euthanasia and genocide, as the German leadership and society did in the 1930s and 40s.[32]

Below, the Code of the American Nurses Association is examined in detail and contrasted with those of the American Association for Respiratory Care (the professional association for respiratory care practitioners) and the doctors' code of the American Medical Association. First examined will be the preambles of each code, and then the segments of each code as they express the values (and resulting law) focused on in this book. [The respiratory care association adopted a new code in December 1994, available from the address below. Does that mean the values (ethics) changed? Or merely the interpretation or wording?]

PREAMBLES OF THE CODES

Nurses: The ANA Code

The ANA Code preamble never says that it is *not* law. (Contrast this with the doctors' and RCPs' below.) This code does not use the word *should* (ethics talk), nor the word *shall* (law talk). This lapse may imply that nurses always do these things, making the code less an ideal than a mandate.

Respiratory Care Practitioners: The AARC Code of Ethics

(American Association for Respiratory Care, 11030 Ables Lane, Dallas, TX 75229)

PREAMBLE

As health care professionals engaged in the performance of respiratory care, respiratory care practitioners must strive, both individually and collectively to maintain the highest personal and professional standards. The principles set forth in this document define the basic ethical and moral standards to which each member of the American Association for Respiratory Care should conform.

Notice that the respiratory care practitioners immediately claim status as "professionals." They seek the highest standards "individually and collectively." The first paragraph gives attention to personal as well as work behavior.

The second paragraph speaks to "ethical and moral"—which, to some, mean the same thing. As noted below under Between Ethics and Law: A Fine Bright Line, the word *should* is important. If *must* were used, it would imply force of law, or at least removal from the organization for violation. The RCP code consistently uses the word *shall*, as does the doctors' code, which usually would imply force of law. Remember, these codes are not law.

Doctors: The AMA Principles of Medical Ethics

The Preamble of the American Medical Association's Principles of Medical Ethics (1980) says some of the same things.

PREAMBLE

The medical profession has long subscribed to a body of ethical statements developed primarily for the benefit of the patient. As a member of this profession, a physician must recognize responsibility not only to patients, but also to society, to other health professionals, and to self. The following Principles adopted by the American Medical Association are not laws, but standards of conduct which define the essentials of honorable behavior for the physician.

—*Source:* **Code of Medical Ethics: Current Opinions with Annotations, American Medical Association, copyright 1994**

Note that this Preamble explicitly states that the doctor's responsibility to the patient is not absolute: that the doctor also has a responsibility to self.

COMPETENCE

Exhortations in codes of ethics to attain and maintain competence reflect the values of doing good for patients, and doing them no harm.

Values Reflected: Doing Good, Doing No Harm, and Freedom

To practice with competence is a basic requisite for Doing Good (Beneficence) and Doing No Harm (Non-maleficence). The doctors' code speaks to maintaining the competence necessary to carry out those values, and refers in a small way to the patient's autonomy ("dignity").

Principle I (below) upholds dignity too; the value expressed is Freedom (Autonomy) for the patient.

DOCTORS.

Medical Ethics: PRINCIPLES

I. A physician shall be dedicated to providing competent medical service with compassion and respect for human dignity.

RESPIRATORY CARE PRACTITIONERS

Respiratory therapy code, paragraph I: *The respiratory care practitioner shall practice medically acceptable methods of treatment and shall not endeavor to extend his practice beyond his competence and the authority vested in him by the physician.*

The reference to the physician's authority makes clear that the respiratory care practitioners practices under the authority of the physician—this is a clear covenant not to compete with physicians. The autonomy of the RCP is derived from the autonomy of the doctor.

Nurses

NURSES

POINT 5 *The nurse maintains competence in nursing.*

POINT 8 *The nurse participates in the profession's efforts to implement and improve standards of nursing.*

Points 5 and 8 (within the above tinted sample) speak to competence and increase of standards in order to do good. Following is the component for the nursing ethic regarding research.

POINT 7 *The nurse participates in activities that contribute to the ongoing development of the profession's body of knowledge.*

Regarding dignity:

POINT 1 *The nurse provides services with respect for human dignity and the uniqueness of the client unrestricted by considerations of social or economic status, personal attributes, or the nature of health problems.*

To increase knowledge and skill is to do good for (benefit) the patient and also to make the practitioner more valued (practitioner autonomy). Respect for the dignity of the patient reinforces the value of the patient's being free (autonomy). An ethical conflict would arise here if a new system of illness care denied treatment for certain health problems (people with AIDS) because the nurses' code says the nurse is to give care unrestricted by the nature of the problem—a direct implementation also of the value, of fairness (justice).

RESPIRATORY CARE PRACTITIONERS

The respiratory care practitioner shall continually strive to increase and improve his knowledge and skill and render to each patient the full measure of his ability. All services shall be provided with respect for the dignity of the patient, unrestricted by considerations of social or economic status, personal attributes, or the nature of health problems.

This is identical to the second sentence of the ANA Code, showing that nurses are not alone in their regard for the individual, although the nurses' code is unique in using the word *uniqueness*.

> *V. A physician shall continue to study, apply and advance scientific knowledge, make relevant information available to patients, colleagues, and the public, obtain consultation, and use the talents of other health professionals when indicated.*

Further regarding competence and increasing standards through research: The underlying value is to increase knowledge through science, which directly increases professional autonomy (value: Freedom) and eventually will do good for the patient.

Value Reflected: Fidelity (Being True to Profession and Employer)

> **NURSES**
>
> **POINT 9** *The nurse participates in the profession's efforts to establish and maintain conditions of employment conducive to high quality nursing care.*

Nurses recognize in their code of ethics that their economic interests are important. This section is often cited as the ethical foundation for collective bargaining. Nursing has several ethics code sections that relate to work, evidence of the conflict nurses experience in being professionals and employees at the same time.

> **POINT 4** *The nurse assumes responsibility and accountability for individual nursing judgments and actions.*
>
> **POINT 5** *The nurse exercises informed judgment and uses individual competence and qualifications as criteria in seeking consultation, accepting responsibilities, and delegating nursing activities to others.*

These can be related to the doctors' item V (above), which speaks to consultation and "use" of other professionals. Nurses have been advised to use these sections of the code of ethics when either refusing or accepting responsibility delegated by physicians. These sections also are used in delegating work to LPNs and nurse aides. Nurse leaders have been adamant that nursing be seen as an independent profession, not under the supervision of doctors. Hence this emphasis in the code—which also reflects the value of autonomy for nurses.

RESPIRATORY CARE PRATITIONERS

The respiratory care practitioner shall be responsible for the competent and efficient performance of his assigned duties and shall expose incompetence and illegal or unethical conduct of members of the profession.

The principle of being true (fidelity) to the employer can be seen here, in "competent and efficient performance," and also doing good (beneficence) for the patient. The whistle-blowing mandate expresses the values of telling the truth (veracity) and doing no harm (non-maleficence) to the patient, above the value of being true (fidelity) to coworkers, coprofessionals, or employer.

"Illegal *or* unethical" is a correctly stated expression. Legal does not necessarily mean ethical. This section could imply—but it is not specifically stated—that the RCP has an ethical obligation to report bad conduct of members of other professions.

Value Reflected: Keeping Promises and Telling the Truth

DOCTORS

II. A physician shall deal honestly with patients and colleagues, and strive to expose those physicians deficient in character or competence or who engage in fraud or deception.

Item II, above, expresses telling the truth, even to the point of being "disloyal" to colleagues who do not tell the truth.

NURSES

POINT 3 *The nurse acts to safeguard the client and the public when health care and safety are affected by incompetent, unethical, or illegal practice of any person.*

This provision of the nurse's code would seem to require the nurse to put loyalty to patient first always. But the words speak only to a threat to the patient from the practice of "any person." For example, this provision would not prohibit the nurse from complying with a scheme to withhold care from old patients, if the state said their care would not be paid. Here the nurses' code properly distinguishes between "unethical" and "illegal" practice—note that incompetent practice is also probably unethical *and* illegal too. Note also that practice, ethics and law are all addressed in this provision.

Value Reflected: Keeping Secrets (Confidentiality)

NURSES

POINT 2 *The nurse safeguards the client's right to privacy by judiciously protecting information of a confidential nature.*

This refers to the requirement of confidentiality, which expresses the underlying value of fidelity to the patient. Confidentiality also is related to doing good and not harming the patient. As is noted in Chapter Six, the ethical value of confidentiality is enforced through statute and case law.

RESPIRATORY CARE PRATITIONERS

The respiratory care practitioner shall hold in strict confidence all privileged information concerning the patient and refer all inquires to the physician in charge of the patient's medical care.

The reference to "the physician" again makes clear the relationship between this occupation and physicians. The new code of this association does not change the relationship.

DOCTORS

IV. *A physician shall respect the rights of patients, of colleagues, and of other health professionals, and shall safeguard patient confidences within the con- straints of the law.*

The doctors' code here expresses the value of freedom for people whom the doctor works with. The code also reinforces, to some extent, the value of justice—noting the "rights" of others. As is discussed specifically in Chapter Six under the value, Being True (Fidelity), the doctors' code unfortunately does not expect the doctor to have a higher value than required by the minimum ethic of the law.

About Money

> **RESPIRATORY CARE PRACTITIONERS**
>
> *The respiratory care practitioner shall not accept gratuities for preferential consideration of the patient. He or she shall guard against conflicts of interest.*

This section deals with economic pressures that might cause the practitioner to put his money interest before the patient's interests. The doctors' code provision below is different. It speaks more to the value Being Free (Autonomy) for the doctor.

> **DOCTORS**
>
> VI. *A physician shall, in the provision of appropriate patient care, except in emergencies, be free to choose whom to serve, with whom to associate, and the environment in which to provide medical services.*

Here, freedom, liberty, and power are valued for the doctor. This provision was changed from earlier days when the code prohibited doctors from being employees. The codes of medical societies formerly prohibited contract work for physicians, because physicians contracted for a number of patients so large as to make care for them impossible.[33] Currently, as physicians contract with and work for HMOs and other managed care organizations, there is again potential for overcontracting, with resultant poor care for patients.

Conflicts between the doctor's loyalty to the employer (making money) and loyalty to the patient (giving care) could cause a change or reversion—*back* to cautions about employment and economic gain at the patients' expense—in the doctors' code.[34]

Value Reflected: Being Free (Professional Autonomy) and Being True (Fidelity)

> **NURSES**
>
> POINT 10 *The nurse participates in the profession's effort to protect the public from misinformation and misrepresentation and to maintain the integrity of nursing.*

In point 10, a little beneficence for the public is mixed with fidelity to the profession. This could be used to justify enforcing nurse licensure laws; it could also be argued that nurse participation in executions, assisted suicide, and dehydration of nondying patients might be seen as threatening the integrity of nursing and the public's trust in the profession.

RESPIRATORY CARE PRACTITIONERS

The respiratory care practitioner shall uphold the dignity and honor of the profession and abide by its ethical principles. He or she should be familiar with existing state and federal laws governing the practice of respiratory care and comply with those laws.

Upholding "the dignity and honor of the profession" is an example of the value of fidelity to one's colleagues and occupation, as well as the value of autonomy in the practitioner's profession. But, to have an ethical principle, which says to uphold ethical principles, is like saying that one of the Ten Commandments is "to obey the ten commandments." The promise to comply with the law seems to be aimed at practitioners who might practice without being licensed, in states that require such licenses.

See what the doctors do with this.

DOCTORS

III. A physician shall respect the law and also recognize a responsibility to seek changes in those requirements which are contrary to the best interests of the patient.

Not the doctor's interest, but the patient's. Of course, one could say the patient benefits when the doctor benefits. This expresses loyalty to the profession and also adheres to the value justice, if law is equated with justice. (See that discussion under Law, the latter part of Chapter One.)

Value Reflected: Doing Good (for the Society) and Being True (to Society)

NURSES

POINT 11 *The nurse collaborates with members of the health professions and other citizens in promoting community and national efforts to meet the health needs of the public.*

The doctors and the RCPs have similar concerns.

RESPIRATORY CARE PRACTITIONERS

The respiratory care practitioner shall cooperate with other health care professionals and participate in activities to promote community and national efforts to meet the health needs of the public.

Sounds familiar!

DOCTORS

VII. A physician shall recognize a responsibility to participate in activities contributing to an improved community.

Role Model Statement for Respiratory Care Practitioners

In addition to their code, RCPs have a role model statement that speaks to research, teaching, public education, and disease prevention programs. In particular, the role model statement admonishes the RCP not to use tobacco, and to hold himself up as a model. The AARC Code of Ethics is politically correct gender neutral (he and she) while the role model is a male.

The doctors' code is gender neutral (*he* and *she* avoided altogether), and so is the nurse code. Both professions have many other pronouncements elaborating on ethical positions taken in their codes, along with divisions to address ongoing ethical problems their practitioners face.

The Committee of Nursing Ethics of the ANA regularly considers ethical problems of the profession and issues interpretive statements of the ANA Code (available from ANA in Washington, above).

Several specialty nurse organizations, including the American Holistic Nurses' Association[35] and the American Association of Occupational Health Nursing,[36] have their own codes.

Ethical issues for nurses are not peculiar to America; nurses in other countries are also active in nursing ethics. The principles of human morals would seem to be universal; if so, ethics cannot be relative (different) from country to country. International conferences in nursing ethics are held, in particular on the ethical theory of caring; discussion is under Feminist Ethics.[37]

Values in Conflict?

When an ethical conflict arises, it is often said that "values are in conflict here." Values have no voices, no thoughts; so, can values be in conflict with other values? *People* with voices express their values; people with values are in conflict with other *people*, who have different values.

In reality, people do not have much internal ethical conflict about what they want to do. They quickly prioritize those interests that conflict and focus on one interest. It is then that they may be in conflict with other people about what they can do.

People act in accord with their interests. Their interests are made visible by what they *do*. What the person values is obvious from the person's actions—not by what the person *says* about belief.

INTERESTS AND EMOTIONS

Ethical conflicts always involve two or more people with different interests (who want different outcomes).

Thinking involves both mental and emotional processes, especially in the nursing profession in which caring (involving emotion) is the major service.

Feminist Ethics as ethical theory and the philosophy of Emotivism also

In any conflict situation, and especially one labeled an ethics conflict, it is helpful to note which people are involved, and then to examine the interest (wishes, wants, biases) of each. If the government has an interest in some ethical problem, such as "costs" or "system reform," remember that the government is a shorthand way of saying "all the people."

If it is an ethical conflict, by definition at least two people have interests (it takes two people to make a conflict). The patient has an interest, the surrogate decision maker (if the patient is incompetent), the patient's family, the hospital, the patient's priest or "ethicist," all have personal interests (a preference for one outcome over another). No one in the midst of an ethical conflict is a neutral person (especially not the patient's nurses). And they all feel some emotion.

People cannot think without using emotion, except perhaps those who are neurologically damaged or those diagnosed as sociopaths. Being *without* emotion about an ethical issue is pathological, it is not a "higher" or better way to be. Ethical conflicts are personal; people decide what they think about an issue (they decide what should be done) by their personal emotional reaction. It can be seen that people project themselves personally into an ethical conflict; for example, when they say, "*I* wouldn't want to live like that" or "I wouldn't want that done to me" or "I wouldn't want to have to do that to a patient."

People identify with others in the situation of an ethical conflict. People who demonstrate in favor of abortion rights, or in opposition at abortion clinics, feel personally about those issues; these are not situations for calm, distant reason. Ethical conflicts personally affect people because they have been or could be in the same kind of situation—or they empathize with people who are. The phrase, "walk a mile in my shoes," and the mother's admonition "how would you feel if that happened to you?" are both appeals to be personally involved (to feel the emotion of another) in order to decide what is the right behavior.

The recognition of the validity of emotion is especially important for nurses. The essence of nursing is caring, and caring incorporates emotion (see Feminist Morality, below, for discussion of caring as ethical theory). Emotivism in ethical behavior is a very old and respected theory[38] that holds that emotion is the basis of right action.

It seems almost unnecessary to say that nurses experience, use, and must cope with emotions raised in their practice with patients. But that emotion has been denied in some instances. Critical care nurses and nurses in small communities (who know patients as friends and neighbors even prior to caring for them) are very prone to emotional involvement.[39]

Ethicists in one case were able to abstractly, objectively counsel that a ventilator be removed when a competent patient requested it. But they had difficulty actually doing the "plug-pulling"—something nurses could face any day. There is a difference between intellectually, logically believing something should be done, and physically, personally, emotionally doing it.[40]

Too much emotion, and emotion alone, can cloud thinking; emotion alone should not determine decisions. But nurses must recognize the emotion (the personal preference) and that it motivates people in one direction or another. Thinking and feeling are intertwined; they are not separate activities. Once one recognizes the emotion felt, one can then think reasonably about the issue. The first emotional response should be analyzed as to whether it is valid or helpful.

Perhaps a nurse is emotional about a violation of patient autonomy—for example, inserting a patient's central line under local instead of general anesthesia as the patient requested. What action should the nurse take? Once she realizes that it's *her* feeling, not necessarily also the patient's, she can think better about the consequences to the patient, to the agency, and to herself. What does the patient want? She then may or may not decide to act, but her action will now be based on more than her feelings.

Nurses may emotionally feel that abortion or euthanasia should be done freely. After recognizing that initial emotion and *thinking* about the consequences of that policy, however, they may realize that some limit on those activities is appropriate. Or, they may emotionally *feel* that abortion and euthanasia should be forbidden, but after considering the consequences, they may realize that some allowance for those activities is appropriate. Either way, nurses must first recognize their feelings.

Closely related to emotivism as a philosophy of ethics and behavior, is intuitionism, the belief that the individual's first reaction to a situation is likely to be the right one or at least worth serious consideration. One writer—countering critics of intuition who say that reason is superior in determining ethical behavior—says it's essentially the same thing, that "reasoning is slow intuition."[41]

PHILOSOPHY AND RELIGION

Ethics is a subset of philosophy; philosophy is metaphysical (can't be physically sensed); ethics are the customs of a people.
   The ethics of a people are based on and reflected in their religions (also metaphysical, also customs).

Philosophy means "love of wisdom." After the middle ages, philosophy included all of knowledge. In the 1400s "natural philosophy," or science, began to be studied separately from "moral philosophy," which then included all the rest of knowledge.

The humanities (history, art, literature) were still included in philosophy, as was ethics and law and religion. Early psychology and the social sciences were part of philosophical studies, too; that was before it became more prestigious to be included (with medicine) in the "hard sciences" along with physics.

All of knowledge that rests on belief, that can't be measured (like ethics and philosophy), is called *meta*-physics, from Greek, meaning "after or beyond, the physical things which are Nature."[42] Anything that is not physical (not measurable or perceivable by the senses) is metaphysical.

The origin of the word *ethics* is from the Greek *ethike tekne*, "the moral art." In Latin the word becomes "morals"; in English, "character." Used in English, it means "character and spirit of a people, or custom." The word *ethics* was commonly used in place of the word *customs* only a few decades ago.[43]

The ethics of a people are their customs. When they say something is not ethical, they mean it is outside their custom. In the United States, a pluralistic society with people of many different customs, it is difficult to say exactly what is the custom of the people (the ethic) in a given situation. As a nation of people with different customs, Americans may need to live with the idea that there is not one "right" behavior (custom, ethic) for all situations.

A basis of Western civilizations, including the United States, is Judeo-Christian religion. The law—and customs that underlie the law—of the West, thus of the United States, is based on the Ten Commandments of the Hebrews. The Commandments do not require people to "do good" (neither does much of modern law, except for those people who voluntarily undertake to do good for pay, like nurses). The Commandments do not speak specifically to being fair. But, all the "do nots" of the Commandments result in the same thing: not being *unfair* to other people by killing them, stealing from them, lying to them.

Another value prominent now, but not so important in tribal life like that of the Hebrews, is freedom or autonomy for the individual. Tribal life, in more difficult circumstances, required more cooperation, less variation from the norm. The current emphasis on individualism is, at the same time: (1) a luxury bought by the degree of material success in the West (modern "success" makes it easier for individuals to survive alone); and (2) a necessity for people of various backgrounds and values to live together with any degree of peace. Americans are of many different "tribes," with different genetics and values.

Religion was the basis of ethics in the past, therefore, much of what is called "ethical" behavior is still reflected in religions. Religions are deontological systems; they express duties that humans have toward each other, in rules for conduct. This religious base of ethics and association with ethics is so strong that some newspapers now headline pages with "Religion and Ethics" (*St. Louis Post-Dispatch*), contrasted with "Religious News" a decade ago.

In an attempt to create a scientific ethical rule for behavior (without using ethics based on religious precepts), Carl Sagan gives his interpretation of different prescriptions for ethical behavior, starting with a *golden* rule (do as you would have done to you, from the Gospel of St. Matthew); a *silver* rule (do not do to others as you would not have done to you, more of a negative, *laissez-faire* philosophy, shared by Ghandi, Martin Luther King, and other nonviolence advocates); and a *brazen* rule (kindness with kindness, evil with justice, taught by Confucius and similar to the Old Testament's mandate, an eye for an eye). Last, Sagan describes an *iron* rule: Be good to the relatives/tribe only.[44] This ethic is developed with computer programs (supposedly without morals or religion). But the machine has all the values of its human programmers and users, subconsciously transferred in programming.

The Christian religion's values of faith (in God), hope (for an afterlife), and charity (kindness prescribed by Christ) were added to the four pre-Christian values of temperance, prudence, justice, and fortitude—a total of seven, a familiar number of spiritual significance to some. The three Christian values have broader meaning, however: Faith (in addition to faith in God) includes a belief that some order exists in the world, so that doing good is ultimately important and not a "random act of senseless kindness"; hope (in addition to hope for an afterlife) is also hope for the self, for patients, children, the future; and charity continues as a part of caring-beneficence, no matter who teaches it.

Nurses have been spiritually motivated through history, from the fourth-century Deaconesses, to those of Kaiserwerth who taught Florence Nightingale and the English modern nurses as well. Nightingale and all the early leaders of the women's and nursing movements saw their work as essentially religious. Indeed, Nightingale said that God had spoken to her personally, calling her to nursing work, in the same way that Joan of Arc's voices spoke to her.[45]

Nurses continue to wonder if they can be ethical without being moral. Some assert that virtue is inseparable from duties and obligations. Prior to

1968, the ANA Code for Nurses referred to "moral purity," and later to private ethics. A concern for moral character is no longer in the code.[46]

It can be postulated that a set of duties (ethics, morals, or religion) higher than law is necessary if civilization is to survive. If law (minimum ethic) becomes the *highest* standard—and the only reason to obey the law is the force of the police—then every person would need a personal police officer to ensure right behavior. (And every police officer also would need a personal police officer. . . .)

THE IDEAL AND THE REAL: TWO VIEWS OF THE WORLD

Major philosophical views of the world underlie ethical issues in nursing, and each nurse's own philosophy is some combination of the major philosophies. The major philosophies can be arbitrarily grouped under either more *idealistic* or more *realistic* views.

Ethics is a subdivision of philosophy. The individual's ethic (belief in what is the right thing to do) is based on a personal philosophy (what life is all about). Some knowledge of philosophy will help to know how the individual's ideas are related to those of the well-known Western philosophers. These same philosophies or ideas are the basis of action for other people, whose actions affect the individual's life, at work as a nurse and as a citizen of her country.

Following is a simplified description of major Western ideas and philosophers, divided arbitrarily into two groups, by whether they focus more on ideals or more on reality. These ideas are discussed as they relate to bioethics in America in the 1990s. If other terms are encountered, they can be researched (the major encyclopedias in the branch library will be of help, and the *Dictionary of the History of Ideas*, New York: Scribners, 1973 is especially good).

Two ways of looking at the world are described as Idealism and Realism. The major philosophies and philosophers are arbitrarily classed into one division or the other (ideas not listed are often variations of one view or the other). There are no "new" ideas in the world, and there won't be until new kinds of humans are made.

EDMUND BURKE ON NEW MORALITY IDEAS

"We know that we have made no discoveries; and we think that no discoveries are to be made, in morality—nor many in the great principles of government, nor in the ideas of liberty, which were understood long before we were born, altogether as well as they will be after the grave has heaped its mold upon our presumption, and the silent tomb shall have imposed its law on our pert loquacity."[47]

A student of philosophy will recognize that great liberty has been taken here with specifics (but a student of philosophy probably didn't need this book).

Idealism

This view of the world is best represented by Plato, the Greek philosopher who lived c. 428–348 B.C. In this view of the world, people are perfectible, or at least society is. In a structured, ordered system—a *utopia*—people are educated for their use to society; some things, values, or people are ranked into a hierarchy—some are better than others.

Plato thought that the four highest virtues (values) an individual could have were justice (fairness), temperance (moderation), prudence (sensibility), and fortitude (courage, endurance). These values are encountered again in this book, proving that the topics in human behavior and philosophy have changed little over 2000 years.

Current examples of Plato's virtues: *Justice* is one of the values on which much of nursing law and ethics is based (the value, Fairness). And, much of nursing practice deals with the results of the failure of patients to *temper* or moderate their actions. The standard in nursing malpractice law is what the reasonable, *prudent* nurse would do. The law, nursing practice, and nursing ethics demand that the nurse have personal *courage*—be an advocate for patient, for self, for profession.

In an idealist's world, thinking is better than feeling, reasoning is valued over emotion; people who *think* are superior to people who *do*, without thinking. The consequence of this idea is that people who do not think at all (anencephalic babies, patients in comas) are less valued, have fewer rights.

Idealists do not focus on specific cases or particulars, but on the generalization (the ideal). The thinking process used is *deduction*, the process of starting with an idea and applying (deducing) to the particular example or case (start with a idea and apply the idea in the real world). In this view, everything evolves, gets better as time passes; the world progresses inevitably from stage to stage. Darwin didn't invent evolution; he applied the idea of progression to species differences. Marx applied the idea of progression to governments, proposing that Capitalism evolve to Socialism to Communism—the planned utopia.

An example of progression in technology would be the belief that every new machine is better than the old. The idea of hierarchy, of evolving and bettering, higher and higher, is the basis of the idea that morality *develops*. (See Kohlberg's theory, later in this unit.) Remember that in the progression of human needs postulated in Maslow's hierarchy of needs, from physical to safety to love to self-actualization, the idea was that some needs are higher than others and that the needs *evolve* as basic ones are met and people get better.)

Thomas Hobbes, an English philosopher of the 1600s, developed an ideal—a social system analogous to the human body: workers the legs, government the brain. (Even now many argue there is a tendency for appointed and elected officials to think they know better what to do than the people who put them in office.)

To focus on the ideal is to be more indifferent to the physical world—somewhat like the Stoics of ancient Greece, whose idea was to live for virtue (good) and avoid vice (evil). Their advice: Be indifferent to transient difficulties, to the opinions of people; trouble has happened to millions in the past and will happen to millions in the future; focus on higher values. (A nurse who puts the value of work above a need for a coffee break fits this description.)

René Descartes, seventeenth-century French philosopher and mathematician, can also be classed under Idealism: He said the mind and body are dual (separate); the mind exists independent of the body. His most famous maxim was "I think, therefore I am." The mind, not the body, is the person. (A physician on a panel, discussing Persistent Vegetative State (PVS) patient Nancy Cruzan, testified for Descartes when he said, "She's not a person.")

Idealism would endorse the idea that something can be known (*a priori*) by mental logic alone, without seeing or touching it or any other sense experience. *A priori* is Latin for knowing something prior to or before any experiment or assessment by observation (by reason alone). (The opposite idea, *a posteriori*, is described under Realism.) Many religious people, philosophers, and some ethicists are advocates of *a priori* thinking. (Scientists use mostly *a posteriori* thinking; see Realism below.)

Immanuel Kant, a German philosopher of the 1700s, believed it possible to reason *a priori*. Kant, associated with the *categorical imperative*, stated that one should judge every act by whether one would choose the same behavior for everyone else in the world. The categorical imperative can be paraphrased as "do only what you would have others do *to someone else*." It is similar to the Christian Golden Rule, but in an objective ("reasonable third person") form. The Christian imperative, in contrast, is subjective (paraphrased): "Do unto others as you'd have them do *to you personally*."[48] When tempted to skip the deep-breathing exercises for the uncooperative patient, Kant would have the nurse consider the categorical imperative.

Kant's categorical imperative has loaned its power in philosophical circles to a other terms: moral imperative and ethical imperative. The word *imperative* means something that must be done or about which there is no choice, no debate, no differing point of view. An act that is termed a moral or ethical imperative might mean there is no argument about it—it's right and that's that! Kant's admirers included Hegel, Engels, and eventually Karl Marx. Kant's philosophy flowed from stoicism, the idea of living for virtue.

Communism and another totalitarian system, Fascism, envisioned a utopia. The Germans under National Socialism (Nazis) visualized an ideal world occupied by a pure, superior Aryan *volk* (folk, people) and worked toward that. (Abortion for genetic reasons might be examined as an ideal at work.) Communism and Fascism were applications of the philosophy of Collectivism, the opposite of Individualism (classed with Realism, next). An illustration of a collectivist philosophy at work is the attempt to shift the healthcare focus from individuals to the community.[49]

Advocates of idealistic philosophies believe humans need ideals—something more than the material world to live in and strive for. Should ideals be imposed (imperative) on people who do not share the ideal?

Christian thought is idealistic, too, valuing the ideal over the real. Christianity advises living for virtue's reward, the afterlife. Material things are unimportant or less important than spiritual ones. Christians added three theological virtues or values—Faith, Hope, and Charity—to the four "highest" virtues of Plato. Faith and Hope might be seen and expressed differently by Christian and non-Christian nurses. (For additional current usage, see Philosophy and Religion earlier in this chapter.)

Of the three, Charity is particularly relevant to nurses, being another way to say Doing Good (Beneficence). Instead of being a voluntary, nonmandatory value that any citizen might express, nurses are paid to do good, to be beneficent, to have charity. This is one value fundamentally different for current professional nursing versus earlier nursing performed for free. Before, doing good (charity, beneficence) was voluntary, performed by some who were encouraged by their religion and ethics. Now, nurses are paid to do good, and in fact mandated to do so. Thus do people turn nursing and other charity over to the professionals who get paid to do it. Instead of "giving to the poor," people may pay taxes to the government, which in turn gives the charity to the poor.

Deontology is a ethical system in which people are considered to have duties toward each other. (The origin of the word is not God, as one might guess, but a Greek word for duty.) These duties give rise to rules that enforce the duties. Doing the duty is considered right. Under this view one adheres to a duty, a set of rules or ideal values; one would "do the right thing" because it's the duty. The nurse might refuse to pull the plug on a patient because one of the Ten Commandments says the duty is not to kill another human.

Some people believe these rules have been developed over thousands of years of human history and should be obeyed even if people see no immediate reason for the rule. They believe violation of these fundamental duties, expressed in the rules, inevitably leads humans into trouble. They would point as an example to the violation of the rule against having babies out of wedlock, the violation having led to many social ills visible only a generation after the rule was violated extensively. (See an explanation of Teleology, which some believe is the opposite of deontological philosophical principles, under Realism, below.)

Jean-Jaques Rousseau, a Frenchman of the eighteenth century, believed the ideal to be the "natural" state of some unspoiled time. He envisioned a "noble savage" as the ideal human and wrote that, under an ideal social contract, people make an agreement with each other to live together harmoniously. Romanticism, the idealization of emotion and the natural world, is closely related.

Natural rights (natural law) is a principle of justice that some philosophers say can be known by logic, *a priori*. The law can be discerned by thinking logically about what it should be, without considering experience. This philosophical principle grew as the influence of religion declined in Europe during the period called the Enlightenment (discussed below in Humanism). Natural law replaces (and in many instances, mirrors) the tenets of Christianity, but it purports to be human law instead of God's law.

Natural law is not written, and it may only be determined by reference to what one believes is "natural." This idea was fully developed by the time of the Revolutionary War. The writers of the U.S. Declaration of Independence evidenced belief in natural rights when declaring

> We hold these truths to be self-evident; that all men are created equal and endowed by the Creator with certain inalienable rights, among them life, liberty and the pursuit of happiness. [Note: "inalienable rights," meaning the rights can't be sold, is another way to say "natural rights."]

The courts have sometimes used the concept of natural law, when no written law was available, to mandate a result they desired or felt necessary. "Natural law" and "natural rights" are invoked when any group or person wishes to bolster a desire for some action with an appeal to law, especially when there is no written law mandating the action they want. There is usually a desire for law to be written to enforce the "natural law."[50]

Realism

Aristotle (384–322 B.C.) best represents Realism's emphasis on the "real world" instead of an ideal in the mind. A student of Plato's, Aristotle produced quite a different philosophy; he strove for the middle (the golden mean, the average). He avoided extremes and advocated realistic moderation. The virtues (values) he espoused were temperance, prudence, and wisdom, all involving rational control over physical appetite and passion. His maxim: Mind over Matter. From these ideas came Freud's id (the physical appetite), ego (human reason), and superego (spirit or passion). Realism is concerned with reasoned behavior as much as Idealism, but reason as applied to the real (not an ideal) world.

In this century, medicine relies more on Aristotle's philosophy. Current scientists are more likely to describe the real world than to invent an ideal one. The *social* scientists, however (sociologists and psychologists), are more likely to *construct* worlds, like Plato's abstract ideal.[51]

Epicureans represent another segment of Greek philosophers whose values, like those of the Stoics, were continued into Roman culture. Still important today, the goal of this philosophy is pleasure (at least, absence of pain). The idea has become associated with hedonism (self-indulgence to excess), but its original writings reflect a more moderate, balanced attempt to enjoy life and avoid pain. Neither Epicureans nor Stoics were much in hope of, nor concerned with, a life after death.

Existentialism—a leap forward in history, to the mid-twentieth century—is a philosophy in harmony with Realism. Popularized by Albert Camus and Jean-Paul Sartre, this philosophy viewed human existence as the basis for all ideas, that humans and their individual existence come first and are the only reality. Camus said, "I know men and recognize them by their behavior, by the totality of their deeds, by the consequences caused in life by their presence." Existentialists would be more likely to say, "I am, therefore I think," reversing Descartes' maxim. The nurse who believes that the patient exists only in the physical body (without other meaning) is more like an existentialist.

Also within the arbitrary classification of Realism are the philosophies of Humanism and individualism. Humanism says that humans are the creatures paramount in the world (in contrast to many religions wherein God is paramount). This idea of Humanism has been rediscovered several times, from the Italian Renaissance ("rebirth" of Graeco-Roman civilization) in the 1400s, to the Enlightenment (new religion of the intellect), which in turn fostered the drama of the American and French revolutions. The latest version is still called Humanism—the religious call it secular humanism.

The philosophy of individualism assumes that the individual is more important than the collective (the society). The individualist will connect "society" to Idealism (above) because the "collective" of people is an abstract idea, while the individual is real. Individualism is an important philosophy in the United States; the nurse who values the autonomy of the patient above all other values is expressing part of the philosophy of individualism.

The philosophy of utilitarianism, also under Realism, borrows heavily from stoicism. Utilitarianism is based on the idea that actions are not good or bad in themselves but only as judged against their outcomes (their *utility*). Actions considered to be good are those that gain the greatest good, for the greatest number of people; in some sense, it is the opposite of individualism. Utilitarianism's advocates would argue the probability that any one individual would be better off, were utilitarianism the prevailing philosophy of society. When planners, government analysts, or epidemiologists consider the effect of any given act on the whole population, they are attempting to gauge its social utility. They seek to measure the act's usefulness to the whole society (not just to an individual), thus giving rise to current controversy about whether this measurement of usefulness can be done accurately or fairly or at all. One example of utilitarianism is Oregon's experiment in Medicaid revision, which will spend taxpayer money for more care for younger and healthy people than for older and sicker patients. Another current example is cost–benefit analysis (for example, screening a whole population for detection of cancer). Both examples illustrate applying "the greatest good to the greatest number."

The names most often heard in connection with utilitarianism are the Englishmen Jeremy Bentham, a philosopher (1748–1832), and John Stuart Mill, a philosopher/economist who lived 1806–1873.

Teleology may be considered the opposite of deontology, described earlier under Idealism as doing something because it is one's duty (because some rule derived from the duty says it's right). In contrast, under the concept of teleology, one does not act because it's the duty, but only for a reason (to get certain results). Teleology might assume that, whatever the end, it is a result of some deliberate process; for example, that people have noses is assumed to be the result of noses being designed (planned or evolved) for some reason, not just Evolution's random mutation. Teleology can also be known as "the end justifies the means . . . the outcome excuses the process." This attitude can be criticized (or praised) as situation ethics.[52]

Another concept related to situation ethics is *casuistry*, a word for going from cases to more encompassing principles. The base of the word is *cases*; the concept is the opposite of absolutism.

The term casuistry is used in a negative way to mean excusing people from the effect of a law one doesn't want to apply, case by case (as in the pejorative use of situation ethics). Critics say casuistry can't be used as a method of finding principles, because people change their principles depending on the cases.

This criticism of deciding case-by-case implies that people wake up in a new world for each case, and it assumes that they don't apply previous experience or learning from prior cases. Contrary to that assumption, a study of nurses showed that nurses with experience in many cases were better at making ethical decisions than those fresh out of school.[53] Casuistry also refers to the system of judge-made law in Britain and in British-founded countries like Canada, Australia, India, Jamaica and the United States, in which a system of decisions in individual cases together compose a body of principles or laws.

Materialism as a philosophy falls under Realism. Materialists say that what exists is the material, not some ideal, and that the highest value is not ideas but material things. A nurse who values the car, house, or income more than ideals is somehow adhering to the philosophy of materialism.

Determinism, also grouped under Realism, is an idea that things are predetermined (that they will happen a certain way no matter what the circumstances). Determinism is maintained both by religious and nonreligious people. This concept is raised when issues of genetics and behavior come up.

Induction, as a method of reasoning, belongs within Realism as the opposite of deduction. Induction works from the case or cases to figure out some big principles (as in casuistry). In practice, people usually think in a combination of induction and deduction; they always start with a case (a real problem) and then induce to the principle above. But, all people have heard or read of some principles (in church or from mother or in the human psyche as part of the collective unconscious—the Jungian theme). It may be that biology (genes) determines human values and ethics to a degree not yet understood. However it is done, induction is never purely "upward" and done value-free without some *a priori* principles already in mind.

The theory of law most related to the classification of Realism is positivism, the idea that people can only know about things that exist (can imagine only what is here and now). Positivism applied to law finds law is just what is written and nothing else (not what it should be or could be, as in the theory of natural law).

Emotivism is a philosophy, explained by Scottish philosopher David Hume (1711–1776) to be this: The emotions of pleasure and pain are the determinants of behavior, and reason is only useful to justify that behavior (which is already determined by whether it is pleasurable or painful).

Intuitionism is an old philosophy that relies on intuition to determine ethical behavior. It is postulated that intuition is actually considered, logical thinking, but done very rapidly; and that seemingly unemotional logic is merely very slowly-done intuition. Nurses often use intuition successfully to solve ethical problems.[54]

After comparing Realism and Idealism, nurses will know that no one is a total realist or total idealist. The philosophies and philosophers represent one view or the other for the reader's convenience; and, perhaps, discussion. The two views are used to organize thinking. The nurse's personal philosophy (view of what the world and life are all about) would more likely be neither *all* Idealism nor *all* Realism.

LAW—Based on Ethics, but Not the Highest Ethic

Law is the minimum ethic, written down and enforced; behavior that is not merely desired but mandated.

Ethics and law are guides for resolving conflict between people; on a continuum from the mandates of law to ethics to manners. Law is the minimum ethic and, therefore, legal behavior is not necessarily the highest ethic.

Laws are proscriptions or prescriptions of extreme behavior.

Law is minimum ethics, written down and enforced. Law is about behavior that is not merely desired but mandated. Some illegal behavior is worse than other behavior; speeding at 57 miles per hour will be punished as wrong (some would say it should not be, that it should be seen as somewhat unethical but not illegal). But speeding at 100 miles per hour through a playground would be considered unethical as well as illegal by most people.

The more severe the penalty for breaking the law, the more strongly the law is enforcing an ethical value.

Ethics and law are guides for resolving conflict between people. Ethics resembles but differs from law; law can be separated from ethics by the effect of each. Law is behavior that people have agreed should be mandatory or prohibited.

Ethics and law are found along a continuum of ways to solve conflicts between humans (the concept of a continuum is helpful in thinking about a number of concepts, from acidosis to ethics). One can arbitrarily draw a line and say "here at this number starts acidosis" (the line is drawn because at that point the condition starts to become lethal). The same thing can be done with law and ethics: The line is drawn exactly (and arbitrarily) when the law is written—there starts law and mandated behavior (it's an arbitrary, human-constructed line).

Both law and ethics play a part in human efforts to live together and hurt each other as little as possible. (As part of that effort, people also help each other, too, at least in some situations.) Law is a very small part of the continuum of control of behavior. Law controls potentially hurtful behavior; it will either mandate (prescribe) that something must be done, or prohibit (proscribe) that something must *not* be done.

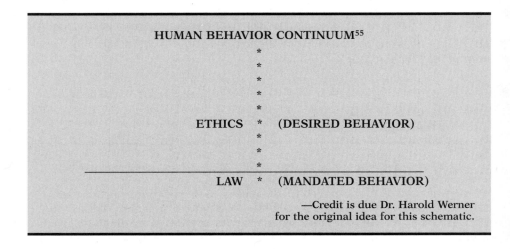

HUMAN BEHAVIOR CONTINUUM[55]

ETHICS * **(DESIRED BEHAVIOR)**

LAW * **(MANDATED BEHAVIOR)**

—Credit is due Dr. Harold Werner
for the original idea for this schematic.

Law usually is about extremes of behavior. People together then decide on certain actions that *must* be done (for example, parents must care for their child); or they decide a certain action must *not* be done and, if done, will be punished (parents must not abuse their child).

People together elect or authorize other people to en*force* the law. The word *force* is important since force is implied in law (as opposed to ethics, which seek to persuade). In statutes and paintings of Justice, she is blindfolded to appear impartial (until the 1600s Justice was portrayed as clearsighted in order to judge). In one hand, she holds a scale to weigh the issue (symbolizes judgment) and in the other hand a sword symbolizing force—enforcement of law. Without force, there is no law. And yet, to live together without fear, people can't allow force to be used by any *except* those with authority of law (authority of law extends to people using force to defend themselves).

Still on the continuum of human action, ethics is higher behavior (desired behavior). It may be wished that people would act ethically, but they will not be made to do so. If there is force, and not mere persuasion, that's law and not just ethics.

Adhering to the legal minimum behavior can be less than fully ethical, since law is a minimum ethic. Under the German law of the National Socialists of the 1930s, judges, lawyers, doctors, nurses, and others performed acts that were legal but certainly unethical by today's standards (unethical by the standards of the time as well). Nurses who say "it's the law—I don't have any ethical choice to make" should realize that nurses in Nazi Germany said the same thing.

> An incompetent patient designates a niece to be surrogate decision maker, and the law says the decision maker has authority to withhold treatment under certain conditions. But the nurse has reason to believe the request for removing the feeding tube is not in the patient's best interest but is done because the niece will inherit when the patient dies. In that situation, the nurse who merely obeys what appears to be the mandate of the law, without any ethical analysis of the problem, does not meet her duty to the patient.

Ethical standards cannot be followed automatically, any more than can law. Ethics (like law) is a guide for resolving conflicts in human behavior, but with regard to law, people as citizens have direct control over which way the law "guides" because they have control over the lawmakers. Laws are made by people with authority, an authority granted by the people who have expressed their demand that laws must be written.

In contrast, people who "make" ethics or "write" ethics, or who establish standards of ethical behavior, are not controlled like lawmakers. Some people would use ethics to get other people to do what they want, putting their wants in ethical terms, in terms of "nurses should." Or they might say that what they want is a moral imperative. Ethics makers have not been elected or appointed to guide behavior; they don't have authority, unless believed and followed.

Morals—Values—Ethics

The words *morals*, *values*, and *ethics* are often used interchangeably. Some authorities regard morals and values as concepts that pertain to what IS, what takes place now. They say that morals and values are the guides existent in human behavior.

They define ethics as what ought to be—the ideal, the goal—a definition or standard to which few people can actually aspire: They can be moral, but ethical behavior would be always out of reach. People would have to strive continually to be better, a familiar idea common in religions in which the individual is typified as unclean (or inferior, or sinful). The individual strives for salvation or nirvana. The end, perfection, is always out of reach. This idealization of ethics assumes that people are not okay as they are. But does it keep people working always to improve?

THEORY OF MORALITY DEVELOPMENT

Moral reasoning (thinking) is distinguished from ethical practice (action) in some theories of ethics (although thinking cannot be observed); some theories (such as Kohlberg's) postulate that people develop morally over their lifetimes.

When tested under Kohlberg's theory of a hierarchy of moral reasoning, women never achieved the "highest" level of morality (the highest value was justice; women valued caring).

Tests of nurses are inconsistent; some research finds nurses "lower" on Kohlberg's morality scale (like most women) while other researchers show that nurses differ from most women (as high as men), valuing justice in preference to caring.

"Justice" as measured on Kohlberg's scale may be actually "social justice." Other research shows nurses with more experience (even with less education) were better at making ethical decisions than those with less experience (even with more education).

Some writers distinguish moral reasoning (thinking) from ethical practice (action). Moral reasoning (moral judgment, moral development) is thinking, they say; ethical practice is the action of ethics, the doing. Since the thinking can't be seen, ethical acting is all that can be known of ethical thinking.

Some writers say this separation can be discerned through tests; for example, the question can be asked, "What do you think the nurses *should* do for the patient in this situation?" That would measure the thinking, the moral reasoning. Then one could ask, "What do you think the nurses *will* do for the patient in this situation?" That answer could tell the interviewer about the ethical practice (the action),[56] if the nurse knew and told the truth to both questions.

Theories are proposed (and accepted by some) that people develop morally as they get older, more experienced, educated. Kohlberg's theory[57] echoes the pervasive idea that people evolve from babyhood (Evolution, the idea of Darwin, Piaget, Maslow, and all the Platonists). Kohlberg thought he could measure stages in development of ethical behavior from lowest ethical behavior to highest; here again, an Idealist idea of hierarchy, ranking, elitism.

Kohlberg believes people develop ethically in stages that are invariable in sequence. People move from simple thought to complex moral reasoning. At higher stages, people use skills that were developed earlier, at lower stages. He constructs three levels of development, each having two stages:

1. Preconventional reasoning. Right and wrong depend on what Mommy (authority) says. "I have to do the right thing because the law, the hospital policy, the supervisor said 'this is right.' "
2. Conventional reasoning. Right or wrong comes from the family or group. The person wants to maintain existing social relationships or order. "I do the right thing because it's the Golden Rule; it's good for my family, my profession, my country."
3. Postconventional (principled reasoning). This person thinks above and apart from the herd and develops a conscience, *a priori*, without referring to her own real situation.

The postconventional level may be classed with Idealist philosophies, above, in that "thinking" alone dictates the right thing to do. Justice is the highest value to aspire to. "I do the right thing because it's good for the whole world, and I have reasoned for myself that it is the ideal right thing to do."

The testing required to measure these stages of ethical behavior is intensive and requires a specially trained interviewer; thus, it is expensive in both time and money to research Kohlberg's theory.

Perhaps Kohlberg saw differences in various people's ethical styles, not differences in the stages of ethical development in one person. He may have measured differences in peoples' interests, values, ways of deciding. He then ranked them according to how he thought people *should* decide things (he arbitrarily classed Justice as the highest value, over caring). People who take the same test, time after time as his subjects did (all men), may seem to progress to higher levels as they learn more of the terms used or learn more what the interviewer expects or wants them to say.

Kohlberg's theory is challenged in particular by feminists. Gilligan criticized the research on the ground that women were not used in the original research, and when women were tested, on average they never reached higher than level 2—that is, not what was defined as the highest level of an adult. Women consistently cared more for family and friends and decided right and wrong on that basis. Gilligan argued that the failure of women to advance to concern about the ideal of justice for all, in an abstract sense, was the result of lack of "care focus" in moral reasoning, in turn caused by exclusion of women from the research.[58]

It may be, however, that women didn't agree with the test's definition of justice as "social justice." The idea measured by justice in such research is not always justice meaning equal treatment under the law. Sometimes the word *justice* as used in ethics research actually means social justice (the idea of abstract equal outcomes for all). Whatever the reason, women in ethics research studies chose caring (relationships with individuals) over social justice (doing good for the abstract collective of humanity).

If women did value relationships and harmony over justice, as some of the research indicates, this has broad implications: The real relationships within the tribe (family) would be more important to women than the abstract ideal of democracy. Women would be more tolerant of authority in the name of harmony, more ready to sacrifice individual freedom (of others and their own) for the sake of peace, which would benefit the tribe.

This genetic or hormonal preference in women for relationships and for the family (*if* it exists), may work to ensure the survival of the species. Perhaps women would intuitively support more intrusions into their lives (socialism) in order to have more benefits for more people. Women might value comfort (representing survival—food and shelter) over the abstract of freedom and equality.

Ethics of Nurse-Women

Using Kohlberg's theory, nurses and nursing students are reported to have "consistently lower than expected levels of moral reasoning."[59] Gilligan criticized Kohlberg's research,[60] but some nurse researchers who have analyzed the original data support Kohlberg's theory. Kohlberg's theory, as applied, finds that women as a group are different from men in their ethical decision making, but Duckett and colleagues dispute that moral reasoning of nurses is lower than men's (see tint, below, for cite).

The review of the nurses who hypothesized that Kohlberg's theory was right found that nurses are not different from men. They found that nurses are good at "justice-based moral reasoning." They believe that little doubt remains that moral reasoning develops (Kohlberg's main thesis). They define moral reasoning as cognitive (thinking, not feeling), assuming that mental processes can be cleanly separated into two different activities. These researchers also believe moral reasoning may not progress automatically with age, but that moral reasoning does increase when people are educated.

BACCALAUREATE NURSE ETHICS?

"Baccalaureate programs for entry into professional practice and graduate programs for advanced practice are likely to produce nurses with higher levels of moral reasoning than one- or two-year programs focused on technical education."[61]

The findings that moral reasoning increases with education is contrary to data showing that nurses with more experience, not more education, make better moral judgments.

These authors distinguish "justice-based" moral reasoning from the concept/ethical value of caring. They do not explicitly say so, but they seem to equate moral reasoning with mental thought processes, and equate caring with emotion.

Research in nursing ethics shows that younger nurses prefer rules for making decisions; older, more experienced nurses seem to need fewer rules for ethical decision making. Younger nurses put "justice" higher on their scale of values; older nurses value care more. Care was more important to nurses with more experience, "justice" less. Many of these "justice" values are about equal outcomes (social justice), not equal treatment under law.[62]

In a study of neonatal ICU nurses and their moral decisions, most (65 percent) of the nurses used the care perspective; 12 percent used the justice perspective; and the remaining 23 percent used a combined care and justice perspective. Again, we are unsure if the "justice" measured is social justice (another version of Doing Good). If so, then *all* the nurses used some aspect of caring to make moral decisions.[63]

Tools to test the ethics of various occupations are helpful in research, but they also may exhibit bias in their assumptions, their design, application, and the conclusions reached. For example, the Judgments About Nursing Decisions (JAND) is an ethics test based on the ANA Code of Ethics.[64] In the questionnaire the nurse is given a hypothetical situation. She decides what a nurse *should* do in that particular ethical case. She then decides what a nurse *would* do in the case. The right answer is decided according to how close it comes to the Code of Ethics (which assumes that all the values in the code are "right" or ethical). Another tool used to test ethics is the Defining Issues Test (DIT).[65]

In practice, ethical research suffers the limitations of all social science research: What people say on a pencil and paper test may be different from what they do in action.

Some say that knowing what to do and doing it are two different things, as in moral reasoning versus ethical practice. They believe that an ethical problem is either *not* knowing what is ethical or knowing ethical behavior and not wanting to *do* it.

If "moral reasoning" exists and if it is a different thing from "ethical behavior," there should be some correlation between reasoning and behaving. Behavior is measured by observing actions; not what people say they will do, but what they actually do—as Leah Curtin writes, "You are the sum total of your value choices."[66]

Beliefs are distinguished from behaviors when it is desired that people behave differently than they do at present. It is wished that people believe differently from how they behave. If that were so, then it is hoped that people can be convinced to behave differently. (It is assumed that they

already *believe* differently.) Some writers say that the ethics of entire generations of providers need reeducation; implicit in that message is that others
need to change, to agree with and act with the writers.[67]

Nurse administrators have a large role in nurse ethics, as leaders, facilitators, and (unfortunately sometimes) hinderers of ethical nursing practice.
The literature reflects this group's attention to the ethics of caring.[68]

Narrative ethics is another term coming into fashion in ethics discussion.
Also called "storytelling," it is more of a technique for discussing issues than
an ethical theory or principle.[69] Another term used is *contextual*, referring
to the need for ethical decisions to be made based on the context of the
problem. Both are related to situation ethics and casuistry, referred to above
under Realism.

FEMINIST MORALITY

Feminist ethics may be defined roughly as whatever is *not*, "western male-
dominated philosophy"; this ethic values caring (relationships, doing good
as in nursing); feeling over logic. Other nurse ethicists postulate nursing as
a variation of a mothering model.

Another approach to ethics is feminist moral philosophy, a philosophy still
in its infancy. No easy definition is possible; in general it is simply whatever
is *not* "western male-dominated philosophy," which seems to hold justice
(one definition or another) as the highest value. Feminist moral philosophy,
in contrast, would hold relationships (caring, doing good) as the highest
value. As noted above, when tested, women on average put a combination
of the values Loyalty (Keeping Promises), Doing Good (charity, caring) and
Doing No Harm (non-maleficence) on a higher level than justice.

Noddings' caring ethic reflects a mothering model,[70] and some feminists
have criticized an ethic of caring. They fear that caring can be exploitative,
with the caring going in only one direction, from *carers* to *cared for*. There
is tension between an ethics based on caring as a foundation for nursing
practice (emotion), versus nursing science (intellect) as foundation.

A good example of the caring–thinking conflict was illustrated in a public
information TV spot in the early 1990s, produced with the advice of the
American Nurses Association. The goal was to get more young people into
nursing (during a nursing shortage) and, concomitantly, to have nursing be
seen by the public as a thinking occupation. The punch line—"If caring were
enough, anyone could be a nurse"—effectively denigrated the value of caring
in order to elevate the value of thinking.

A caring ethic could underlie nursing science. The metaphor (symbol) of
caring differs from other metaphors for nursing, such as a religious calling
or a duty to battle disease, said to be "masculine metaphors that evoke

images of separateness and adversity."[71] The caring metaphor is said to evoke images of women as mothers, nurturers of the young, old, ill, and nurses. The image is one of humans connected, not disconnected; not of duty and a calling, but of caring, freely chosen.

If this caring is a "feminist" ethic, the role of men in nursing may be questioned. Perhaps the essential caring nature of nursing accounts for the fact that, still, relatively few men practice nursing. This is not a new question, nor only an American one.

OLD ITALIAN ATTITUDES RELEVANT?

"The issue of nurse and nursing as feminine concepts and profession was widely debated at the beginning of the century by various professional and political groups and female associations. One of the most accepted positions even among nurses was that women by nature are more patient and kind, therefore born to care for men.

"Women supported this position because they saw in the nursing profession the possibility to have a job and economic independence . . . ."[72]

Of course, "feminine" qualities (example: caring?) are not exclusive to women, nor "masculine" qualities (example: thinking?) to men.

Nurses experience conflict when good care is seen to conflict with good economics (saving resources). Nyberg uses hope for the patient as a factor in her assessment of nurse conflict (see Hope as one of the three Christian values, above). She believes that tending to economics is a form of caring because it enables the agency to support the care. The goals of patient care and organizational survival are interdependent.[73]

Another study found that nurses thought caring behaviors—expressive, nontechnical care—were their most important acts, whereas patients placed more importance on the technical aspects of their care. Neither patients nor nurses thought actions like "offering reasonable alternatives" to the patient were important. One nurse found that the most surprising thing about her return to America and her return to nursing was the intensity of her feelings of caring *about* (not just *for*) her patients.[74]

This "new" feminist philosophy of caring (actually a new priority of values, with caring first) could well serve nurses as a group. At this point the concept is less a philosophy and more a different prioritizing of values. Nurses, as women in the most visible "caring" occupation, will be instrumental in continuing work on the theory.[75]

A theory of caring is a valid part of the formal study of ethics. Knowledge about caring should encourage nurses who believe it, to assert that the value of caring (emotion-based) is at least as important in their ethical decisions as the value of justice (reason-based).

ETHICS COMMITTEES

Ethics committees are common in illness care agencies; they may give advice on individual cases, assist in making policy, and help educate patients and staff on ethical issues.

Ethics committees are common in hospital and other illness care agencies. Many hospitals and other institutions that care for patients instituted these committees in response to the Joint Commission for Accreditation of Health Organizations (JCAHO) mandate that the agencies it surveyed have some kind of ethics procedure for ethical problems.

JCAHO MANDATE FOR ETHICS MECHANISM

". . . the right of the patient or the patient's designated representative to participate in the consideration of ethical issues that arise in the care of the patient:

"RI.1.1.6.1   The organization has in place a mechanism(s) for the consideration of ethical issues arising in the care of patients and to provide education to caregivers and patients on ethical issues in health care."

—JCAHO Accreditation Manual for Hospitals, Patient Rights, 1993, p. 106.

This directive did not say that ethics committees were mandatory (an ethics consultant could also serve as a "mechanism") but a cheaper and, in some ways, better method is to have an ethics committee.[76]

Members of ethics committees include staff of the agency (doctors, nurses, and administrators, usually), community representatives, and perhaps a lawyer and clergy. Such committees write bylaws and procedures; they may set policy for staff to use in situations of ethical conflict, and they educate staff and the public about ethics.

They use the same process to resolve conflicts as do ethicists. Nurses, too, can use the decision-making process for ethical issues in their practice; below are suggestions for such a process. Committee members ask questions, gather information, clarify interests (values), and act as mediator. If people in conflict can't agree after that, some committees decide the issue for them.

The members of the committee may have no special qualifications in ethics, but they may develop a consensus (a "conscience"?) of opinion. (But, Margaret Lady Thatcher has said that consensus is the negation of leadership.) In that sense they are making ethics, and those ethics may become law. Such committees were recommended in the *Quinlan* case, discussed in Chapter Seven. The court in that case mandated the use of ethics committees in "right to die" or withdrawal of treatment situations.[77]

Some type of case review may be done by the committee, in which the committee hears from some or all people involved. When recommended by a court of law, this case review by ethics committees is delegation of the court's decision-making power to informal courts of citizens who are closer to the situation.

Like the continuum from law to ethics, the formal law court gives way to a less formal committee, which often defers to the informal family/patient/physician decision. Government or law or ethics, usually all work better when decisions are made by people close to the problem.

Some have questioned whether ethics committees should themselves initiate investigation into cases, or should wait and be available to any patient or staff member who wishes to appeal to them. Some authorities prefer that an ethics consultation (face to face with the patient or family) be accomplished, before the committee considers the matter. In that case, the patient is not necessarily present at committee decisions.[78]

Other writers insist that the patient must be involved when committees deliberate.[79] Some form of patient/family participation, somewhere, is indicated by the JCAHO requirements, noted above.

Some authorities criticize any committee review of individual cases. They think the committee should be a forum for abstract discussion of ethical issues, not for advice on real cases; that the committee should make policy and educate, but not do clinical analysis of cases. They believe that advice to the patient's family and nurses should be given by an ethical consultant.

Some physicians believe an ethics consultant should be a physician/clinician who has an interest and skill in ethical decision making. Equally, some fear the authoritarian role that an "ethicist" might take on, and prefer the joint decision making, increased experience, and information available in committee.[80]

A study from Massachusetts General Hospital showed that consultations by ethics committees have risen in recent years. The committee decided in more cases to advise that Do Not Resuscitate orders be written, even against the wishes of family.[81]

Ethics committees may have some fear of lawsuit for their actions; thus far, however, lawsuits against committees are rare (one is the *Elizabeth Bouvia* case discussed in Chapter Seven: Life).

In some cases court-made law has required the "ethics court" be the ethics committee. Another law, the Patient Self Determination Act (PSDA), will also make more work for ethics committees. The act mandates that the agency have a policy on informing patients of their right to refuse treatment. The law requires the institution to decide if it will honor advance directives.

The ethics committee should help decide whether the agency will participate in honoring advance directives when they are used to end patients' lives. The law also mandates that staff and community be educated about advance directives, and the ethics committee should be involved in that education also. The PSDA is discussed more fully in Chapter Four, Freedom

(Autonomy). The ethics committee may also be an "AIDS committee," deciding policy for HIV-infected workers in the agency.[82]

One writer, with several years of experience in case consultation by ethics committee, saw a tendency for providers to quit too early. His committee was asked more often to uphold the wishes of the practitioners to stop care, against the wishes of family and friends. Larger societal issues of money and fairness loom also; he sees in the next decade that ethics committees may be less concerned with protecting the autonomy of the individual, and more concerned with defining the limits of the patient's freedom against the demands of the society (and the demands of providers of care).[83]

Ethics Committees in Research

Ethics committees to protect research subjects (animal and human) are mandated to review research that is funded by or controlled by the U.S. government: Institutional Review Boards (IRBs).

U.S. law to protect research subjects, both animal and human, mandates that another type of ethics committee, Institutional Review Boards (IRBs), review patient consent in advance, in research studies funded or supervised by the federal government. In consent for treatment that is not experimental, review of consent may happen only if a malpractice suit is filed as a result of the procedure.

The power of IRBs is delegated by the Congress—not to government regulators, but to the people on boards in each institution; this avoids the necessity of the government agency making decisions on the safety of all research subjects. As with ethics committees, there is delegation from a formal government body to a less formal body, the IRB of the agency. Again, a more local decision, instead of a national one.[84] (The issue of protection of research subjects is discussed in Chapter Three, on Doing No Harm.)

ETHICISTS AND DECISION MAKING

As noted, some institutions provide a mechanism for ethical discussion by employing or contracting for the services of an ethicist. Ethicists are a classification of philosophers (but, most true philosophers are usually so designated after death). In one sense, all people are ethicists; all have a philosophy and decide every day on the right things to do. People who are identified as *ethicists* and *philosophers* usually work in a position in which that word is part of their title, or the subject they teach.

Authorities recommend that people who teach ethics have a degree in the field, profession, or area in which they are going to work (for example, in illness care), plus one year of ethics training. Or, as an alternative, the teacher can qualify with an advanced degree in philosophy, and one year in the field of interest (illness care).

The person teaching ethics should be knowledgeable about the theories of ethics and philosophy, which is different from being ethical. (Any person can be ethical.) But ethicists in illness care can ask questions, gather information, and help people see various interests in a case. (Is a formal "ethicist" title necessary?)

People formally labeled ethicists seem often, like journalists, more likely to be politically liberal. There are few conservative ethicists.[85] This remark, attributed to an ethicist, assumes that "liberal" and "conservative" is a meaningful label. Often people so labeled agree with each other more than they disagree; usually discussing issues is more helpful than expounding ideology. The original meaning of "liberal" was a person who valued the freedom of the individual over group thinking.[86]

Ethicists' decisions start with preferences. Human beings have built-in preferences, genetic and environmentally formed. Lawyers have preferences; when the nurse enters the office to hire one, the lawyer has a preference for the nurse's position even before any facts are heard. Computers too have built-in preferences, those of their human program writers.

Judges decide cases the same way; they hear the facts, decide the case on the facts, and then they find the written principles (law) to use as base. But, deep within their decision on the facts, they are applying unspoken, unwritten principles—the ethics with which they were born and grew up learning.

Ethicist preferences can be detected by careful reading and listening. One ethicist cited positively a number of cases that resulted in patients' deaths, and said, "The *progressive* California decisions just cited were followed by a small number of extremely *conservative* rulings in New York, New Jersey, and Missouri." (EMPHASIS ADDED).[87] His characterization of decisions that resulted in death as "progressive," while describing rulings that kept the patient alive as "conservative" (unprogressive), reveals his preference.

The terms "bioethicist" and "medical ethicist" are distinguished; it is asserted that the study of medical ethics is not a value-free discipline (meaning that it has preferences that reflect the preferences that doctors have).[88] Does that imply that bioethics (as different from "medical ethics") has no particular values, that it is a pure field of study, objective, without innate values?

Decision Process Used by Ethicists and Nurses

The ethicist's/nurse's first step is to be sure there is an *ethical* problem: Sometimes an "ethical problem" is really a nursing practice problem (or a labor relations problem). Suppose a patient refuses to eat or take medication, and says, "Let me die." That may be the occasion for the nurse's first using her nursing skills, and only if that intervention is not successful will the nurse consider the *ethical* issue of allowing the patient to die.[89] If there's a nursing action to be tried, it usually *should* be tried before labeling it an ethical issue.

Approaches to ethical decision making—other than the one recommended in this book—start with gathering of information about the case by seeking outside information. The different recommendation of this book is virtually to do the opposite: to start with the nurse's own values, the information "inside" oneself.

As an example of the usual, "outside information" approach, one writer suggests this formula:

1. Determine medical treatment goals.
2. Determine patient preference.
3. Look at quality of life (only if item 2 is not available). This has to be done by a person other than the patient since the patient would assess his own quality of life subjectively, if capable.
4. Examine externals (family, impact on others, money issues). This process looks at externals only if item 2, patient preference, is not available; meaning, if the patient is incompetent. This process fits medical treatment to what the patient wants. That's rarely a problem; rarely do providers treat a competent patient who doesn't want treatment.

The usual problem that raises ethical conflict is the situation in which there is no patient preference stated, because the patient is not competent. Then the problem is to assess the quality of life for someone else, "objectively." Quality of life can in fact only be assessed subjectively, by the person who decides whether life is worth living or not. The conflicts come from item 4, those "externals," who turn out to be daughters, one who wants to let her father die, and one who wants him to live.[90]

Another approach to ethical decision making puts heavy emphasis on *medical* decisions first; after that the wishes of the patient are considered and other values are examined and ranked.[91] In both the decision processes, the ethicist starts with a value, implicit or unstated: Both processes start with the *medical* aspect of the patient's care, external information. By medicine's being considered first, it can be assumed that the medical part is considered the highest value (though that is never stated aloud).

Specific techniques for administrative decision making are variants on the "gather information and assess" theme (so familiar to nurses as "the scientific method").[92] Others simply apply the nursing process—assessment, planning, implementing, evaluating—to the ethics process (again, the scientific method).[93]

Another writer follows the same procedure, but adds "argument" about each possible solution identified. Then she's "ready to engage in ethical decision making" but doesn't say exactly how. She nicely points out that nurse managers' ethics must reflect that their first duty is to patients, second to employees, and third to the institution.[94]

A different way to approach ethical conflicts is to start with the nurse's *own* values, the nurse's internal information. This can be identified with the advice parents give to children before they cross the street: A warning to *stop, look, and listen—and add one more stop*.

Stop, Look, Listen—and Stop Again

PROCESS FOR ETHICAL DECISIONS

STOP and decide whether it's an ethical issue and not a nursing practice problem. Immediately (without further information), decide what should happen in the case (this alerts the nurse to her personal preferences).

LOOK AND LISTEN now. Gather information about the case, realizing that the personal preference already identified will affect what information is sought and found.

STOP again, separating personal and professional interest from the patient's interest, the agency's interest, and the family's interests. The problem will be solved, or else the solution will be clear; it remains to help others through the process.

Stop. When confronted with an ethical conflict (any conflict that involves values), stop and realize it for what it is; then begin this process: The nurse should think about personal values and use them. The nurse should allow intuition, feeling, and emotion free rein and decide what she thinks should happen in the case (what the nurse wants to happen). Once this unconscious information is conscious, the nurse can acknowledge that gathering data, looking, and listening will be practiced from that point of view.

Nurses must admit their values (their preferences) to themselves first. The old cliches are helpful: Know yourself, to thine own self be true. In discussion of the philosophy of Realism, it was noted that one of the ancient virtues was prudence—and note further that Prudence is portrayed in works of art as a woman with a mirror, the mirror to see herself, to know herself first in order to act prudently. (And note that the standard of care in malpractice is what a reasonable *prudent* nurse would do).

Many histories of values have been written for patients to use in identifying their own values, so that they can make decisions about their own care. It is just as important, possibly *more* so, for *nurses* to explore and recognize their own values, the feelings used in giving care (or not giving care) to so many people. Below is a Values Assessment for nurses, adapted by the author from Rushton's values history *for patients*.[95] Nurses who answer the questions therein may surprise themselves with what they learn.

NURSE VALUES ASSESSMENT: FIRST STEP
IN ETHICAL DECISION MAKING

Describe your current health or illness status.

What do you plan for the future? (can make happen)

What do you hope for, in the future? (can't make happen, but wish would happen)

What do you fear?

What is most important in your life now?

Is your life worth living?

What would make your life better?

What would make your life not worth living?

If you knew you were dying, what would be most important?

Where do you want to die?

How would you feel about life-sustaining procedures if you were dying? In a persistent vegetative state? If you had a chronic, irreversible illness, like diabetes?

How important are family and friends to you?

How important is your work?

How do you make decisions about your life? Your illness care?

What is your religion?

Does your religion affect your beliefs about death and illness?

Who would you want to make decisions for you if you could not?

Have you informed your family, friends, or practitioner about your values? Have you made an advance directive? Why or why not?

What would you do if you won the lottery?

Nurses project their own values onto patients, so they must be aware of their own preferences. Once the nurse is aware of the influence of personal values in an ethical conflict, the easier part of the process follows.

Look and Listen. This part is easy for nurses; they're used to gathering information, along with listening to overt and hidden communications. In looking and listening in order to make an ethical decision, they look at the person and condition, and listen to wishes. They look for others who are interested, and listen to their wants. By having admitted personal preferences before gathering data, they are able to assess if they have all the information, or just the part they wanted to hear (the part that supported their preference).

Then STOP again. The nurse should separate personal and professional interest from the patient's, the agency's, the family's interests, and other providers' interests. It may help to write down such assessments of interests, for private use.

At this point, the most important interests may become apparent. The more information gained about the conflict, the better; more information yields a better outcome (at least the result is more likely based on reality). But nurses must be prepared to deal with the information sought; for instance, finding the patient's living will reveals a revocation of it, signed and sealed at the back. Or, the terminal patient may have answered "yes" to a question as to whether intubation and ventilation is wanted.

Often this process of stop, look, listen, stop, is enough; but usually there is someone who didn't hear or know some information (perhaps the nurse). The time involved in the process of gathering all the information may solve the problem; the patient may die anyway on the ventilator, or get better; the relative may change her mind, or the doctor may decide to try a different treatment. The nurse will want to help others in the case to work though the process in this stop, look, listen, stop again, method, probably enlisting at some point the help of the agency's ethics committee or consultant.

Allowing time to gain information and reflect is always better than a quick decision based on inadequate information (and, as asserted above, sometimes unrecognized personal preferences). Obviously nurses shouldn't create problems if they don't exist, there being plenty of problems without creating them. There's no need to get a court order for treatment or non-treatment if the doctors, nurses, patient, and family agree. Some hospital lawyers have not gone to court in years on an ethical conflict case for their facility. When the real conflict between people cannot be resolved with information, mediation, and persuasion, the courts exist as final venue for conflict resolution.

Fear of Courts

When the process of STOP, LOOK AND LISTEN, STOP AGAIN has been fully completed in a given situation, but conflicts remain, the only venue left for conflict resolution may be the court system. Despite beliefs of illness care ethicists to the contrary, courts do well at ethical decision making in illness care.

Many say that courts are inappropriate places for making ethical decisions; they say the courts are inadequate to decide because they can't know the wishes of family and patient, and don't have the medical knowledge. But, courts exist to resolve conflicts of interest between people. Courts decide for people who cannot decide among themselves on an action.

The anger that some feel toward court "interference" in ethical decisions may be in reality a preference for local, informal decision making at the bedside, in preference to formal decision making in a distant courtroom. But conflict resolution at the bedside has already failed when the court is asked to decide. Much of this anger may also be a projection onto the court of what some actually feel toward the other people who will not agree. People who say that the court is meddling may really feel the other people in the conflict are meddlers.

Some people dislike court involvement in illness care simply because courts decide: Somebody wins and somebody loses. As lawyers know, people should try to stay out of court as long as possible, even when dealing with people thought to be meddling. Voluntary compromise, they know, means that everybody wins at least something they wanted—in court, somebody may lose completely.

The court, then, is a last resort for solving an ethical conflict that the parties cannot resolve themselves. Courts are remarkably good at this, despite bad press. Illness issues are no more difficult to understand than any other area of human activity. The special area of ethics conflict expertise may seem mysterious, but engineering, finances, trusts and wills, all require expert testimony and evidence from families, just as issues about illness care do.

This endorsement of the judicial system as conflict resolver of last resort presages the next section, the formal, written, and enforced part of ethics—the Law.

RESOURCES

American Association Critical Care Nurses (101 Columbia, Aliso Viejo, CA 92656) has position statements on patient advocacy, and on withdrawing treatment.

American Nurses Association has a Center for Ethics and Human Rights, which develops and disseminates information; provides resources and consultation to guide nurses and state nurse associations on application of the ANA Code of Ethics; and guidance for implementation of the Patient Self Determination Act to nurse managers, faculty, journals, law firms, individual nurses, and human rights organizations (such as Amnesty International): ANA, Center for Ethics and Human Rights, 600 Maryland Ave., SW, Suite 100 West, Washington, DC 20024-2571.

National League for Nursing offers the following publications on ethics, all published in June 1990:

Creighton, H., *Should Nurses Report Negligence in Medical Treatment?*

Letters to the editor of *Nursing Outlook*: re. the *Tuma* case.

The nurse-physician relationship: II. Somera and Tuma.

Fagin, C.M., *Nurses' Rights*.

Feliu, A.G., *The Risks of Blowing the Whistle*.

The Nurse as Advocate: Concepts and Controversy

Muyskens, J.L. *The Nurse As a Member of a Profession*.

Witt, P. *Notes of a Whistleblower*.

Other published resources include the following:

American College of Physicians Ethics Manual, Third Edition. Published in *Annals of Internal Medicine*, 1992; 117(1):947-960.

Bioethics Research Notes, P.O. Box 206, Plympton, S.A. 5038, Australia. Good section of journal abstracts and references and balanced relief from pro-death, anti-religious views in some other ethics journals.

Trends in Health Care, Law & Ethics, Robert Wood Johnson Medical School, 675 Hoes Lane, Piscataway, NJ 08854-5635

LAW

▽

"I'd give the devil benefit of law, for my own safety's sake."
—CHANCELLOR SIR THOMAS MORE,
in Robert Bolt's play, *A Man for All Seasons*
(New York: Random House, 1960)

△

LAW THE NURSE NEEDS TO KNOW

Legal topics considered important for nurses to know are covered in this book, but nurses who practice good nursing using ethical standards needn't know all the specifics of law (indeed they cannot).

Natural law as a philosophy of law asserts that law cannot be known by studying the law that exists now; law is not only what is, but what ought to be. Positivism as a philosophy of law focuses on what law is in the present (not what it was or should be).

"Legal aspects" of nursing have become such an accepted part of nursing knowledge that it threatens to become dogma (something taught just because it's always been taught, not necessarily because it is the truth or is needed). This book covers the legal topics considered important for nurses to know,[96] and it does something more radical: It suggests that nurses who use ethical standards to practice good nursing do not need to know all the specifics of law.

Nurses cannot know all the law affecting them; the law is written after practice develops. It is impossible to know in advance, with certainty and in every case, what is "legal" and what is not. The lawyer's main job is to give an educated guess as to what the law will be; but the law in a specific instance will not be known until a court rules on it.

For example, the nurse who calls the daughter of a 90-year-old patient and says that her father has refused to take food and water, that he wants to die, may theoretically violate a law of confidentiality. But it will not be punished if the circumstances dictate it was good practice (in the patient's best interest overall) and if it is the ethical thing to do. The statute or case law on confidentiality will speak in vague terms; the application of the law to the specific facts will depend on the circumstances. When asked about inconsistent application of rules, Grandmother used to reply: "Circumstances alter cases."

Nurses must use some basis for their action other than what is narrowly "legal." Even if there were a known statute exactly on point, the statute might not be applicable to a particular situation. Nurses must know the basis for the law; if they do, they will be able to anticipate the legality of their actions.

Admittedly, the farther lawmakers stray from making laws to enforce a minimum ethic, the harder it is to predict specifics. It is hard to predict that 55 miles per hour is lawful, while 56 is not. But it is not hard to predict that running a red light and killing someone is illegal, because it is immoral to kill anyway. The harder it is to predict an action is illegal, the less likely the action will be seriously punished, even if illegal (for example, driving 56 in a 55 mph zone).

PHILOSOPHIES OF LAW

The two major philosophies of law are *natural* and *positivist* law. The difference between them is best illustrated by describing the focus of each. Positivists focus on what law IS; they believe that law can be determined and studied and enforced without reference to ethics and morality. Proponents of natural law believe that what law IS cannot be considered without thinking at the same time about what law OUGHT to be (that law cannot be defined and enforced merely with scientific study, without reference to ethics and morality).[97]

The difference is important; a natural law judge might say, "This law is not fair; I won't send this nurse to jail," while a positivist might say, "The law is clearly written and this nurse clearly violated it; off with her head!" Or, the positivist judge: "No technical violation; innocent," but the natural law judge: "It *should* be illegal; off with her head!"

While philosophers debate about what law *is*, this book must delineate at least what law is *not*. Sought here is the fine bright line that differentiates law from ethics.

As can be seen consistently in this book, the line between law and ethics is a fine one; it moves, and it's not bright at all. Using ethics (what OUGHT to be done) as a guide is easier, safer, and more helpful than trying to pin down exactly what the law IS in every case, and following that narrow path.

This section outlines law according to the following:

1. law's basis in, but difference from, ethics;
2. the distinction between rights and entitlements;
3. the divisions of law into criminal and civil, and
4. the kinds of law, according to source.

Before a discussion of the kinds of law, it is important to understand what law is and what it is not.

Because humans have a born need to classify, and because law is a very old, complex system, law has been divided into classifications easier for people to learn. In addition, division has made easier the task of legal analysts to classify rules about the laws—rules that apply to certain classes of law and not to others.

> *Divisions of law:* Criminal or civil; federal, state, or local; administrative, case or statute law; procedural law or substantive law.

Large divisions in the subject of law are made on the bases of whether

1. Law is criminal law or civil law. These depend on whether the law punishes wrongs against the group (criminal law) or wrongs against individuals (civil law).
2. Law is federal, state, or local law. These depend on which level of government makes the law and enforces it.
3. Law is administrative, case, or statute law. These depend on which group of law-making people at any level makes the law and determine how much force the resultant law has.
4. Law is procedural or substantive law. These depend on whether the law is about *how* to decide (the process that must be gone through) or *what* to decide (the actual decision). The concept can be confusing even to the lawyers and sometimes the distinction is not useful, but an analogy to football can be illustrative: Procedural law is like the rules of the game (for example, four downs, eleven players); substantive law is the reality of the game (the players' sizes and skills, and the eventual score).

The divisions of law into criminal and civil law, and by whether it is rule, case or statute, are discussed separately below. Divisions of law into procedural and substantive, or into federal and state, are not addressed separately here, but are in each section on values as the law of that value is discussed. In addition, some history of law is woven into the discussion of the divisions of law.

HISTORY OF LAW: A BRIEF OVERVIEW

> Systems of law are as old as the existence of humans living in groups; religion is the basis of much law (or perhaps, much law is reflected in religion).

Law in some form must have originated about the time humans began to live in groups; some kind of "law" is necessary in order for people to live within rock-throwing distance of each other.[98] For example, the Code of Hammurabi is a very old set of laws; another, the laws of the Egyptians. These laws look strange to modern eyes, but they served the purposes of the people who wrote them, as laws usually do today.

The major source of law (and ethics) is religion; or is religion's basis a human need of ways to solve conflict? Regardless, much of the basis of Western law can be traced to the Hebrew Old Testament Ten Command-ments. The Commandments (don't kill, don't steal, don't lie) are the basis of Western ethics and law—expressed positively, they are the values earlier discussed individually. Some sections of the Old Testament sound very much like statutory tort law: Punishment is listed for trespassing, damage to personal property, and damages listed for torts. The Christian church law (based on Old Testament tribal law) continued the traditions, using Roman civil law as a separate law of the Roman Church following the Roman Empire's collapse. European countries thereafter used local customs as law, interposing and mixing the Roman-based Church law as needed; the code of Napoleon was a written-down mélange of this kind.

In the year 1215, England's King John was forced by his nobles to sign to some basic principles in the Magna Carta, one of history's many examples of a people changing their law, whether peacefully or not. One of the most important principles in the Magna Carta was that the people (the nobles) had rights that even the King couldn't abrogate. This basic premise—that the people have rights the government can't take away—continues in Ameri-can constitutional law and in the laws of other countries with law systems based on Britain's. (More about the U.S. inheritance from English law is discussed under Case Law, below.)

Nursing Law

Even a short history of nursing law would be longer than this book. Nursing law has not developed separately from other kinds of law, but it has paral-leled the development of the law of medicine. Malpractice law (the case law of negligence done by professionals) has been developing for several hun-dred years, first in England (the origin of the U.S., Canadian and British Commonwealth systems of law) and now in America and English-based legal systems around the world.

Nursing malpractice law develops further as nurses begin to be seen as individuals responsible for patient care, and to be seen as people with enough money or insurance to make them worth suing (and, nurse liability is a route to get to the employer-agency's money or insurance). In the past, most hospitals had charitable immunity, a concept under which a hospital that was a "charity" (one operated to take care of the poor for free) could not be sued. Today, taxes pay for care of the poor, not being considered a "charity" because it is compensated (some hospital administrators would argue with that).

Between Ethics and Law: A Fine, Bright Line?

> Law can be distinguished from ethics in that law is written, by people with authority, and uses mandates like "should" and "must," while ethics seeks to persuade.
>
> Laws are either cases, regulations, or statutes (or constitutions, made in the same manner as statutes).
>
> If "ethics" are written into law, they are no longer merely desired behavior but mandated behavior, and thus law.

To anticipate the consequences of their actions (to anticipate whether a given nursing act is ethical and thus legal) nurses can find the line that separates ethics from law.[99] Depending on the situation, finding the line separating law and ethics may be important; because, although violating their ethics may make nurses feel guilty, violating the law may make them actually *be* guilty (and jailed).

Like ethics, law is a concept (an abstraction); although different, the difference is a fine one. Both are part of one continuum of guides for resolving conflicts in human behavior.

Law is usually negative (Thou shalt *not* . . .). Several reasons for that exist (including Hayek's, below). One practical reason for law written as "don't" instead of "do" is that it is very difficult to force everyone to do a positive thing. It is much easier to punish someone for doing something that is forbidden (negative).

ON NEGATIVE LAW

"[P]ractically all rules of just conduct are negative in the sense that they normally impose no positive duties on any one, unless he has incurred such duties by his own actions . . . "[100]

—Sir Friederich Hayek

Nurses do incur positive duties by their own actions, by getting licensed and going to work. (The positive legal duty of Doing Good is discussed in Chapter Two.)

In order to find the line separating law from ethics, this is the first question to ask: Is the contemplated act good nursing practice? If it is, it's probably ethical. If it's ethical, it's probably legal. Ethical actions are those society *wishes* people would take, not action believed to be necessary. So, if the nurse does a desirable act, she will probably do the minimum necessary as well.

In order to know whether there is a writing in law or an ethical guide for the contemplated act, there are further tests.

Law uses words like "must" and "shall," whereas ethics says "should" and "may." To know the difference between what "should" be done and what "must" be done, the law can be recognized by its source. In a country like the United States, if a writing does not come from one of the following sources—the three branches of government: legislative, executive, and judicial—it is not law. Only the representatives of society can write into law (as statutes, regulations, or cases) the will of the people.

Statutes are written by the legislative branch—in the United States, the Congress or state legislatures. As an example, in most states the legislature has written a "living will" statute that mandates nurses and doctors respect patients' wishes about illness care. The statutes vary, but many of them allow patients to refuse all forms of treatment except the provision of sustenance, which is what a feeding tube provides.

Regulations. The second of the three kinds of law are regulations, written by people in the executive branch of government (headed by the governor of the state or by the president of the country). Examples are regulations written by the people who work for the Board of Nursing, the administrative agency that enforces the Nurse Practice Act written by the legislature.

Case Law. The third and last type of law is case law, written by judges after deciding appeals of lawsuits. A lawsuit results when people in conflict with each other cannot compromise. Case law starts with a lawsuit, a trial, a decision by a jury or judge, then an appeal of the decision, wherein the case becomes precedent. At that point it is written law, binding on future cases in lower courts under the appeal court's jurisdiction.

Case law is sometimes referred to as "common law" and "unwritten law" because it is written by judges *after* they make a decision in a case, instead of being written in advance of cases, as statutes are written by legislators. But case law is finally written and must be, else it could not be used as precedent in other cases.

Constitutions are "super statutes" that set up and limit governments. Listed within constitutions are rights, actually limits on the lawmakers' freedom to make law or apply it in some cases.

An easy rule is: Any written document not a statute, a regulation, or a case, is not a law. Law must be written. A document may be a writing used in enforcing law, such as a patient's living will, standing orders, standards of practice, or agency policy, but such writings themselves are not law. Laws are statutes, regulations, and cases (and constitutions) written by people with authority to do so, and anything else is not law—that is the bright line.

The problem (sometimes the opportunity) is that the law changes. The line moves. Missouri legislators made over 150 changes to that state's laws in 1995 alone—think of that, multiplied by 50 states, and don't forget the U.S. Congress. The reason that being legal and *not* ethical is not safe practice? What is ethics today well may be made into law tomorrow.

Ethics is desired behavior, neither mandated nor prohibited (not law). Some examples of ethical behaviors are in the codes of ethics of professions (ANA Code of Ethics, AMA Code of Ethics), standards of practice (ANA or agency Standards of Nursing Practice), or the Patient's Bill of Rights of the American Hospital Association. All these may be used as guides for ethical behavior.

Sometimes desired "ethical behavior" is written into statute, as in Florida's regulations for a mental health patients' bill of rights,[101] or when a state board of nursing prescribes rules. Texas nurses as well as nurses in other states can be denied licensure for unprofessional conduct and failure to meet standards of nursing practice, which incorporate what some might consider in the area of unethical, not illegal, behavior.[102]

If nursing board rules (these are law, too) about professional conduct did not address skill, but what was once considered merely "desired ethical behavior," the behavior so addressed will be not just "desired" any more—it is law then, and it's mandated. The American Bar Association suggests ethical behavior for lawyers, and this turns into law when the state supreme courts make rules (law) that mandate that behavior.[103] Lawmakers can change ethics into law, which may or may not be a good idea, depending on one's view of the world and the role of law. But it is reality.

Lobbying

> Nurses can change laws by lobbying in the legislature, lobbying with rule makers, or making case law; and they can influence ethics by making decisions about issues and speaking out on them.

The certainty is that law (unlike its ethical base) will change; it might as well change to be more efficient, gentle, tough, or whatever is more in accord with nurses' and patients' values and needs. Nurses can influence changes in the law.

Statutes written by legislators are easily influenced: Nurses can run for office, vote for a particular legislator, or campaign for one; nurses can testify at hearings about proposed laws; and nurses can support organizations whose lobbyists work to influence state and national law.[104]

Rules and regulations made by people in the executive branch can be changed at public hearings (held before the rules are published), or proposed rules can be changed during the time for public comment (after publication). Lobbyists for nurse organizations influence people who write regulations, too. Ultimately, a state's governor and the U.S. President are responsible for regulations made by their employees—and nurses can work for their election or defeat.

Case law also changes; nurses change it by bringing lawsuits, as nurses in Missouri did to prevent the Board of Healing Arts from stopping their practice. Their case affirmed the nurses' right to practice, even to practice what looked like Medicine to the doctors.[105] Nurses can directly influence case law by sitting on a jury (and shouldn't pass up a chance for this exercise in citizenship). And nurses can generally speak up. Nurse comments contribute to "public opinion," and a distillation of that opinion is what lawyers, plaintiffs, defendants, and juries believe—and ultimately what judges will write into case law.

Speaking out leads to public opinion, and strong public opinion may become ethics. Ethical behavior is the consensus/consciousness/conscience of what people think is desirable behavior. All people may never agree that a particular behavior is desirable, but nurses can compare observed human behavior to what they think it should be, and speak out. They can sit on ethics committees in their community and hospital; the *Quinlan*[106] court actually mandated the use of ethics committees.

Nurses' opinions are valuable because nurses know the reality of the problem facing their patients and themselves. The *Cruzan*[107] case was not over when the patient's feeding tube was withdrawn. And the case is not finished for the nurses who cared for her as she dehydrated and died, nor for other patients as they are euthanized or as they live on and on. The law and the ethics matter to patients and matter to their nurses. Law can't be left solely to the lawyers, nor ethics to the philosophers—those who *write* abstractly about human action. Nurses are the ac*tors*.

The fine, bright line is fine indeed, and it moves. There *is* a difference between law and ethics—between what is mandated and what is desired— and law can be identified by its source.

The nurse can identify what is ethical behavior (good nursing practice) and recognize that behavior as also legal; and also can identify whether a writing is a law or not. These concepts are useful for nurses in making decisions; the nurse's actions, in turn, contribute to shaping both ethics and resulting law. Whether the nurse's acts toward the patient are ethical and/or legal depend on whether those acts are consistent with good practice.

Part of that practice is acting consistently within the limit: The nurse has neither the authority nor the responsibility to make decisions for patients. This can limit the nurse in the practice role, but the nurse's role in the wider world as a thinking, speaking person remains as broad as desired. For the nurse who knows her own values, the final question will be: Is this act or omission consistent with my own beliefs, whether it meets anyone else's ethical or legal code?

RIGHTS—Limits on Government Power

Rights limit the power of the lawmakers to control the actions of individuals. Rights guarantee an individual's ability to perform an action. The guarantee of a good or service is properly called an entitlement.

Proponents and opponents of various causes use the word "rights" freely, and the concept is frequently misunderstood.

Rights are a guarantee of an individual's ability to perform an action. Rights are not a guarantee of the individual's ability to have something (a good or service). If what is being called a "right" causes one person to have to give something to another, then it's not a right, it's an entitlement. The root of the word *entitlement* is "title," a proof that one owns a thing, some kind of property.

The individual has a right to speak (an action) under the U.S. Constitution (that is not the case in all countries). But individuals do not have a "right" to a job, a car, food, housing, or illness care, things that belong to people. Whether one can obtain an entitlement (title) to any of those things depends on one's willingness and ability to work, or on the individual's (group's) lobbying power in the government.

> Rights to life, liberty, and property are guaranteed in the United States in the federal and in most state constitutions; in addition, many state constitutions guarantee a right to privacy and other rights.
>
> More fundamental than "which rights" is "who decides the rights?"; whether the legislative or the judicial branch should decide what limits on government protect individual freedoms.

Under the Fifth and Fourteenth Amendments to the U.S. Constitution, citizens have a right to keep property they have earned or otherwise gotten legally (the keeping is an action). This is not the same as being entitled to be given the property of someone else. Against that right to *keep* property, is the government's power to *take* property (taxes).

In legal terms, rights are limits on the freedom of the lawmaker, legislator, regulator, or judge to make laws, that deny citizens the freedom to act in some way. The U.S. Constitution lists certain rights that limit the law that states and the federal government can make. Rights (limits on government) do not often limit private action; for example, a private employer may violate the employee's freedom of speech without penalty (but a government employer must not). The Thirteenth Amendment forbidding slavery is the only one applicable to private parties (the private employer can silence the employee but can't enslave the employee). Private citizens are less limited than government because they don't have police power as the government does.

The Ninth Amendment to the U.S. Constitution, among the Bill of Rights, says that the list of rights is not all-inclusive. This means that there may be certain additional rights beyond those listed in the Constitution. Someone must decide what those other rights are.

In 1803 the Supreme Court decided it had the authority to review whether laws passed by Congress or the states were in keeping with the Constitution;

in other words, whether rights listed or implied in the Constitution were being undercut.

Each state constitution also has a list of rights, usually more numerous than the federal. State courts also decide if lawmakers have exceeded limits (violated rights) in the state or federal constitution. In recent years, state constitutions have been used more often to protect people from lawmakers. For example, several state constitutions specifically list a right of privacy.[108] A state law that limited abortions was struck down as violating the Florida Constitution's listed right of privacy. In addition, Florida state courts have held that a law that prevented feeding tube removal also violates the right of privacy.[109]

In the U.S. Constitution there is no specific "right to die" listed, nor right to abortion, nor right to suicide. In the past, however, a right of privacy has been implied in the Constitution by the Supreme Court. The Court used that implied right to limit the state legislatures' ability to make laws that restricted abortion and birth control.

The present Court does not write opinions that speak of an implied right of privacy. Instead, when they want to limit lawmaker power in those areas, they have relied on the right of liberty, guaranteed in the Fifth and Fourteenth Amendments. These two amendments also guarantee a protection of life (and property). The Court has not ruled that a fetus at all stages of life is a person; therefore states may not prohibit abortions completely as long as the fetus is not "viable" (implication: not a person).

The Supreme Court declined to find an unlimited "right to die" implicit in the right to liberty in the *Cruzan* case (noted above and in Chapter Seven: Life). The court did allow states to make their own decisions on that issue. In the *Cruzan* case the court did find, for the first time, that the right to refuse treatment is based on the Constitution's guarantee of the right of liberty in the Fourteenth Amendment. Refusal of treatment can include refusing food and water. Finding a constitutional right to refuse treatment means that no state law can override the right; many state "living will" statutes may be unconstitutional under this standard, since they prohibit the withdrawal of food and water even if requested in advance, while the patient is still competent.

The debate on a "right" to physician-assisted suicide is more important to nurses than it is to doctors. If clinics provide assisted death, or perform euthanasia on involuntary patients, nurses—not doctors—will be hired to do the actual "assisting to death" or "killing" (the word used, depending on one's view of the activity).

The issue of whether states may prohibit such activity can be argued under the issues of a right of liberty/privacy. *Cruzan* held that people have a right to refuse treatment under the right of liberty; it could be argued that they also have a "right" to actively end their lives. In that case, then, state laws punishing suicide attempts and assistance, would be held unconstitutional. The state's interest in protecting the citizen's life, even protecting her from killing herself, would then be subordinate to the right to do what she wished with her life. These are precisely the issues in the abortion and *Cruzan* cases: The individual's liberty (autonomy) ends and the people's interest in protecting life (sanctity of life) begins at some point—but where is that point?

These questions confront the issue of what is it to be human (to be a person); the point at which a fetus becomes a baby (a person); when a woman becomes a vegetable (a nonperson/dead); and finally when (if ever) the government (the state, the society, the "we") have an interest or a duty to intervene.

Should Courts or Legislatures Decide "Rights"?

A more fundamental question than those above is whether these issues should be decided by courts—the judicial branch of government—or by legislatures—the executive branch of government. Ultimately, rights (limits on government action) are decided by the will of the people; either they are written in an original Constitution or in amendments to the constitutions, by the elected representatives of the people.

As Justice Oliver Wendell Holmes, Jr. said, "All rights tend to declare themselves absolute to their logical extremes." But rights are never absolute. The right of free speech does not extend to telling defamatory lies about another, and the right to practice religion does not extend to sacrificing children in the ritual. How far rights extend is interpreted by the courts under the present system.

"The multiplication of rights can carry us only so far. . . . Obviously a structure of rights is necessary to protect us all . . . but when you are manufacturing, distributing and handling rights, as when you are handling any other sharp cutting instrument useful in aggression, prudence is in order."[110]

A right granted for one person usually means a limit or a duty on another. Rights are designed to protect the people, usually an individual or the minority, from the laws of the those in power in government (elected by the majority).

Are rights that prevent the lawmakers from *forcing* people to act or not act in some way, better made by judges or legislators? Arguing in favor of the legislative process, one might conclude it has more input of information and therefore should make laws more likely based on reality. But lawmakers—unlimited by a Constitution with rights for a minority—can result in a tyranny of the majority. A majority can be legal and at the same time unethical (the Germans and Austrians who voted overwhelmingly for Hitler's National Socialist Party are the example).

As with any part of the system of government, the present system, in which judges seem dominant as laws are tested in courts, can be changed if the electorate chooses to do so. And citizen-nurses will participate in that vote.

The American Nurses Association has published a statement on the relationship of human rights and ethics. The ANA statement relies on Kant's philosophy, defining human rights as originating in the philosophy that human beings are ends (that is, valid or important) in themselves and not just means to an end (goals and purposes) of other people.[111] The statement assumes that the value, "justice," is interpreted as meaning "social justice." (The concept of social justice is discussed in Chapter Five, Fairness.)

Power in the American Lawmaking System

> Power in the American system of government originally resided in the citizen, who ceded it to the state government, who ceded some of it (originally in limited fashion) to the federal government.

To understand the fights that occur when a minimum ethic is made into law (for example, abortion law), nurses must understand who has the power to make laws. Under the U.S. system of government, the people have original power, which through elected representatives they gave to the various states; originally, the states held complete power. All the powers of the federal government were granted to it by the states (the 13 original colonies—literally "states"—were independent countries).

Through their eighteenth-century federation (joining together) the states granted some power to the federal government. They also put limits on federal power—the Bill of Rights of the U.S. Constitution. Under the Constitution and through their legislatures, the people of the states have the power to make all laws except those specifically granted to the federal government in the Constitution. So, it is the state legislatures that, in the first place, turn the minimum ethic into law—for example, allowing abortion.

The federal power over abortion law derives from the U.S. Constitution, as decided by the Supreme Court. The Court decided in a landmark case that the Bill of Rights allows women to have abortion on demand during the first trimester (first three months) of pregnancy; thus were state laws restricting abortions made invalid. (The abortion issue is further discussed in Chapter Seven.)

RESOURCES

Australian Human Rights Commission (Box 9848, Canberra, Australia, ACT 2601, Australia), *Human Rights: A Handbook*, Canberra: Australian Government Publishing Service, 1983.

United Nations Universal Declaration of Human Rights (New York, NY 10017), New York: United Nations, 1948.

Divisions of Law: Criminal and Civil Law

Law may be broadly divided into criminal law and civil law. Nurses who know the basis for the distinction can then anticipate whether a law encountered will be considered a crime or a tort; they will know generally the punishment for each and why the difference; and they will be able to estimate how serious a violation of either kind of law will be.

For example, if the nurse lets the license lapse negligently, she'll know that violation of licensure statute law is a crime, and that the possible punishment is jail. But she will anticipate that, because the basis of criminal law is to revenge wrongs (to get "even"), she can estimate that such a violation would result in a fine instead of a sentence; a board or judge will make the punishment fit the crime. If the punishment were worse, the sentence could be overturned on appeal to a higher court as being unfair (uneven).

To quickly distinguish criminal law from civil law:

CRIMINAL LAW

Wrongs are called crimes, either misdemeanors or felonies (if penalty is more than a year of jail). The case name will be something like [*state* or *U.S.*] v. [*defendant's name*]. The punishment is fine or jail.

CIVIL LAW

Wrongs are called torts, either intentional or not (negligence/malpractice). The case name will be [*plaintiff/patient name*] v. [*defendant/nurse name*]). The punishment is money damages.

Occasionally the judge will order an injunction, an order to make someone do something or to prevent someone from doing something—for example, an injunction to keep a nurse from practicing medicine. An injunction is one of the few positive mandates in law to prevent harm, distinct from negative prohibitions that punish harm already done.

Criminal Law

Underlying criminal law and the power to punish is the grant of the wronged citizen's right to get "even" (revenge), to the state.

Due process (appropriate procedure) under Anglo-Saxon law starts with the premise that the accused is innocent until proven guilty.

Criminal law deals with people who are accused of committing wrongs. Wrongs against the state or society (deemed as against the people as a whole instead of people as individuals) are defined as crimes. The criminal law affects nurses, too; many of the statutes that govern nursing practice provide for a criminal penalty, either a fine or imprisonment (as in nursing licensure law, child abuse reporting, nursing home neglect, Medicare fraud for improper charges, or manslaughter or homicide, if a patient dies from neglect).

The wrong done in criminal cases is usually against another individual. But some wrongs against individuals are considered crimes (wrongs against the whole people) because they "disturb the peace." In the old days, all "crimes" were against individuals, and the crimes/wrongs were punished by individuals and their families.[112] This resulted in fights (feuds) between families and tribes, with revenge, counter-revenge, counter-counter revenge, on unto the seventh generation (as in the blood feuds of the Mafia and the Hatfields and McCoys). Some family feuds have lasted well into the twentieth century (for example, among Albanian clans in Kosovo, formerly Yugoslavia).[113] Constant warfare was not and is not good for the health or lives of any involved, nor for the economy of the rest of the people. Therefore, through the millennia, people began to turn over revenge to a more neutral authority.

Some now say that criminals are to be punished to deter them from repeating crime and to prevent others from following their example. Although these may be motives also, the basic human emotion behind punishment is revenge. When the law fails to exact revenge on behalf of the people harmed, some of them take the law into their own hands; they may kill or cut someone they believe has harmed them or harmed their child. Then it can be seen that the motive for punishment is not initially to deter or prevent crime but, rather, to revenge the wrong.

Even little children who are wronged say they want to *get even* with the one who has hit them. Justice makes the harmed and the harmer "even" again, so the harmer has to get some pain, too. Inherent in this process is a notion of evenness (balance), of putting things back into harmony (revenge for the wrong, as in the tribal situation).

Criminal law is founded on the need of people to punish, to see that people who harm others get what they deserve for such acts. Legal philosophers have written extensively on the subject.[114] Kant wrote about the *jus talionis*, the right of retribution, giving like for like; and he defended the state's right to punish and to pardon.

Usually people relinquish to the state their right to revenge; they let a "neutral" party prosecute and judge. If needed, the state takes the individual's place in punishing the wrong. The people have more peace.

The first step in the state's revenge in behalf of the individual harmed is the indictment. An indictment is the paper that says in essence "the state thinks someone did a crime and they are going to prosecute." In Texas the indictment must always say that the crime is *"against the peace and dignity of the state."* The value demonstrated here is revenge in behalf of a member of the tribe; thus, the value, Being True (Fidelity) is involved. The secondary value is peace, necessary as an economic factor. Fairness in the process is also a value underlying criminal law, but the punishment is for violating the ethical principle of doing no harm.

The state tries to be fair (to do justice, be impartial) in criminal cases—its purpose is to make the parties "even" again. If the state (the people's stand-in) is not fair, the state sinks to the status of a non-neutral participant in the feud. If two gangs fight and the state takes the side of one gang because the prosecutor's son is a member of that gang, the state sinks to the level of one of the gang; the purpose of a neutral decider is lost, and the war goes on.

There is one major difference between criminal and civil law: In civil cases like malpractice, people lose only their money. Under criminal law, they can lose their money (fine) or their life (part of their life in jail or all life, by being *executed*, the euphemism for killing a person convicted). In a criminal law proceeding for licensure revocation, the nurse could lose her career, which to some nurses is almost their whole life.

Nurses' Rights to Due Process

Due process is a somewhat archaic phrase that translates as "appropriate procedure." Due process is not invoked to protect "criminals" but, rather, to protect anyone accused of a crime.

Nurse licensure law is classified under criminal law. Before the state takes a nurse's license, some due process is mandated. This is the same due process the accused gets in a murder trial (perhaps appropriately, the nurse gets quite a lot less due process in losing a license than a convicted person gets before execution).[115] (Due process in a licensure context is described below, under Regulations.)

Under the civil law, the wrong is still against an individual. There the state's peace and dignity (the group) are not considered to be harmed, just the two parties involved. Instead of dueling or casting spells on each other as in some old days, they go to court and let the impartial decider to decide.

Anglo-Saxon law (that is, from Britain and its former colonies, including America) is distinguished from law that originated in continental Europe in this assumption: The accused is innocent until proven guilty. This assumption means that the prosecutor must prove the accused is guilty; the accused need prove nothing and has the right to remain silent. That right *not* to speak is fixed in the U.S. Constitution (the Fifth Amendment says the accused may not be forced to incriminate him or herself) in the Bill of Rights. It was placed in the Constitution because in past times (and still occurring in other places) people were tortured into confessing (speaking against themselves) and *not* allowed to remain silent. An American jury is instructed not to draw any implication of guilt from the fact that the accused does not testify. If they could imply guilt from silence, then the accused's "right" to remain silent would be a sham.

Sources of Specific Laws

Nurses can know a lot about a law by knowing the source of the law (either statute, case, or regulation). Knowing the source, the nurse can then know how a law can be challenged, how it can be changed, and to some extent the power of the law.

STATUTES

The categories of statutory law discussed here do not cover all the state statutes that may affect nursing practice. (A book with all of them would be at least a thousand pages long, specific to the nurse's state only, and be out of date the moment it was written.) The nurse who is interested in specifics can go to the library and find the state statutes, looking in an index under Nursing and reading some of the statutes specific to the state. The nurse who practices good nursing will be "legal" 99 percent of the time (the one percent of practice possibly technically "illegal" will still be right). Further, the nurse who does read all the statutes must still practice good nursing; knowing the law is not the same as doing good practice (legal practice).

General Information. Statutes are the source of most law that affects nurses. Licensure, patient abuse laws, consent to treatment (and refusal of treatment), Medicare and Medicaid reimbursement (source of much of nurse salaries in former times), employment law—all are largely controlled by statutes, not by cases or regulations. The nurse who finds the statute on a specific nursing topic has found most of the law on that topic. Statute law is now the most common source of law.

For much of the history of the United States, statutes were less important than law made by judges' decisions. But that is changing. More law is now made by statute—by legislators sitting in state capitals and in Washington, D.C. They write prescriptions for behavior ("do it") and proscriptions ("don't do it").

Some experts say that making law by statute is a good thing. They point out that problems are solved more quickly by the legislature passing a statute, than if judges made a decision on a case. The advocates of statute law say it's fairer to have representatives of all the people make decisions about what the people must do.

Other people prefer less statute law, and would like more law made by judges instead; that is, by case law or "common law." The people who prefer that law be made by judges worry that the people who have the majority in the legislature can act as tyrants, enforcing their will on the minority.[116]

One could argue that statute-made law can may be seen as "common law" expressed faster. In that view, statutes are the new "common law," the will of the people. Whichever side is right, application and interpretation of statute law will always require judges and juries to examine individual facts in particular situations to see if they fit the statute as written. No legislature can write a statute so specific that it will fit every situation without interpretation.

No Law May Be Good Law. As one reads statute law or hears of bad statutes, it may be seen that some statutes harm instead of help a situation. That's because all laws have intended consequences *and* unintended consequences that can't be known until the statute is enforced. Sometimes, if the solution to a problem does not require a legal solution, the best action is *not* to legislate. The problem may be better solved with private action than with state force.

State Law: The Source of Most Nursing Law

> State statutes are the source of most law that affects nurses, and it is the law most accessible to nurses.

For nurses, state statutes are the most important of the three sources of law. (Federal statutes are less important.) This is because the states still have the power to govern most of the areas that concern nurses. (This may not always be so, if more power is transferred to the federal government.)

Examples: The state grants the license to practice nursing, the nurse's economic base. The state says who can consent for whom, or refuse treatment for whom. The state legislature decides what constitutes the crime of patient abuse, and what diseases or injuries must be reported. A state statute specifies how long an injured patient can wait to sue a nurse, and where, and many conditions of malpractice liability. (Some of these are also discussed in Chapter Two, Doing Good.)

The legislative process, or how an idea becomes a law, is fascinating. Nurses who plan to be involved in the legislative process can obtain specifics about their state's process from the state nurses association or the League of Women Voters. (Call the state capital for the phone number of either group.)

Nurses also have lobbyists to tell them what they need to know about the legislative process. (They're called lobbyists because they used to sit in the lobbies of the legislators' hotels and the legislative chambers, waiting to talk to the lawmakers.) Lobbyists can explain exactly how a bill gets to be a law, at the state or federal level. In general, a bill goes from introduction in the house (or senate), to committee, to the floor (debate, amendment, and vote by the whole group); to the other body of lawmakers, to a committee there, to the floor of that second body for a vote; to a conference committee of lawmakers from both groups for final compromise, and then to both groups for the final vote. The law is really the product of committees.

The governor or President will sign it (if so, it's now a law) or veto the bill. If the governor or President vetoes the bill, the legislature can still pass it, over the veto, by another vote. Nurses in Missouri accomplished the first override of a governor's veto in 138 years when they obtained their liberal nurse practice act, passed in 1976.[117]

People who want a certain law passed almost always hire a lobbyist; good lobbyists know the steps in the process, and where information or influence by nurses can help. Lobbyists may know the procedure better than the legislators.

At the request of the members of a special interest (like nurses) who have hired him/her, the lobbyist will write (or have someone write) a proposed law (bill). The lobbyist solicits sponsors for that bill, trying to sign up influential members of the legislature and of the committee that will first consider the bill.

The lobbyist provides information to the legislators: why the bill is needed, and what it will do and how. State legislators do not have big staffs of people to gather such information. Even the federal legislators, who have more staff, can't possibly gather as much information on an issue as the many and varied lobbyists can provide. The lobbyist's goal is to convince the legislators to vote for the bill and, to that objective, the lobbyist provides as much convincing information as possible. People who oppose the bill likewise have lobbyists who present information unfavorable to the law.

Those "special interests" and their lobbyists maximize the information the legislators receive to make decisions; maximum information is the basis of the free market. Limited information works badly, in markets or in legislatures.

This plural and maximal information input is the basis of the legal system also, since judges or juries use information gained through the adversary system of law (in Britain and countries with British-derived law). Because people with different and opposing interests furnish information, the most accurate information possible is obtained and the likelihood of accurate or correct decisions being made is increased. Such decisions are more likely based on reality than if less information about reality were available.

The lobbyist also provides information on other bills, particularly on bills that a "special interest" group opposes. In this way the legislator, hearing what sounds like a good law, may be informed of the harm to a special interest group's position. That knowledge minimizes the unintended consequences of that legislation. Killing a bill containing potential bad consequences may be the best work lobbyists do.

SPECIAL INTEREST FAILURE TO LOBBY:
A NEGATIVE EXAMPLE

The medical association in Massachusetts did not lobby against a law that forced physicians to accept minimum Medicare payment (called "assignment"). The well-*intended* consequence of the law was to provide cheap medical care for the elderly. Despite this good intention, the doctors' group knew that the result would be bad for doctors. But the association didn't want to be seen as a "selfish" special interest group, so they didn't lobby against this popular bill. Instead, they quietly challenged the law in court after its passage. Their court challenge failed.

The *un*intended consequence of the law was seen afterward; doctors left or did not come to the state because of the law. There were fewer doctors to care for the elderly (the people the statute was supposed to help). The association didn't advance its members' interests at first, and the unintended consequence (foreseen but not acted upon by the medical association) was bad for all, patients and doctors.

Nurses can learn the specifics of the legislative process in their state, if they're interested in influencing the legislature on a special bill or on a regular basis. As mentioned above, the League of Women Voters is a good source of information; the organization fought for women's right to vote in the 1920s, and won after approximately 100 years of work. Changes in the law don't always come quickly or easily.

And the nurse's state legislator, or the lobbyists for the nurses' organizations in the state, can immediately bring the nurse up to date on where a particular bill is in the legislative process. They can also tell the nurse what can be done to help or hinder the bill, along with any other details wanted.

Determining Whether a Statute Is Federal or State

Federal statutes have the initials "U.S." somewhere in their designation; state statutes will have the initial of the state.

State statutes can be found in public libraries (central or perhaps branch); federal statutes and regulations and state regulations are available from law libraries, as are federal and state cases. Lawyers may be of assistance in locating this law, as will lawmakers on the state and federal level.

The nurse who has a copy of a law, or the number of a law, can know whether it's a statute, a regulation, or a case, but first must determine whether it is federal or state law. Federal laws, made by Congress, or federal courts or federal regulators, have the initials *U.S.* in them, as in "48 USCS 3397" (United States Code Service)—which means it's in the set labeled United States Code Service, in Volume 48, at section 3397.

A state law will have the initial of the state in it, such as "17-86-102(2)A.S.A. (1987)." The A.S.A. here stands for *Arkansas* Statutes Annotated (at that volume and section and number is written the definition of nursing in Arkansas). In the Revised Statutes of *Missouri*, at Chapter 335.016.8 (1987) RS*Mo.*, will be found the definition of nursing in Missouri.

If the piece of law is a federal regulation, it will have the designations CFR (Code of Federal Regulations) or FR (*Federal Register*) somewhere in the numbers and letters. A case will have the name of parties at the front (like

Jones v. Smith). (See the sections on Regulations and Case Law, below, for specific information.)

Finding Statutes Affecting Nurses

Some specifics of state statutes that affect nurses are outlined under the various chapters. Most statutes are attempts to enforce the value, Doing Good and Doing No Harm, and so are discussed in those chapters. If the specific wording of state law is needed, it's easy to find. Each state's law is different from one of the other states; the statutes in all states are similar because human behavior is similar everywhere, but 50 different legislatures can certainly come up with 50 different ways of solving a problem.

Neither this nor any other book can be relied upon to tell exactly the specifics of the law that affect any individual's practice. This chapter has informed in a general way about which statutes affect nurses; the nurse can find what such statutes usually say in chapters on specific values. If specific information is needed, the state statute should be found. No textbook can possibly tell as much as will be known by finding and reading that law.

Every state publishes (prints) its statutes. To be considered and enforced as law, statutes must be written. If they're published, the people are presumed to know what the law is. The nurse is responsible for following the law, even if she hasn't read it. If the laws aren't published, the people can't be held responsible. Federal statutes are less accessible; a law library or the nurse's federal legislator (Congress or Senate) may be able to help with the text of a federal statute.

If one is needed, a state statute can be found easily, starting with the most certain source, a law library. In any city of some size one may find a law school library connected to a university. A court will also have some kind of law library. In a rural area, the county, circuit, or district court, located often in the county seat, will have a library and a set of state statutes.

Every lawyer has a set of state statutes (or access to one), and many will be glad to help. (The nurse is a potential client, or a possible expert witness.) The lawyer should not be asked to look up the law (that costs time, which is money); the lawyer should merely be asked to use the statutes. Lawyers' secretaries are also sources of help, especially on basic procedure.

Nurses who work in a big institution may have an "in-house counsel," a lawyer who works only for the institution. That lawyer will have a set of statutes, and perhaps much more. Even if the agency doesn't have a full-time counsel, outside counsel can help. Or the administration may have a set of statutes somewhere in the hospital library or administrative offices. Most reliably, the public libraries (even many branches) have a set of state statutes in the reference section.

Among the "sets" of statutes available are both annotated and non-annotated statutes (most common), both of which set out all the language of the statutes as passed by the legislature. Annotated statutes have notes after each section of the statute. The notes tell of cases (decisions by judges) about that section. The case may modify the meaning of the statute. The annotated sets of statutes are usually only found in a law library or law office; reviewing only the nonannotated version is often sufficient, however, since only occasionally will a case have modified the statute significantly.

The statute wanted can be found in the index, which is alphabetized. The numbers of the several statutes under the heading Nursing might be copied, since those statutes specific to the state may affect nursing practice, and are good to have for future reference.

Legal indexes may use "legalese" in the headings. Several related words may be tried, and the librarian's help enlisted. For example, the Missouri living will statute is indexed under Medical Procedures, Right to Refuse—not the first place one would look, but findable.

The numbers in the index under Nursing Licensure refer to the volume, or statute, or section, or chapter number of the actual words of the statute. The statute can be located under that number, copied, studied, and kept for future reference.

Pocket Parts Are Imperative

The legislature changes the statutes every year in most of the states; new laws are added, old ones modified, and some repealed and removed. Most states don't revise and print the whole set of statutes with changes every year; they may print a new version in 1987, one in 1990, and then one in 1993.

The statute book will have a date on the cover, on the spine, or in the front (the year the whole set of statutes was published). In the years in between the printing of the hardcover books, in most states the legislature still continues to make new law. Those newly made statutes are published in softcover supplements.

These supplemental laws are separate volumes in paperback, or in a pocket at the back of the hardcover volume. They set out the language of the laws that are all new, or that modify or amend a prior law. Once the statute is found, it is imperative to look under the same statute number in the supplement to see if the legislature passed any new law amending that statute.

The legislature may even have *repealed* the statute or part of the statute just found. If there's no later law in the supplement, the original law is still effective as written.

One last, best, and easiest way to obtain the law (the latest law) is to ask the legislator. The state senator and state representative both have offices somewhere near, and they also have offices in the state capital (call information in that city, or ask the librarian for the names and phone numbers and addresses). Write—or faster, call—and ask the secretary or the legislator to send or fax the statute on the subject wanted. Ask also for any bills that would affect the law requested, which have been introduced into the legislative process to become a law. The current law and any potential law on the subject may be obtained, along with a contact who may be of help some time.

Before analyzing the statute found, read the short section in this chapter, Case Law (below), listing the rules of statutory interpretation. Those are the rules that courts use when they read a statute in order to apply it to a particular case.

REGULATIONS AND RULES

> Regulations (rules or administrative law) are made by the executive branch of government, to carry out the statute law made by legislators.
> Rulemakers must not act outside the power granted by the legislators (the rule cannot be *ultra vires*) and rules must be made and enforced according to procedural due process.

Situation: The state board of nursing in the state has made a rule that nurses must have 15 hours of mandatory continuing education each year for relicensure. *Legal?* Jane Nurse did not document 15 hours of CE last year. The board has taken away her RN license. *Can they do that?*

Regulations are made by the executive (or administrative) branch of government and are called administrative law. The state board of nursing is an administrative agency, part of the executive branch of government.

The rules and regulations that the executive branch make as they administer the law are actually law, too. The administrators make law, just as surely as legislators and courts do. Rules and regulations are enforceable in court and with police power, just as any statute or court decision.

Regulators have two general functions at least. One is a *rule-making* function, analogous to the legislature's lawmaking function. Administrative people also have a *decision-making* function when they investigate and enforce rules that are broken; this function is analogous to the courts' decision-making function. Boards investigate, prosecute, and decide individual cases; for example, denial of licensure for failure to document mandatory CE.

Rules made by administrators (bureaucrats, regulators) differ from statutes made by legislators. Rules must be made *pursuant to* some statute. The statute is made by the legislature, and then the rules can be made to implement (to pursue) the statute. The administrator has no authority to make rules unless the rule implements a statute. Rules made by administrators may be challenged in court by alleging that the regulation is not made under the authority of a particular statute—a charge that the administrator has acted *ultra vires* (Latin for "outside the power") of the office.[118]

Was the mandatory CE rule, in the situation above, made *ultra vires* by the state board of nursing? It depends (the lawyer's favorite answer).

Regulations (rules) differ from statutes in that decisions or actions by an administrator or board can be further appealed in court. Statutes are harder to overturn.

The board of nursing's act, in making the CE rule, can be protested as being *ultra vires*. Or, a case filed in court can protest that the act (or rule) did not follow due process, either substantive or procedural—another division of law: whether the issue concerns procedural (process) issues or substantive (real) issues.

The board would assert that its mandatory CE rule was not *ultra vires* if the nursing statute specifically gives them the authority to implement mandatory CE. And they'd be right. Even if the legislature has not written mandatory CE into the statute, the board could still assert its rule was not *ultra vires* because the board has a broad duty to protect the citizens who receive nursing care, and this rule comes under that duty. Nurses opposing the rule would say that the duty to protect the public is not so broad that it gives the board license to write any rule it wants, without the legislature having indicated its wishes. The court would decide which is right.

The question of whether the administrator followed *procedural due process* falls under the area of procedural law. Was the rule published in a timely manner, were the people concerned notified about the problem, was a hearing held on the matter, was procedure appropriate to the action followed? Under *substantive due process* is the question of whether the board had some rational basis for their acts or rules. They cannot act arbitrarily.

Due Process

"Due process" requirements come from the U.S. Constitution, from the Fifth and Fourteenth Amendments' requirements that no person shall be "deprived of life, liberty or property without due process of law." The procedural due process needed before the board can legally revoke the nurse's license are, for example, procedures like notice of the charges, opportunity for hearing, right to counsel, and unbiased decision makers. Regardless of the details, the issue in both rule-making and decision-making administrative law is fairness. (Due process is also discussed above under Criminal Law and in Chapter Five, Fairness.)

Did the state board's rule on mandatory CE violate procedural or substantive due process? Did the revocation of licensure?

Procedural

The board would not have violated procedural, *rule-making due process* in making the rule about CE, if it complied with the procedures used to make such rules. Each state has a process that agencies must use for rule making and decision making, sometimes a statute called an "administrative proce-dure act." The act will specify what must be done before a rule can have the force of law; for example, publish the proposed rule, hold hearings open to the public, allow time for comment, and publish the finally adopted rule in a state register of rules.

The administrative procedure act (and the rules adopted by *its* adminis-trative agency!) would also specify exactly what procedural, *decision-making* process was due to the nurse whose licensure was in jeopardy. The board must comply with the state administrative procedure act, as well as the federal requirements of due process that arise from the Fifth and Fourteenth Amendments of the U.S. Constitution:

> "No person shall . . . be deprived of life, liberty or property without due process of law . . . ." (Article V)
> "No state shall . . . deprive any person of life, liberty or property without due process of law . . . ." (Article XIV).

The nurse's license is considered to be a property right, and the nurse's ability to work at an occupation is a liberty right.

Substantive

> Substantial due process has been met if the administrative act has a rational basis (that is, if the act had a reasonable relationship to the duty imposed on the agency by statute).

Substantive due process is an easy test for lawmakers to meet. This is one of the bases for challenging statutes made by the legislature as "unconstitu-tional"—as not meeting the constitutional test set out in the Fifth and Fourteenth Amendments, above. As long as the administrative act has any rational basis, if it bears any reasonable relationship to the duty of the agency, then the rule or act will be considered constitutional.

The nurse whose license was threatened for nondocumentation of CE would argue, for example, that there was no rational basis for the mandatory CE to protect the public. She could assert that no data exist that demon-strate that mandatory CE reduces nursing malpractice, or reduces licensure discipline for incompetence, or makes any other increase in competent practice or any decrease in incompetent practice.

She would argue (her attorney would argue) that no data exist that mandatory CE has any effect on nurse behavior, other than to produce attendance at CE in the required minimum amount. In other words, the nurse could argue that the rule has no rational relationship to the goal of protecting the public. Its purpose and effect is not to make safe nurses, but to increase attendance at CE. She would argue that mandatory CE *does* have the effect of increasing the cost of nursing care to the public through the lost time, cost of travel, food, lodging, and registrations required.

The court hearing this case might decide that the minimal test of rational basis for the rule had been met, and uphold the board in taking the nurse's license. For example, even a licensing requirement that nurses must swear that they have paid their state taxes, has been upheld in Massachusetts as being reasonably related to their competence and safe practice. (More discussion of mandatory CE and legal challenges will be found in Chapter Three, Doing No Harm.)

Administrative Law

Any law proceedings that are not in law-deciding court, nor in the lawmaking legislative session, can be classed as administrative law. This area of law encompasses all of the process involved with regulatory bodies that make rules and enforce them—the rule making, investigation, and decision making that bureaucrats do.

As noted above, each state has some kind of administrative procedure, and many set up a kind of "junior" judicial body (perhaps called the Administrative Hearing Commission) to make decisions at a level just above a regulatory board such as the nursing board. Some lawyers specialize in representing clients in these fora, before boards and quasi-judicial administrative law courts. The administrative procedure law will specify due process requirements for those bodies. In this forum will come, for example, hospital challenges to the state agency's Medicaid reimbursement rate.[119]

If the person aggrieved by a decision of a board takes the case to the administrative law court/commission and also loses there, there remains the option of continuing the disagreement in court. As taxpayer money becomes a more important part of illness care budgets, decisions by bureaucrats in Medicaid and Medicare agencies are challenged in court.[120]

Over-regulation is a danger that tempts administrative regulators, sheltered as they are from re-election and oversight of the electorate. Forcing more regulatory burdens on people can result in their obeying the letter, but not the spirit, of the law. Forcing motorists to have insurance and inspections, for example, results in a black market in windshield stickers. The sticker (form) becomes the focus of the motorist, not the insurance and inspection (substance). An analogy to mandatory CE can be made, where the importance becomes the form (the certificate for *X* hours of CE sitting time), instead of quality of the education or resulting competence of the nurse.

Finding the Regulations

Regulations of the state and federal governments are published in some form so that the people may know what duties they have under the law. Regulations are less accessible than statutes, but can be obtained from "depository" libraries, law libraries, and lawmakers.

To be enforceable by law, regulations must be written and published so the public can find them. U.S. federal agency rules are published in the *Federal Register*, published daily (on some days, it is hundreds of pages long). Again, note that it is impossible for anyone to know *all* that "law," so some shorthand way of knowing the law is needed. Knowing the values and ethic underlying the law may obviate the need to know all the latest specifics.

But if the actual words of the regulation are needed, the *Federal Register* is found at any library that is a repository of federal documents, listed by the date on which the regulation was published. A library in each city or area is designated as the one to have a copy of all federal documents (the branch librarian will know where that library is). In addition, other libraries and some medical libraries subscribe to the *Register*, including a cumulative monthly index, organized according to the name of the agencies that promulgate the regulations. Most regulations of interest to nurses will issue from agencies like the Department of Health and Human Services and the Federal Drug Administration (look at the list of agencies and estimate which agency issued the regulation sought).

Each year regulations are indexed and printed on a staggered quarterly basis, into a new *Code of Federal Regulations* under the proper area of the law. "Staggered" means that one-fourth of the "regs" are reissued with changes incorporated in January, the next one-fourth re-done in April, and so on. If the reference the nurse is seeking has a particular "CFR" number, that code is what must be found; the *Code of Federal Regulations* is found at law libraries and the federal depository library.

Look to see if there is a new rule that has modified the original code section, since the last CFR was printed. (In the same way it is necessary, when finding a statute, to check for any addition made to the statute since the printing.) The date of printing is at the front of the Code; check for the rule's CFR section and number in the index of *CFR–List of Sections Affected* (published in the *Federal Register* each month; check each month since the Code was printed). If this CFR rule has been modified, the index will give the date the modification was printed in the *Federal Register*, a date needed to find the modification of the regulation.

State rules are handled in much the same way but with less volume. The state will print a state register (list and text of rules) perhaps weekly or monthly, which is provided to some libraries and subscribers. Then, periodically the newly published regulations are indexed and the code of state regulations is updated. If the nurse is serious about legal research, a lot of help is available from Stephen Elias's *Legal Research: How to Find and Understand the Law*, from Nolo Press, 950 Parker Street, Berkeley, CA 94710—and from the ever-helpful law librarian.

CASE LAW

THE CASE OF THE UNRAISED RAILS

Familiar scenario: It's 11:00 P.M. and the nurse raises Mr. Johnson's bed rails. He complains and wants them down. He gets up, falls, is hurt, sues. Now that attention is focused . . .

Case law is made on a case-by-case basis. Case law was called common law in England because it was made by the king's judges, considered "in common" to all the people of the country ("common" in contrast to the local law made in each county by its lord). Common law is different from civil law on the European continent (France, Germany, Spain), where societies did not make law on a case-by-case basis but by canon (church), by king or emperor (Caesar or Napoleon), or by statute (French Revolution).[121] Continental civil law systems were not really sprung full-blown from the forehead of a king, but were based on customs of the local people (remember that *ethic* too means "custom"). Thus, continental civil law is not as different from the English system as anglophiles might like to believe.

Case law in the United States is based on English law; most states have "inception statutes" that make the law of that state, the law of England at about the beginning of the nineteenth century.

Much of U.S. and Canadian case law is inherited from England and the long tradition of judge-made law in that country; the Magna Carta is often mentioned as the start. But long before King John was forced to sign the Magna Carta, the tradition of the tribes who settled England, from Anglia and Saxony (Anglo-Saxons), was that their king or leader was merely first among equals. This accounts for the attitude of individualism and equality so prevalent in English-based legal systems. People are assumed to be autonomous equals, each person as smart as any other about personal affairs. This is the basis of "freedom" as many know it.

The various states in the United States of America (the other "United States" in North America is the United States of Mexico) used the case law of England as their base. Most adopted such statutes soon after their inauguration as states, in law known as "inception statutes."

Inception statutes say something like: "The law of England as of the year 1804 will be the law of this state." Then the legislature of the state and the judges of its court add on, extend and sometimes delete, and change the law as received from England. The basis of statute law in the United States is case law from England; and the basis of case law in the United States is English law, too. (U.S. malpractice law is based on concepts first established in English case law).

Case law is less important in the U.S.A. than in times past, but it is still important. In no way can legislatures make laws so clear and so specific that they could cover every conceivable conflict situation. Judges, juries, and courts are necessary now, and will continue to be; the case (the controversy) is the actual application of a statute, if one exists on the subject.

Statutes are often made deliberately vague in order to get them passed. If two sides on an issue are deadlocked, a compromise may be worked out in which the language is vague enough so that both sides can claim that their interpretation is correct; and therefore both sides can "win." When a real conflict comes up (when the statute is to be applied), the courts will have to decide what the legislature meant. Courts decide; that's their strength—and that's the danger of going to court: Somebody wins, but somebody loses, too.

Case Procedure

STEPS TO MAKING CASE LAW

Conflict (not resolved)

Plaintiff files complaint (petition)

Defendant(s) respond (answer)

Discovery (interrogatories, depositions)

Trial: Opening Statements
- Plaintiff's Case
- Defendant's Case
- Closing Statements
- Verdict

Post-trial motions

Appeal to higher court

Decision: Case law

Case law in the making: Patient and nurse have a conflict. Patient says nurse negligently failed to put up the side rails of his bed; patient got out of bed and fell, hurting himself, and nurse owes him $50,000 for his trouble. Nurse says an attempt was made to put up the rails, patient said not to do so, and nurse hasn't got $50,000. Neither of them can or will compromise enough to settle the conflict.

They didn't listen to Abraham Lincoln, who said:

> Discourage litigation. Persuade your neighbors to compromise whenever you can. Point out to them how the nominal winner is often the real loser. Fees, expenses, and waste of time. As a peacemaker the lawyer has a superior opportunity of being a good man. There will still be business enough.[122]

The Process: Patient-plaintiff sues nurse-defendant. The reality: Plaintiff's lawyer files a piece of paper (*complaint, petition*) at the courthouse and sends a copy to the nurse (and invariably sues the nurse's employer, too, when possible). The nurse's lawyer (malpractice insurance will provide one) and the employer's lawyer file answers and send copies to the plaintiff's lawyer. The defense may request the court to dismiss the suit on a variety of grounds.

The Process: The lawyers conduct *discovery*. The reality: *Interrogatories* (written questions about what happened, how much insurance is available, etc.) are sent and answered; *depositions* (spoken questions in an interview under oath, recorded by a court reporter) are conducted. Often cases are settled after discovery; the attorneys can hear the witnesses, judge their credibility and the facts, assess the chances of winning/losing before a jury, decide what the case is worth, and settle if warranted. A tiny percentage of cases filed actually go to trial.

To Trial: If the parties cannot agree on a settlement, there's eventually a *trial*, perhaps after many years.

The jury is selected through a *voir dire* questioning about their attitudes about the case and defendants. (Black's Law Dictionary says *voir dire* is Old French for "speak the truth.") This process is used by lawyers for both sides to introduce some points to the prospective jury; for example, a question like "Do any of you believe that a nurse is responsible for injury which the patient in fact caused to himself?" The case could be tried before the "court" only, meaning that the judge acts as the fact finder (no jury is used). In most malpractice cases, both sides have a right to insist on a jury.

The patient-plaintiff's lawyer and the nurse-defendant's lawyer make *opening statements* explaining their version of the case, what evidence they will use to prove that version, and what they hope the outcome will be.

Then both introduce *evidence*. The patient-plaintiff will have the burden of proving some things (such as how the nurse was negligent in letting the patient out of bed). The nurse-defendant will have the burden of proving some things (how the patient assumed the risk of falling when he got out of bed alone against instructions). (Further discussion of malpractice law is in Chapter Two: Doing Good.)

As defendant, the nurse testifies (tells her story).

ADVICE TO NURSES WHO TESTIFY

Nurses who testify as defendant, expert witness, or witness to some incident in a case, are given the following advice: Listen to the lawyer's counsel before testimony and take her advice.

The writer's advice (to be followed if it is not contrary to what the lawyer in this case says): Be yourself, wear a blue suit, not sexy (even if that IS yourself), look the jurors straight in the eye, and tell the truth.

Do not *ever* lie to the court, even about a small thing; if the nurse is caught in a little lie, the jury/judge will assume the nurse is lying about everything. Lying is corrosive to the individual's opinion of herself as well.

The nurse was not negligent and knows it; she should tell the jury and convince them of that. The nurse is the good guy in the white hat to most people and will lose only if she somehow fails to communicate that.

If the nurse thinks she *was* negligent: As long as human beings and not machines are doing the nursing, mistakes will be made. If that is the case, she must tell THAT to her lawyer and why. The lawyer will either be able to explain how under the law a mistake was not made (that legally the nurse is not responsible) or the lawyer will wisely attempt to settle the case before trial.

Either or both the plaintiff and defendant will use *expert witnesses* and various other evidence to prove the standard of care, that it either *was* or *was not* breached. The nurse who is not a plaintiff or defendant may be asked to be an expert witness at trial or on depositions, or could be called as a "fact" witness, a person with some knowledge of the circumstances (for example, the nurse who worked the same shift when the incident occurred).

In this situation, the plaintiff-patient testified as to his version of events. Then the testimony of the nurse-expert for the patient was that, in the situation described, the nurse defendant had the duty to do good for the patient (beneficence) by protecting him and that a reasonable prudent nurse would put the rails up, even if the patient objected.

The patient was disoriented, the patient's expert witness concluded from the chart and the patient's testimony.

Then the nurse-defendant testified to her version of events. A nurse expert for the nurse-defendant was of the opinion that, in this case the nurse initially had a duty to put the rails up but that, if the patient insisted, a reasonable prudent nurse would assess the patient and honor the patient's autonomy by allowing the patient who so insisted to sleep with rails down. The patient was *not* disoriented, this expert witness concluded from the same chart and the nurse's testimony.

After both sides have presented their cases, each attorney will make a *closing argument* (which is what it sounds like). The jury will deliberate and come back with a *verdict* (Old French for "say the truth"). This process is the adversary system of justice, which assumes that two sides will make their strongest arguments and efforts to bring out the truth for their side. More information, and more likely the truth, will result.

Inquiry/Inquisitory Vs. Adversary/Advocacy

In continental European systems, there are fewer "lawyers" and more "judges." In those systems there is more of an investigative role played by an administrative-type judge, who asks questions and develops the case slowly (whereas, in the United States, the parties' advocates present the case). Under investigative-inquiry systems, case files become very thick; the judge will take a long time to resolve the case. In the United States a decision may be made by the jury in as little as one day, once the case gets to trial.

In the hypothetical side-rail case, by the way, the jury found for the plaintiff-patient and awarded him $200,000. (Should the defendant have settled for the original $50,000 offer?)

Making Case Law

To turn a trial-level verdict into established case law a further step is required: the *appeal*. There are some intermediate procedural steps the lawyers will do—motion for a new trial, ask the judge to overturn or reduce the verdict—but such requests are often denied. The lawyer (either or both sides) can then ask the next-higher court to change the decision made by the trial court, alleging that a mistake was made.

Either or both sides can appeal to a court of appeals. (The nurse in the hypothetical case will appeal, because of the loss at the trial level. The patient may appeal, because the amount of damages wasn't high enough.) Some or all of the record of the trial will be sent to the appeals court with the allegations of mistakes. "Briefs" will be written containing legal arguments and listing legal precedent in this and other jurisdictions that decided the way the advocate wanted. There may be oral argument by the attorneys in front of the court.

Some months later the appeals court will issue an *opinion*. If individuals have an opinion, it may not be binding on anyone or anything. But the court's "opinion" becomes the law for similar situations.

If the court is being asked to interpret a statute, they use a set of rules to analyze it.

RULES FOR ANALYSIS OF STATUTES
State judges follow generally accepted rules of statutory interpretation to analyze state statutes. Guidelines are particularly useful when the statute is

vague, or when two statutes appear to conflict. That is true most of the time. The following guidelines are common:

1. Attribute plain and ordinary meaning to the words used in the statute.
2. Look at the general purposes (intent) of the legislation.
3. Identify the problem the legislature probably sought to remedy and as nearly as possible the conditions existing at the time of enactment.
4. Interpret amendments to statutes on the theory that the legislature intended to accomplish some substantive change in the law. A later written statute or amendment rules over an earlier one. The annotated statutes with dates of enactment are often necessary for correct interpretation.
5. Try to harmonize (as the courts will do) the various statutes that are applicable.[123]

In the hypothetical raised-rail case, the nurse (through the lawyer) appealed on the ground that the patient-plaintiff sued later than two years after the incident occurred, so that the statute of limitations precluded the lawsuit. The court interpreted the statute of limitations the way the nurse (through the lawyer) asserted that it should be read, so the appellate court *reversed* the trial court, because the case was filed later than the statute of limitations allowed. This illustrates the point that the case law decided may not be at all about the substance of the case itself, but about some procedural point. Depending on the state, a further appeal step may be possible, to a supreme court (in New York, the Court of Appeals is higher than its supreme court).

When finally issued by the highest court, the decision *is* case law, binding on all lower courts in that state. It need not be followed (is not binding) in any other states or jurisdictions, but often cases are used in other courts in other states to try to convince that the principle of the case law is sound.

Now the case will be published in a set of books called "reporters" and made accessible on computer; now it can be called "law," enforceable and mandatory, *only* in the state of the court that decided it. If it is a federal case, it is binding on all lower courts in that circuit; if it is a U.S. Supreme Court case, it is binding on all federal courts and state courts, depending on the issue decided.

Finding Case Law

Case law is harder for nurses to locate than statutory law, but fortunately is not needed as often. If the annotated version of the licensure and other statutes is found, some cases will be mentioned, with usually a short explanation of the holding in the case. The nurse won't have to find the actual case. The full text of the case can be found in a law library. The local library can network with a law library or, as in the statute search, the local lawyer may help. Depending on type of practice, the lawyer may have only the cases decided in one state, those cases within the state the lawyer practices in. However, the lawyer might have access to a computerized database; the law library will certainly have one. Computer access works something like Medline, but better: Every word in every case and statute and rule in the database is indexed. A computer search of the database will cost something, so inquire beforehand.

Lawyers

To correct some misperceptions: The U.S. population does not contain 70 percent of the world's lawyers nor does it spend $300 billion per year on 18 million lawsuits. The 18 million number is skewed, for it includes routine cases like small claims, probate routines, and divorce matters. The correct number of adversary proceedings is about 2.5 million (still perhaps enough to maintain the charge that Americans are the world's most litigious people).

The United States has about 25 to 35 percent of world's lawyers (not 70 percent); and if people didn't patronize lawyers, there would simply be no market for lawyers. The $300 billion cost is casual speculation and not derived in any sense from investigative or statistical analysis.[124]

> "Lawyers are blamed for a whole Pandora's box of social ills: for the endless proliferation of government rules and regulations, for national litigiousness, for a lot of things—for crime itself. Nevertheless we ultimately are thankful for you, and look to you, because you, along with the government, are the standard-bearers of the Constitution. It is a sacred trust, and I know you view it as nothing less."[125]
>
> —George Bush, then U.S. Vice President

The famous quote (from Shakespeare's *Henry VI,* Part 2, Act IV, Scene 2) must be put in context: Jack Cade, rebel leader, has plans for when he becomes king. He'll establish a utopia where all have free food, identical clothes and live in harmony, worshipping him. Co-rebel Dick the Butcher interrupts, with an a practical caution: "The first thing we do, let's kill all the lawyers."

They commence their work, however, by hanging a teacher because he can read and write.

RESOURCES

Sources of current cases:

Dahanayake, C., "The nurse and the law (Part 1)," *Medicine & Law*, 1991; 10(3):249–267.

Tammelleo, A.D., "Legal case briefs for nurses," *Regan Report on Nursing Law*, published monthly, 1231 Fleet National Bank Bldg., Providence, RI 02903.

In the following article, sources of legal authority are explained and the essential components of one case presented in detail; computer and manual searching strategies are also identified, and along with the citation system discussed:

Weiler, K., and Rhodes, A.M., "Legal methodology as nursing problem solving," *Image—the Journal of Nursing Scholarship*, 1991; 23(4):241–244.

Nursing journals offer continuing update on law, changes and particulars. Having read this book, such updates can be better understood.

Fiesta, J., "Legal update for nurses, Part I, II and III," *Nursing Management*, 1993; 24(1):16–17, (2):14–16, (3):16–17. But read with caution: in Part III, p. 17 of Fiesta: ". . . the individual staff nurse satisfies his or her legal accountability by discussing the issue with the nurse manager." As Fiesta correctly goes on to say, at that point the nurse manager also has a duty to act. But if the manager does not act, the staff nurse may still have responsibility to act until help is obtained for the patient from up the managerial chain, the physician hierarchy, or public officials, if finally necessary.

ENDNOTES

1. Steppe, H., "Nursing in Nazi Germany," *Western Journal of Nursing Research*, 1992; 14(6):744–753.
2. Rawls, J., *A Theory of Justice*, Cambridge: Harvard University Press, 1971.
3. Mill, J.S., *On Liberty*, originally published 1859, Chicago: Great Books of the Western World, 1952, vol. 43, p. 271.
4. Bennett, W.J., *The Book of Virtues*, New York: Simon and Schuster, 1993, p. 9.
5. Von Mises, L., *Human Action*, New Haven: Yale University Press, 1949, p. 99.
6. Pellegrino, E., in Cassell, E.J., *The Place of the Humanities in Medicine*, Hastings-on-Hudson, NY: The Hastings Center, 1984, at p. 30.
7. Harkness, E.G., and Pallikkathayil, L., "Ethics in the nursing curriculum for all levels of education: Baccalaureate, masters' and doctoral," *Medicine & Law*, 1989; 8(2):191–198.
   The Teaching of Ethics in Higher Education, A Report, Hastings-on-Hudson, NY: The Hastings Center, 1980.
   Cassell, E.J., *The Place of the Humanities in Medicine*, Hastings-on-Hudson, NY: The Hastings Center, 1984; quoting Pellegrino, E., "The humanities in medical education," *Mobius*, 1982; 2:133–141.
   Coutts, M.C., *Teaching Ethics in the Health Care Setting*, Washington, DC: Kennedy Institute of Ethics, September 1991.
8. Hall, J.K., "Ethics for Patient Care," CE Course, Text, Graduate Course, National City, CA: California College for Health Sciences, 1993.
9. Todd, J., "Health care reform and the medical education imperative," *Journal of the American Medical Association*, 1992; 268(9):1133–1134.
10. Rosen, D.H., "Inborn basis of the healing doctor-patient relationship," *Pharos*, 1992; 55:17–21.
11. Densford, K.J., and Millard, S.E., *Ethics for Modern Nurses*, Philadelphia: Saunders, 1946; p. 181.
12. Reich, W.T., *Encyclopedia of Bioethics*, Washington, DC: Kennedy Institute of Ethics at Georgetown University, 1978, p. 1138.
13. Smith, W.B., and Lew, Y.L., *Nursing Care of the Patient*, Sydney: Dymock, 1968, p. 2.

14. Dolan, J.A., *et al.*, *Nursing in Society: A Historical Perspective*, Philadelphia: Saunders, 1983, p. 45.
15. Helmstadter, C., "Robert Bentley Todd, Saint John's House, and the origins of the modern trained nurse," *Bulletin of the History of Medicine*, 1993; 67:282–319, at pp. 315–316.
16. *Ibid.*, at 317.
17. Densford and Millard, *op. cit.*, p. 98.
18. Johnstone, M.-J., *Bioethics: A Nursing Perspective*, Sydney: Harcourt Brace Jovanovich, 1989, p. 18.
19. Steppe, H., *op. cit.*, pp. 744–753.
20. Pound, R., *The Lawyer from Antiquity to Modern Times: With Particular Reference to the Development of Bar Associations in the United States*, St. Paul, MN: Western, 1953.
21. Friedman, E., "Troubled past of 'invisible' profession," *Journal of the American Medical Association*, 1990; 264(22):2851–2855, 2858.
22. Gideon, J., "Registered Nurse bargaining units: Undue proliferation?" 45 *Missouri Law Review* 348 (1980).
23. Smith, S., "When ethics and orders conflict," *RN*, 1991; 54(9):61–62, 64, 66.
24. Yocke, J.M., and Donner, T.A., "Floating out of ICU: The ethical dilemmas. Part I: The ethical case. Part II: The case analysis," *Dimensions of Critical Care Nursing*, 1992; 11(2):104–107.
25. Rushton, C.H., and Hogue, E.E., "Confronting unsafe practice: Ethical and legal issues," *Pediatric Nursing*, 1993; 19(3):284–288.
26. Telephone information from Mike Palmer, American College of Pathologists, 11 March 1994.
27. Ducanis, A.J., and Golin, A.K., *The Interdisciplinary Health Care Team*, Germantown, MD: Aspen Systems Corporation, 1979.
28. Davis, A.J., Aroskar, M.A., *Ethical Dilemmas and Nursing Practice*, Norwalk, CT: Appleton-Century-Crofts, 1983, p. 49.
29. Dickstein, E., *et al.*, "Ethical principles contained in currently professed medical oaths," *Academic Medicine*, 1991; 66(10):622–624.
30. Densford and Millard, *op. cit.*, p. 154. But the writer does suggest some "good rules" for nurses to follow, at p. 157!
31. Cianci, M., "The code of ethics and the role of nurses: An [sic] historical perspective," *NursingConnections*, 1992; 5(1):37–42.
32. Freitas, L., "Historical roots and future perspectives related to nursing ethics," *Journal of Professional Nursing*, 1990; 6(4):197–205.
33. Densford and Millard, *op. cit.*, p. 167.
34. "When finances may influence physician decision making," *Ethics Case Studies, 1990–91*, Philadelphia: American College of Physicians, 1992.
35. "Code of ethics for holistic nurses," *Journal of Holistic Nursing*, 1992; 10(3):275–276.
36. "Code of ethics and interpretive statements," *American Association of Occupational Health Nursing Journal*, 1991; 39(10):470A-D.
37. Davis, A.J., "New developments in international nursing ethics," *Nursing Clinics of North America*, 1989; 24(2):571–577.
    Davis, A.J., "Ethical similarities internationally," *Western Journal of Nursing Research*, 1990; 12(5):685–688.
38. Stevenson, C.L., *Ethics and Language*, New Haven: Yale University Press, 1944, p. 33; in Johnstone *op. cit.*, p. 57.
39. Sigsby, L.M., "Crisis and ethical dilemmas: Who will care for the rural nurse?" *Heart & Lung*, 1991; 20(5 Pt 1):523–525.
    Rushton, C.H., "Care-giver suffering in critical care nursing," *Heart & Lung*, 1992; 21(3):303–306.
40. Edwards, M. and Tolle, S., "Disconnecting a ventilator at the request of a patient who knows he will then die: The doctor's anguish," *Annals of Internal Medicine* 1992; 117(3):254–256.
41. Goldberg, P., *The Intuitive Edge*, Los Angeles: Jeremy Tarcher, 1983, p. 37; in Johnstone, *op. cit.*, p. 60.
42. Partridge, E., *Origins: A Short Etymological Dictionary of Modern English*. New York: Greenwich House, 1983.
43. For example, Cutter, E., "Address on dietetics—Medical food ethics now and to come," *Journal of the American Medical Association*, 1893; 20:239–244.

44. Sagan, C., "A new way to think about rules to live by," *Parade*, 28 November 1993, p. 13.
45. Cecil, W.-S., *Florence Nightingale, 1820–1910*, London: Constable, 1950, p. 17.
46. Fowler, M., "Ethical issues in critical care: Ethics without virtue," *Heart & Lung*, 1986; 15(5):528–530.
47. Burk, E., quoted in William Buckley, "Redefining Smart," *Playboy*, January 1985.
48. For a discussion of the *un*ethics of imposing a single imperative on a diverse, free people, see Engelhardt, H.T., "Medical ethics for the 21st century," *Journal of the American College of Cardiology*, 1991; 18(1):303–7.
49. O'Neil E.H., Director of the Commission, "Healthy America: Practitioners for 2005, an agenda for action for U.S. Health Professional Schools," speech 28 Oct. 1992 at the University of Missouri, reported in *Missouri Alumnus*, Winter 1993, p. 46.
50. For a discussion of natural law in nursing literature, see Nolan, M.T., "Natural law as a unifying ethic," *Journal of Professional Nursing*, 1992; 8(6):358–361.
51. Edelstein, L., "Platonism or Aristotelianism," *Bulletin of the History of Medicine*, 1933; 7(6):757–769.
52. Fletcher, J., *Situation Ethics: The New Morality*, Philadelphia: Westminster Press, 1966.
53. Cassells, J.M., and Redman, B.K., "Preparing students to be moral agents," *Nursing Clinics of North America*, 1989; 24:463–473.
54. Allmark, P., "The ethical enterprises of nursing," *Journal of Advanced Nursing*, 1992; 17(1):16–20.
55. Hall, J.K., "Law vs. Ethics," COPE: Working in Oncology, Sept.–Oct. 1994, p. 22.
56. Ketefian, S., "Moral reasoning and ethical practice in nursing," *Nursing Clinics of North America*, June 1989; 24: 509–521.
57. Kohlberg, L., *The Philosophy of Moral Development: Moral Stages and the Idea of Justice*, San Francisco: Harper & Row, 1981.
58. Gilligan, C., *In a Different Voice: Psychological Theory and Women's Development*, Cambridge: Harvard University Press, 1992.
59. Nokes, K.M., "Rethinking moral reasoning theory," *Image—the Journal of Nursing Scholarship*, 1989; 21:172–175, at p. 172.
60. Gilligan, *op. cit.*
61. Duckett, L., *et al.*, "Challenging misperceptions about nurses' moral reasoning," *Nursing Research*, 1992; 41(6):324–331.
62. Corley, M.C., and Selig, P.M., "Nurse moral reasoning using the Nursing Dilemma Test," *Western Journal of Nursing Research*, 1992; 14(3):380–388.
63. Chally, P.S., "Moral decision making in neonatal intensive care," *Journal of Obstetric, Gynecologic, & Neonatal Nursing*, 1992; 21(6):475–482.
64. Ketefian, S., "Moral reasoning and moral behavior among selected groups of practicing nurses," *Nursing Research* 1981; 30:171–176.
65. Rest, J., *Development in Judging Moral Issues*, Minneapolis: University of Minnesota Press, 1979.
66. Curtin, L., "On writing a column on ethics," *Nursing Management*, 1993; 23(7):18,20.
67. Vladeck, B., "Editorial: Beliefs vs behaviors in healthcare decision making," *Public Health Policy Forum*, 1993; 83(1):12–22.
68. See, for more information:
    Milner, S., "An ethical nursing practice model," *Journal of Nursing Administration*, 1993; 23(3):22–25.
    Nyberg, J., "Teaching caring to the nurse administrator,"*Journal of Nursing Administration*, 1993; 23(1):11–17.
    Morath, J.M., and Manthey, M., "An environment for care and service leadership: The nurse administrator's impact," *Nursing Administration Quarterly*, 1993; 17(2):75–80.
    Corley, M.C., and Raines, D., "An ethical practice environment as a caring environment," *Nursing Administration Quarterly*, 1992; 17(2):68–74.
    Biordi, D.L., "Nursing error and caring in the workplace," *Nursing Administration Quarterly*, 1993; 17(2):38–45.
    Jacques, R., "Untheorized dimensions of caring work: Caring as a structural practice and caring as a way of seeing," *Nursing Administration Quarterly*, 1993; 17(2):1–10.
    Smeltzer, C.H., "The impact of prospective payment on the economics, ethics, and quality of nursing," *Nursing Administration Quarterly*, 1990; 14(3):1–10.
    Nyberg, J., "The element of caring in nursing administration," *Nursing Administration Quarterly*, 1989; 13(3):9–16.

69. See Bowman, A., "Teaching ethics: Telling stories," *Nurse Education Today*, 1995; 15(1):33–38.
70. Noddings, N., *Caring; a Feminine Approach to Ethics and Morals*, Berkeley: University of California Press, 1984.
71. Condon, E., "Nursing and the caring metaphor: Gender and political influences on an ethics of care," *Nursing Outlook*, 1992; 40(1):14–19.
72. Dimonte, V., "Una finestra sul passato: la donne e piu adatta alla cura degli infermi?" ["A window on the past: Are women more adapted to care of the sick?"], *Rivista dell Infermiere*, 1992; 11(4):219–227.
73. Nyberg, J., "The effects of care and economics on nursing practice," *Journal of Nursing Administration*, 1990; 20(5):13–18.
74. Hall, J.K., "Coming back to America," *RN*, February 1991, p. 112.
75. Bunting, S., and Campbell, J.C., "Feminism and nursing: Historical perspectives," *Advanced Nursing Science*, 1990; 12(4):11–24.
76. Ross, J.W., *Handbook for Hospital Ethics Committees*, Chicago: American Hospital Publishing, 1986.
77. *In re. Quinlan*, 70 N.J. 101, 355 A2d 1647, *cert denied* (1976).
78. Agich, G.J., and Youngner, S.J., "For experts only? Access to hospital ethics committees," *Hastings Center Report*, 1991; 21(5) 17–25.
79. Veatch, R.M., "Advice and consent," *Hastings Center Report*, 1989; 19(1):20–22.
80. Siegler, M., "Ethics committees: Decisions by bureaucracy," *Hastings Center Report*, 1986; 16:22–24.
81. Brennan, T., "Ethics committees and decisions to limit care," *Journal of the American Medical Association*, 1988; 260(6):803–807.
82. "New law creates challenges for hospital ethics committees," *Medical Ethics Advisor*, December 1991, pp. 148–150.
83. Andereck, W.S., "Development of a hospital ethics committee: Lessons from five years of case consultations," *Cambridge Quarterly of Healthcare Ethics* 1992; 1:41–50.
84. See generally, Agich, G., "Human experimentation and clinical consent," in Monagle, J., and Thomasma, D., (Eds.) *Medical Ethics*, Rockville, MD: Aspen, 1989.
85. Murray, T.H., Director, Center for Biomedical Ethics, Case Western Reserve, in "Physicians, journalists, ethicists explore their adversarial, interdependent relationship," *Journal of the American Medical Association*, 1988; 260: at 757.
86. Hayek, F.A., *The Road to Serfdom*, Chicago: University of Chicago Press, 1994.
87. Raffin, T.A., Withholding and withdrawing life support," *Hospital Practice*, 15 March 1991, pp. 133–155, at p. 141.
88. Singer, P., and Siegler, M., Letter to editor, *Journal of the American Medical Association*, 1988; 260:789.
89. Lund, M., "The heart of the matter," *American Journal of Nursing*, 1992; 92(4):22, 24.
90. Hildreth, E.A., "Workup for a bioethical problem," *Hospital Practice*, 25 January 1990, pp. 86–100.
91. Thomasma, D.C., "An ethical workup," *Forum on Medicine*, December 1978, pp. 33–36.
92. Sullivan, P.A., and Brown, T., "Common-sense ethics in administrative decision making. Part I, Preparatory steps," *Journal of Nursing Administration*, 1991; 21(10):21–23. And "Part II, Proactive steps," *Journal of Nursing Administration*, 1991; 21(11):57–61.
93. Miedema, F., "A practical approach to ethical decisions," *American Journal of Nursing*, 1991; 91(12):20,22,25.
94. Curtin, L., "When the system fails," *Nursing Management*, 1992; 23(8):21–25.
95. Rushton, C.H., "Advance directives for critically ill adolescents," *Critical Care Nurse*, June 1992, p. 36.
96. Northrop, C.E., "Legal content in the nursing curriculum: What students need and how to provide it," *Nursing Outlook*, 1989; 37(4):200.
97. Fuller, L., *The Law in Quest of Itself: Beacon Series in Classics of the Law*, Boston: Beacon Press, 1940.
    Also see Nolan, M.T., *op. cit.*, note 50.
98. Levi, E.H., *An Introduction to Legal Reasoning*, Chicago: University of Chicago, 1972.
99. Hall, J.K., "Understanding the fine line between law and ethics," *Nursing*, 1990; 20(10):34–40.
100. Hayek, F., *Law, Legislation and Liberty: The Mirage of Social Justice*, Chicago: University of Chicago Press, 1976, p. 36.

101. Rule 10D-28.110(9) F.A.C.
102. 22 Tex. Admin. Code §217.13(22), defining unprofessional conduct as failure to repay a student loan.
103. For example, Chapters 4 and 5 of the rules regulating the Florida Bar.
104. For more information:
    Takach, M.B., "A recipe for political action," *Nursing Economics*, 1989; 7(5):273–275.
    Sharp, N., "The path of legislation: Best opportunity for nurses' input," *Nursing Management*, 1993; 24(9):28–34.
    Bushy, A., and Smith, T.O., "Lobbying: The hows and wherefores," *Nursing Management*, 1990; 21(4):39–41, 44–5.
105. *Sermchief v. Gonzales*, 660 SW2d 683 (Mo. 1983).
106. *In re. Quinlan, supra.*, note 77.
107. *Cruzan v. Director, Missouri Department of Health*, 497 U.S. 261 (1990). In the aftermath of the Supreme Court case, nurses were ordered to allow the patient to die of dehydration.
108. Section 23, Article 1, Constitution of the State of Florida, adopted 1980.
109. *In re. Guardianship of Browning*, 543 So2d 258 (Fla. Dist. Ct. 1989).
110. Will, G.F., "For the handicapped, rights but no welcome," *Hastings Center Report*, 1986; 16:5–8.
111. Hockenberger, S.J., "American Nurses Association philosophical statement on ethics and human rights," *Plastic Surgical Nursing*, 1993; 13(1):41, 44.
112. Maine, H.S., *Ancient Law; Its Connection with the Early History of Society and Its Relation to Modern Ideas*, Boston: Beacon Press, [first published 1861], 1963.
    Hoebel, E.A., *The Law of Primitive Man*, New York: Atheneum, 1968.
113. Stein, P., *Legal Institutions: The Development of Dispute Settlement*, London: Butterworths, 1984, p. 22.
114. Cohen, M.R., and Cohen, F.S., *Readings in Jurisprudence and Legal Philosophy*, Boston: Little, Brown, 1951, pp. 280–366.
115. Henry, P.F., "Your due process rights in a disciplinary action," *Nurse Practitioner Forum*, 1991; 2(4):210–210.
116. Hayek, F.A., *op. cit.*
117. Hall, J.K., (as lobbyist for the bill), personal reminiscence.
118. Oxhorn, V., and Rosen, S., "Understanding the regulatory arena," *Association of Operating Room Nurses Journal*, 1992; 55(2):623–623.
119. Jordan, D., "Medicaid issues at the administrative hearing commission," *Journal of the Missouri Bar*, 1993; March–April, 135–144.
120. "Arkansas Medical Society wins Medicaid lawsuit," *Arkansas Medical Society News*, 29 April 1993, pp. 1,2.
    "MSMA again successful in court case," *Missouri State Medical Association Progress Notes*, April 1993, p. 6.
121. Stein, P., *op. cit.*
122. Lincoln, A., lecture notes, 1 July 1850, *The Harper Book of American Quotations*, New York: Harper, 1988.
123. See, *e.g., Sermchief v. Gonzales, supra.*, note 105.
124. Miner, R., U.S. Court of Appeals judge for the 2d Circuit in New York, in an October 1993 speech to the Association of the Bar of the City of New York, quoted in Reske, H., "In defense of lawyers: Conservative judge challenges Quayle statistics," *American Bar Association Journal*, 1993; January, p. 33.
125. Reske, H., *ibid.*

TWO

Ethics and Law of
Doing Good (Beneficence)

TOPICS COVERED

General explanation of the value, Beneficence (basis for the law)

Malpractice: The law that enforces the ethic, Beneficence

Essentials of malpractice
DUTY • STANDARD • INJURY • CAUSATION

Defenses
COMPARATIVE NEGLIGENCE • CONTRIBUTORY NEGLIGENCE

Malpractice insurance

General tort law
VICARIOUS LIABILITY—RESPONDEAT SUPERIOR • STRICT LIABILITY—ASSUMPTION OF RISK—PRODUCT LIABILITY • IMMUNITIES • JOINT AND SEVERAL LIABILITY—CONTRIBUTION AND INDEMNITY

Good Samaritan laws

Malpractice statutes of limitation

Tort reform

Avoiding lawsuits (includes documentation)

BENEFICENCE (DOING GOOD): THE VALUE AS BASIS FOR THE LAW

$\triangledown$

"They shall lay hands on the sick, and they shall recover . . . ."
—MARK 16:18, New Testament

$\triangle$

Bene in Latin means "good"; *ficence* means "to do or make." The value of doing good for the patient is above all others for nurses.

Other values, notably the value placed on life, are also promoted by doing good for patients.

Doing good for others is in the individual's self-interest, since it enhances self-esteem and the odds that others will do good in return.

People working in occupations *other* than illness care may not have the legal mandate to do good, as do nurses.

Licensure law and malpractice law enforce (mandate) the ethical duty to do good for patients.

In Anglo-Saxon words, the value discussed in this chapter is simply Doing Good. In Latin-derived terms, the word for this important nursing value is *beneficence*. Much of English is Latin-based (academics tend to use Latin-derived words, and William the Conqueror added some French (a form of Latin) to the English after his conquest of England in 1066.

Bene in Latin means "good" in English; *ficence* is Latin for "do" or "make." Nurses act for the good (the benefit, the health) of another—the patient. This value above all others characterizes nursing; sometimes above the freedom, and even the life of the patient. Beneficence is another way of describing what nurses do: Caring.

Other Values Involved

Most of caring (doing good) for patients promotes the patient's life. Care extends the length or improves the quality—or better, both. Indeed, some of the issues discussed in Chapter Seven, under the value, Life, could as easily have been discussed here, under beneficence. In particular, the issues arise about whether care is actually doing good or harming. The benefit (beneficence) weighted against the burden (the harm) could be addressed under the value, beneficence, instead of where it is, under the value, Life. The use of ordinary versus extraordinary treatments is also discussed in Chapter Seven, although such treatments also involve beneficence.

For clarity of organization, this book groups the ethics and law around one value—the value predominating a particular illness care issue or situation. But when beneficence or another value predominates, human actions and law usually are based on several values at once.

Doing good for others is in the individual's self-interest, too. As people care for others, they feel good about themselves. They value themselves. They believe they are seen as good people (their self-esteem rises).

Nurses adopt a system that places the value of beneficence above all others in "professional" behavior. They assume that helping other people now, increases the odds that they themselves may get help when they need it.

The work of people in occupations *other* than illness care may not be practiced directly as doing good for other people. The act of doing good is desired as a goal for all (ethical behavior), but doing good is not mandated for all (law-enforced). But for people who undertake a duty to nurse, doing good by caring for another person is both desired *and* mandated. Nurses are paid to care. They are professionals at caring, while other people are not paid (and, so, are "amateurs," from the French word meaning to do the work for love instead of money).

Nurses assume a legal duty to care. The law will enforce that duty to care if the nurse does not voluntarily meet the duty. Licensure could also be discussed under the value of beneficence; licensure law is the one major area of law, other than malpractice, that mandates the nurse actually do good. That ethic and that legal mandate are: To care for the patient.

PATER/MATERNALISM

Paternalism describes acting in a parental way toward patients; it assumes the nurse knows best what is good for the patient.

Since patients are becoming more autonomous, they are less willing to leave decisions to providers of care; and practitioners are more reluctant to make decisions for patients. Practitioners now are increasingly unwilling to take responsibility for another's choices.

Doing good to an extreme is called paternalism (the origin of the word is *pater* or "father," in Latin—of course, *mater*, means "mother"). Paternalism in the extreme connotes acting in a father-like or mother-like (maternalistic) way toward patients and, at times, virtually ignores the patient's autonomy. Nurses wish to obtain some good for the patient. They believe they know best what is good for the patient. The patient's freedom to choose is valued secondarily.

Total paternalism ignores the patient's freedom to choose her own action. The assumption is that one can do good for patients by doing what is best for them, no matter what the patient wants. Very paternalistic nurses believe they know more about what the patient needs than the patient does because they have more education, knowledge, and information.

Now more than formerly, nurses and doctors seem to be more respectful of patient freedom (autonomy), thus less paternalistic. Have nurses suddenly become better people? The more likely reason is that patients have begun to refuse to trust practitioners to make decisions for them, different from the time when people knew each other better.

One writer postulates that there are different models of practitioner-patient relationships: One is a paternalistic model, in which the practitioner decides what is best for the patient. At the other extreme is the informative model, a kind of relationship in which the practitioner merely informs the patient about his condition and options, without offering interpretation or assisting in deliberation.[1]

In earlier times—and even at present in places where people are not so accustomed to freedom—people were more likely to obey authority. They were not so insistent on their autonomy. In addition, they knew each other better, could trust each other more readily. (Other parts of this book discuss other consequences of the fact that people are more like strangers to each other now.)

Practitioners now are increasingly unwilling to take responsibility for another's choices. They see themselves as technicians or advisors whose patients make their own decisions. Practitioners do not see themselves as trusted father or mother figures. Current attitudes mean the patient, not the practitioner, has responsibility for the decision.

Malpractice: Law Enforcing the Value

> More law is written to enforce the ethical value to do good than is written to enforce any other value (possibly excepting the value, Life), and the largest segment of that law is malpractice law.
>
> Malpractice law demonstrates clearly that good practice is ethical and lawful. Bad practice is not merely unethical; it also violates the law (resulting in monetary liability or criminal penalty).

The value of doing good is the highest value for nurses. That value (caring for the patient) underlies all of nursing law. No other value in nursing, except perhaps the value, Life, has as much law written to enforce the moral duty. Beneficence, the value and duty in this chapter, is enforced by laws that operate after the fact. One difference between law and ethics is that laws mandate, while ethics request. But laws cannot prevent wrongs; they can only punish after the fact, the failure to do good.

The largest area of law that enforces the value of beneficence is malpractice law. Malpractice law doesn't force the nurse in advance to do good for the patient, but the law may punish the nurse afterward, if she fails to do good for the patient. Even if the nurse doesn't value the ethic of doing good for the patient voluntarily, the prudent nurse will do good to avoid malpractice and possible punishment.

Some malpractice law is governed by statutes made by the state legislatures. But the larger part of malpractice law is made by cases (judge-made law), not statute (legislature-made law). Most of the rules about malpractice liability come from case law.

In malpractice law it can be seen clearly that good practice is ethical and lawful. Bad practice is not ethical, *and* it violates the law (resulting in monetary liability or criminal penalty).

Brief History of Malpractice

Malpractice ethics and law have a long history, predating the Greek civilization more than 2000 years ago.

Much malpractice law is made by cases when judges review a lawsuit after it is appealed. Malpractice (also called professional negligence) is an unintentional tort (wrong); if the person intended the act, the wrong is classed as an intentional tort.

Intention can be inferred from the act; it is not necessary to intend the *harm* (only to intend the *act*).

The history of malpractice ethics and law is too long for this book, but as in all areas of law, the concept has a long history. Note below the words of two of the ancient Greeks about right treatments and judging professional practice. Remember that practitioners are not automatically liable just because the patient dies or has a bad result from therapy.

Plato writes that lack of intent should excuse malpractice:

and also with physicians, if the patient dies . . . *against the will* of the physician, the physician will be held pure in the eyes of the law. [EMPHASIS ADDED].[2]

This principle would excuse any harm the physician caused, except intentional harm.

Aristotle wrote on the need for expert witnesses to testify in malpractice cases:

. . . it might be held that the best man to judge which physician has given the right treatment is the man who himself is capable of treating and curing the patient of his present ailment, namely the man who is himself a physician.[3]

This is the principle that even today requires testimony of an expert witness to prove malpractice.

Case law is made by judges in the review of a lawsuit, after it is appealed. For convenience of study, case law is divided into different areas. One area is tort law (*tort* is an Old French word for "wrong"), for the kind of lawsuit in which the plaintiff (the patient) seeks to be compensated for a *wrong*. Tort law can be further classified by degree of intent present in the wrongdoer's act. If the person intended the act, the wrong is classed as an intentional tort. It is not necessary to intend the *harm*; only to intend the *act*. A quasi-intentional (half-intentional) tort falls between intended and unintended acts. The two classes of torts of intent are discussed in Chapter Three, on laws enforcing the ethic of "doing no harm" (non-maleficence).

Since intentions can be inferred from certain acts, for centuries people have made tort law that deals with actions and intentions. If the person performs an act knowing the consequences that will follow the act, law assumes the person intends the consequence of the act, and the law holds the person responsible. Omissions can be "acts" also, such as *not* feeding or watering a dog with the knowledge he will die without care.

TORT LAW SCALE OF INTENTION

Negligence (Malpractice)	Quasi-intentional Tort (Defamation, Invasion of Privacy)	Intentional Tort (Battery, Assault, False Imprisonment)

At the "accident" end of the intent scale, torts (wrongs) that are not caused by intentional acts are described as being caused by negligence. Some association with accident is implied. Negligence law includes car wrecks and falls in supermarkets. A subdivision of negligence law is malpractice law—regarding the negligence of professionals like doctors, nurses, and lawyers, which causes injury to their patients or clients.

FOUR ESSENTIALS FOR MALPRACTICE

The essentials for malpractice (in order to hold a nurse liable): The nurse must have had a *duty* to another person and must have *breached* the standard of care, which *caused* an *injury* to the person.

Over the centuries, case law decisions have developed four requirements for a successful lawsuit by a patient against a practitioner: duty, breach, causation, and injury. To successfully hold a nurse liable, the nurse must have had a *duty* to another person, must have *breached* the standard of care, which must have *caused* an *injury* to the person.

Duty

> Duty is established when the nurse has (or should have) undertaken to care for the person in question—acting in the capacity of a nurse or holding out as a nurse.
>
> Law imposes a duty on everyone (nurse or not, paid or not), to avoid harming other people, but law imposes the duty to do good only on people who voluntarily assume it.
>
> Nurses have a duty only to the person whom they can foresee they might be responsible to.

Duty encompasses the question of whether the nurse owes a duty to the person in question: Was this person actually a patient of the nurse? Did the incident happen on the nurse's unit, or in the cafeteria, or in the nurse's backyard, or did the nurse give free advice of a casual nature?

If a nurse is not acting in the capacity of a nurse (not getting paid to practice, or representing herself as able to give professional care) the law seldom imposes a duty to do good for another person.

The law does impose a duty on everyone (nurse or not, paid or not) to avoid harming other people, if possible. The law of negligence in the area of car wrecks, dog bites, or icy steps is about *avoiding* harm to others.

The duty to do good is only imposed if the individual is identified as a person whose job or other situation requires doing good; for example, a nurse. Courts almost never uphold a suit for damages against a volunteer or Good Samaritan who had no duty to act, even without a protective statute. And Good Samaritan statutes do not protect paramedics from suit, because it's the paramedic's job (duty) to rescue. There's no affirmative duty to do good placed on the general public; the parents of a baby run over by a truck cannot sue the bystander who stood idly by and let it happen.

A few states have written legislation to suggest that citizens have a duty to rescue others if the proposed rescuer is at no risk to herself. Such laws contradict thousands of years of tradition, which say that citizens don't owe each other a positive, legally enforceable duty to do good (beneficence). People merely owe each other the negative legal duty not to harm (nonmaleficence).

But once individuals take a job *or* represent themselves as being willing and able to do good in a professional capacity, they may have a duty to do so. For example, the nurse working in a free immunization clinic for no pay still represents herself as a nurse, with some assurance to the public that citizens will be well served. This is also the situation in giving "free" advice to one's neighbors, if the nurse knows the neighbor will rely on the nurse's advice alone. A court, however, would have to consider the circumstances. The court might find that, since the nurse was not paid for the advice, the nurse actually had no duty to the neighbor.

> In what is said to be the first malpractice case argued in the state of Illinois, Abraham Lincoln was the attorney for the defendant sued![4]

Even when nursing for pay, the nurse has a duty only to a foreseeable plaintiff. If the nurse can't foresee that someone will be hurt by some action, there is no duty to them. This is usually not an issue in malpractice, except possibly in case of a family member who witnesses harm to a patient and sues for her *own* "injury." The nurse *can* foresee that the patient might be harmed by negligence; but it's unlikely that the nurse can foresee that the patient's relative would be upset and have a heart attack.

If the nurse puts someone in danger, the person who acts to rescue the endangered person also is a foreseeable plaintiff, in addition to the person put in danger. The volunteer rescuer, injured at the scene of an accident, can also sue the person who caused the accident. Further, in some states a duty of care is owed to a viable fetus, but possibly not to a "non-viable" fetus (before the stage of life at which the fetus is able to survive, if born).

As noted above, there is usually no duty to act unless one assumes a responsibility, such as going to work as a nurse. But if a person negligently puts someone in peril, the person may have a duty to rescue the endangered. Airlines, bus companies, and innkeepers have a special duty to protect passengers and guests. One may have a duty to control a third person, if one has charge of the person and knows there is a need to control (this could be a liability in the care of the mentally ill).

The duty (relationship) to the patient is harder to establish without person-to-person contact. For example, a consulting doctor who spoke by phone with the ER doctor, but who never spoke to the patient, may not have a duty to the patient who the ER doctor called about.

Breach of the Standard of Care

> The second requirement for liability for malpractice is breach of the standard of care; failure to act as a reasonable, prudent nurse in a particular circumstance.
> The reasonable prudent nurse standard is objective, not subjective; the nurse's personal problems or shortcomings are not an excuse.

The standard of care that the nurse must meet can be established in a malpractice case by expert nurse witnesses, standing orders or protocols, equipment instruction books, ANA and JCAHO standards, quality improvement program documents, standards of specialty nursing organizations, the ANA Code of Ethics, nursing textbooks, physician-expert witnesses, statutes written to protect patients (especially nurse practice statutes and regulations), and nursing journal articles and texts.

Once established that the nurse has a duty to the person injured, the second requirement of liability for malpractice is that the nurse breached the duty. The definition of *breach* for nurses is failure to act as a reasonable, prudent nurse in that circumstance (an old value: Prudence was one of the four main values of the ancient Greeks). If the nurse has a *duty* she is obligated to treat the patient according to the standard of care (nursing as done by a reasonable prudent nurse). Evidence of the breach is failure to act in accord with accepted nursing practice (not meeting a standard, or violation of statute, or *res ipsa loquitur*—discussion below).

The reasonable and prudent nurse standard is objective, not subjective; this means the law doesn't care about the defendant/nurse's age or tiredness or particular stupidity. Nurses are judged according to what they should be and do as a reasonable, prudent nurse, not what they actually are. The law stands the nurse up in an abstract reasonable prudent nurse's shoes—not the dirty shoes run over by the portable x-ray machine as the nurse looked in disbelief at the supervisor who said the nurse would be charge nurse (first charge experience) on a second straight shift with 20 sick patients and one aide!

The law does care about the plaintiff/patient's particular characteristics. If the nurse knows a patient has particular physical handicaps or mental conditions, the nurse is expected to be careful of them. This may seem unfair, but the patient is sick, helpless, and has an expectation of safe care. The nurse is assumed to have options; the patient does not. The nurse's bad work situation is not the patient's fault. Nurses work in such conditions by choice (choice because the Thirteenth Amendment to the Constitution abolished slavery).

The law holds the nurse to an objective standard (what a reasonable prudent nurse should be), while the patient's condition is measured subjectively (what this patient's situation actually is). That policy reality is that the law will not shift the nurse's problem to the patient, by asking the patient to assume the risk that the nurse is deficient.

Evidence of this breach of a standard can be testimony by an nurse-expert witness; the nurse-expert might say that the nurse's behavior was not that of a reasonable, prudent nurse, in the expert's opinion.[5] Agency policy is another evidence of the standard of care against which the nurse's behavior could be measured (a good reason to know policy it and make sure it conforms to what is actually being practiced).

Standing orders or protocols, if those are in use in the workplace, can be used as evidence to establish breach of the standard of care as well. Nurses don't have to follow such guidelines if there is good reason to deviate, but they must document why the guidelines were not followed. Nurses should be aware of national nurse association *practice guidelines* and recognize that they can be used as the standard of practice in malpractice actions.[6]

Equipment instruction books can also be introduced to establish proper use and care of equipment. Nurses should know how to use the equipment and that it is in good working order. It's the nurse's job to make sure the equipment is safe for the patient, as far as can be determined, and to refuse to use equipment that doesn't work. If the faulty electric bed causes a fire or shocks the patient, the jury will not be sympathetic to the nurse's excuse that the maintenance department was overworked and so the nurse didn't report an unsafe condition. Other departments that fail to do their jobs must be responsible (notified). The patient deserves safe care.

Other standards of care that could be used to establish breach of the standard of care are those of the American Nurses Association. Such standards are usually written in such general terms that they may be difficult to apply to a specific situation, but plaintiffs might seek to hold all practitioners to such professional organizations' fairly vague statements.

Standards for nursing services established by the Joint Commission on the Accreditation of Health Organizations (JCAHO) might be introduced to prove breach. This use of their standards in a lawsuit could hurt the nurse worse than bad marks on a survey ever could (surveys rarely if ever result in hospital decertification by the JCAHO).

Standards of care can be evidenced by some of the documents developed in quality improvement programs such as "critical pathways" and "total quality management" documents. If the nurse doesn't meet the standards, this could be evidence of malpractice; if the standard was met, it is at least evidence of some minimal quality of care. Such written statements all describe what should happen to the *average* patient, almost never what should happen to the *individual* patient. If individual circumstances indicate deviation from the standard, the reasons should be documented.

Such documents may be "tools" for lawyers and courts; they could be used to prove that *not* following them breaches the standard of care. As written, they have many names—critical paths, practice guidelines/parameters, clinical guidelines, clinical protocols/algorithms. Nurses, therefore, should recognize the potential liability they may provoke. (Among the other terms used are anticipated recovery paths, clinical outcomes, collaborative care tracks, key processes, outcomes management, program evaluation, service strategies, standards of care [!] target tracks, uniform data systems.)[7]

Still other standards are set by specialty organizations, for example the American Association of Nurse Anesthetists, regarding IV conscious sedation. Nurses who practice new and unusual procedures should look for any such guidelines done by specialty organizations.[8]

The JCAHO revised standards regarding nursing care, say nursing care plans go into the permanent medical record; that the nursing assessment, patient needs, interventions, outcome, and discharge will "be permanently integrated into the clinical information system (i.e., the medical record).[9] This record could be evidence that the standard of care was breached, or was not.

The ANA Code of Ethics also could be used as a standard, although as ethics it should be seen as an ideal behavior, not a minimum required by law. Nursing textbooks can be used in some states, and physician-expert witnesses can testify against nurses (but usually not vice versa). The standard of care for nurse practitioners who practice medicine is often the behavior required of a reasonable, prudent doctor doing such procedure. Practice guidelines or protocols are increasingly used to set practice standards; they will be used also in malpractice cases to prove whether the nurse breached or met the standard of care.[10]

EXAMPLES OF STANDARDS AND RESPONSIBILITY FOR CARE

Nurses who are not Nurse Practitioners (NPs) seem to be liable for a *medical* standard of care. A 1991 Pennsylvania case said the hospital may be liable for a plaintiff paralyzed because the doctor failed to monitor her heart disease therapy. The court said that hospital employees have a duty to "question a physician's order which is not in accord with standard medical practice. . . ." This would mean that nurses not only must know and practice standard[11] nursing practice, but also must know "standard medical practice" and enforce it.

The Ohio Supreme Court held RNs to a lower standard, saying that their only duty is to inform doctors and follow orders. The Ohio Nurses Association objected to the court, and the court dutifully amended its conclusions, saying that "nurses are persons of superior knowledge and skill" and that they share responsibility for patients' care. They may also now share *liability* in future cases, because of the amended ruling.[12]

Statutes themselves can be very weighty standards of care. Breach of a statute that prescribes a certain behavior intended to protect the class of person who has been harmed, is called *negligence per se*. If the nurse practice act in the state says that nurses shall observe the patient, and the nurse fails to do so, the statute itself can be admitted as evidence of the standard of care that should have been met. The statute establishes the duty and standard of care. In some states it is a *conclusive* presumption, meaning no other standard of care need be used to show the standard of care. But the opposite evidence, showing that the nurse complied with the statute, is not conclusive presumption that the nurse took due care. Under *negligence per se*, it is possible that no expert witness would need to testify to the standard/duty of care.

As do boards of nursing in many states, the Texas Nursing Board wrote regulations specifying nurse standards of practice.

Example of Texas regulation used by plaintiffs in malpractice cases

[The RN shall] accurately report and document the client's symptoms, responses, and status. . . .

—22 Tex. Admin. Code §217.11(7) (1992)

The regulations written by boards of nursing are often used against nurses in malpractice suits, as well as in licensing discipline.

If the nurse is a defendant, any of these evidences of standards (for example, nurse-expert, agency policy, ANA or JCAHO standards) can also be used in defense, to establish that the nurse's actions were in accord with good practices of nursing care.

Nursing journals are another source of advice on new standards of practice applicable to nursing malpractice. The law's standard of care is the standard of good nursing *practice*; keeping up with what is good practice actually also keeps the nurse current with what is good law. Journals also regularly update the latest legal cases and statutes that apply to nurses.[13] These articles are interesting and helpful, but not a substitute for knowing that the basis of the law is ethics and good practice. The changing cases and statutes are merely variations and examples of the principle: Good practice is good ethics is good law.

Damage—Injury

The third requirement for liability in a malpractice case, *injury* can be proven by testimony of the patient, current doctor, or expert witness. Patients without expensive injuries may have difficulty finding a lawyer to pursue the case.

Injury is the third requirement for liability in a malpractice case. Physical *injury* and damages are usually not a problem for the plaintiff to prove; the patient and current doctor or expert witness can testify as to injuries. If the patient can't prove injury, no liability exists, even if the nurse had a duty to the patient and breached it.

A patient who has not been injured seriously is unlikely to find a plaintiff's lawyer willing to take the case. The case would not be brought if damages were not fairly large. Small damages are usually not sued on since the cost of prosecuting a small claim exceeds the possible recovery. Plaintiff's lawyers work on a contingency fee, which means that whether the lawyer will be paid is contingent on whether the patient-plaintiff wins.

Such cases are expensive to bring to trial and win (defendants win a large percentage of the time). The lawyer usually can't take a malpractice case unless it is likely to result in (1) victory and (2) enough damages to pay for time and expenses. That means the patient-plaintiff's injuries (damages) must be substantial.

Other systems for paying lawyers exist: In the British system, plaintiff's lawyers do not receive a percentage of the damages contingent on winning (instead, they are paid by the patient or a legal aid system, by the hour). The loser of the lawsuit (plaintiff or defendant) must pay the winner's lawyer. The advantages of that system are that it increases out-of-pocket costs to the patient-plaintiff, discouraging frivolous lawsuits. The disadvantage is that poor people with injuries due to malpractice may not be able to afford to get a remedy for the wrong done to them.

Damages can be sought and awarded for past, present, and prospective injury. They can be special damages (in malpractice, usually for specific expenses incurred as a result of the harm) and general damages. Whether the damage was foreseeable is not an issue in determining the *amount* of damages (foreseeability *is* a factor in determining whether there's a *duty* to a particular person). Once duty to a particular person is established, it doesn't matter if the nurse couldn't have anticipated a particular kind of *injury* from the act.

Damages usually do not include interest that would have accrued on the monetary damage award from the date of injury, only from the date the court awards damages; nor are specific amounts awarded for attorney fees (they're taken from the total amount of damages received). Punitive damages are not usually awarded unless the defendant was grossly negligent, sometimes called "wilful and wanton" behavior.

The plaintiff has a duty to mitigate damages. The patient who gets bad advice from the nurse, injuring his leg, will not receive further damages for letting the injury further deteriorate to the point of loss of the leg. He can only recover damages for the original injury. The patient has a duty to prevent further damage when possible. In most states, the plaintiff's damages are not reduced by collateral sources, which means the patient can recover the cost of medical care incurred as a result of the malpractice, even if insurance has already reimbursed. The policy reason: the defendant should not be helped, nor plaintiff hurt, by plaintiff's foresight in providing personal insurance or other protection.

Damages for lost earnings potential and for anticipated medical expenses can be proven by experts. In some states with tort reform, damages for pain and suffering are limited to a certain dollar amount (for example, $250,000 in California). The plaintiff's lawyer calls it pain and suffering; the nurse's lawyer calls it "non-compensatory damages," to reduce the emotional tone.

Damages for nonphysical, psychological pain are harder to prove and are not awarded in some states unless they are intentionally caused.

Causation

> The fourth essential for malpractice liability, causation, is established when it is proven that the patient's injuries would not have occurred *but for* the nurse's failure to act as a reasonable prudent nurse.
>
> Another standard of causation used in some states is whether the nurse's failure is a *substantial factor* among other factors causing the injury.
>
> Intervening forces that could have been foreseen do not excuse the negligent person; as example, a negligent driver could foresee that a negligent doctor might harm the person run over.
>
> But the negligent person is not liable for unforeseen criminal acts, and intentional torts done by a third party.
>
> Loss of chance for life (even if less than 50 percent) is sufficient to sue in some states.
>
> In some states the defendant needn't prove a specific individual liable under *res ipsa loquitur* (when the injury couldn't have happened except for someone's negligence).

The final requirement for liability is *causation*. Causation is established when it is proven that (1) the patient's injuries would not have occurred *but for* the nurse's failure to act as a reasonable prudent nurse; and (2) the nurse could *foresee* that failure to act in such a way would result in injury (the exact kind of injury needn't be foreseeable). The "but for" test is really a test of what is the proximate (close) cause of injury—"but for" the first event, the second would not have occurred. Several states have adopted this test.[14]

Under a lesser or looser standard of causation, used in some states, liability exists if the nurse's failure is even a *substantial factor* among other factors causing the injury. If there are joint causes of injury (the nurse and doctor are both negligent), there may be liability if the act was a "substantial factor" in the injury. If alternative causes of the injury are alleged, each defendant must prove his or her negligence was not the proximate cause. If the defendant nurse is to win, there must not be a direct connection from defendant's act to plaintiff's injury.

For example, if the nurse fails to assess, or suspect, or fails to report, obvious child abuse in a minor patient in the ER, the nurse may violate a criminal statute. In addition to being a crime, the failure to assess and report may be negligent and a "substantial factor" in the child's death, if the child returns to the abusive situation and is killed. The nurse's failure is not the direct cause of the death; the abuse is. But the failure might have been a substantial factor in the death (the abuse might not have occurred if the nurse had acted correctly).

If the negligence was an indirect cause of the injury—if a person slightly injured in a car wreck dies as a result of malpractice—the rule is that intervening forces that were foreseeable do not exculpate the negligent person, whether the negligence occurs at a car wreck or in a patient's room. Some examples of foreseeable intervening forces (sequelae that can be predicted from a situation), are medical malpractice, negligent rescuers, predictable reactions to an event, subsequent diseases, actions of people protecting property, and even subsequent related accidents.

On the other hand, the negligent defendant will not be held liable for *unforeseeable* intervening forces that cause harm. Two things that are not foreseen (anticipated) as a result of a negligent act are criminal acts and intentional torts of third persons. (Note that both are intentional acts of a third person, not accidents.) Intentional abuse of a child is a crime, but the act can be foreseen; a pattern of abuse means that the criminal intentional act *is* foreseeable in these cases.

Some states now allow a causation theory called *loss of chance*. This allows patients/plaintiffs to recover damages if the practitioner's negligence caused them to lose even a chance of cure. For example: Suppose the patient died of a brain tumor, a patient whose nurse practitioner failed to discover the tumor earlier when the patient had a 30 percent chance of recovery. The damages are calculated and then the survivor (who is now suing) is given 30 percent of the calculation.

A peculiar version of proving causation is *res ipsa loquitur* (Latin again, literally meaning the "thing itself speaks"). The thing (the injury, the incident) tells its own story and proves negligence. In other cases, the plaintiff has to prove that one or more specific defendants was negligent. For example: The patient goes to the OR for a hysterectomy and comes out with a dislocated shoulder, and no one "knows" or will admit what happened. The patient can't prove specifically who injured her (who was negligent), so the law of *res ipsa loquitur* presumes that anyone with an opportunity and control of part of the procedure could have been negligent. In this example, any and all of the OR staff will share negligence. In the real world, the hospital's liability insurer will pay—and possibly the physician's and nurse's, if there is one.

In a majority of states, if more than one person is a defendant, the plaintiff still has the burden of proving "who did it." In other states, the example given above would be the outcome; the burden is on each defendant to show innocence, or else share the blame.

DEFENSES IN MALPRACTICE LAW

Consent is not a defense to a charge of malpractice (but it *is* a defense to a suit for battery).

Defenses to malpractice may be denials of one or all of the four necessary elements to establish liability for malpractice: no duty, no breach, no causation, and/or no damage.

Any negligence on the patient/plaintiff's part (contributory negligence) was a defense to a suit for malpractice against a nurse or doctor in earlier days.

Comparative negligence has been instituted in place of contributory negligence in most jurisdictions, either by case law (the courts changed the law) or by statute (the legislators changed the law).

Under a system of comparative negligence, the percentage of each party's fault would be decided, damages established, and judgment given accordingly.

A signed consent is not a defense in malpractice action; it may be a defense to a charge of battery, classed as an intentional tort. Some writers speak of a "negligent" failure to inform or "negligent" failure to get consent, and a suit on that ground would be classed under negligence law and not under battery (intentional tort law).

If a lawsuit alleges that the practitioner was "negligent" in not getting informed consent, then establishing a valid informed consent *would* be a defense.

The defenses to malpractice are, in one form or another, denials of one or all of the four elements necessary to establish liability for malpractice: duty, breach, causation and damage. These can be encapsulated as "arguing in the alternative."

ARGUING IN THE ALTERNATIVE: AN EXAMPLE

Defendant is charged with borrowing a pot and returning it broken. Defendant can plead at the start of the case, alternatively *and at the same time*,

1. "I never borrowed the pot," *and*
2. "The pot was already broken when I borrowed it," *and*
3. "The pot was not broken when I returned it."

Pleadings can be asserted even though they are contradictory. The defense can present evidence on any of the theories, but must pick one theory by the time the case goes to the jury.

The plaintiff must establish all three things: (1) the pot was unbroken, (2) the defendant borrowed it, and (3) the defendant returned it broken. If the plaintiff fails to prove all three (if the defense can refute any one of the points), then plaintiff loses. Defendant wins. The policy is similar to that in criminal law, that the prosecutor must prove the positive case against the defendant; it is not the defendant's job to prove the negative.

A limit on the defendant's pleading is that lawyers cannot assert any claim *not* made in good faith; the lawyer must have some reasonable belief that the claim is plausible and, if not, faces sanctions by the court. The defendant asserting alternative theories also runs the risk of appearing foolish and/or untruthful (as in the broken pot example).

Alternative theories can be pled by the defendant in a malpractice case. Since the patient-plaintiff has to prove all four elements of malpractice (duty, breach, causation, and injury), the defendant may deny that any or all of the allegations of the plaintiff are true.

No Duty

The nurse's defense may be that no duty existed; the patient was not the nurse's. This defense will not excuse the nurse if the defendant was a patient of the agency, the nurse was on duty, and a reasonable prudent nurse would have assumed a duty. For example, a nurse who refused to assist a patient who arrested in the lobby of the hospital may be liable.

No Breach of the Standard of Care

Or, the nurse can say that no duty existed; and, even if it did, the nurse can deny that the standard of care was breached. If the person *was* the nurse's patient (and so the nurse had a duty), the nurse denies that the standard of care was breached. The nurse asserts that she acted as a reasonable and prudent nurse. This assertion is the most common defense: In order to prove it, the nurse will present evidence to counter the plaintiff's evidence; for example, the nurse may present a nurse-expert to testify on his or her behalf.

No Causation

The nurse can say there was no duty, but if there were, the standard of care wasn't breached (the nurse was reasonable and prudent). If the standard of care was breached, the nurse still may defend by proving that the breach did not cause the patient's problem. This could be proven if there were some independent, unforeseeable cause of the injury, such as the patient's being attacked by a visitor who caused further damage. In another situation, if the nurse gives the patient negligent advice, but the patient doesn't follow the nurse's advice and later takes negligent advice given by a doctor (even if it's the same advice), the nurse may not be liable.

As noted under Causation above, the courts are reluctant to let defendants off the hook if they find malpractice. In some states they may use the "substantial factor" reasoning and hold the nurse partially liable.

No Injury

The nurse who had a duty *and* breached it *and* caused the problem, can still seek to defend on the ground that the patient has no injury resulting from the breach. A nurse might successfully argue that her nursing action caused the patient no physical injuries. However, as punishment for using a racial slur against the patient, the court might say the nurse was "unprofessional" in language, and find that the nurse had committed malpractice that could be sued upon, even if the injury was not physical.

Contributory Negligence

Before the last few decades of tort law, *any* negligence on the patient/plaintiff's part was a defense to a suit for malpractice against a nurse or doctor. For example, if the nurse misapplied a cast or failed to warn the patient to check toes for circulation, the nurse committed malpractice. But if the patient was also negligent (for instance, noticed symptoms and failed to seek attention for them), the patient would have been contributorily negligent (was negligent and contributed to his own injury). Under contributory negligence theory: No matter how bad the malpractice of the provider, *any* negligence by the plaintiff was a good defense for the provider. In the past few decades, in most states, this doctrine has been modified into some form of comparative negligence by case or statute law.

Contributory negligence was imputed from the actual negligent party to the party vicariously liable. A master (employer) would have the servant's negligence imputed to him; a partner, the *other* partner's negligence; a person in a joint venture, *another* joint venturers' negligence. But husband and wife are not in such a vicarious relationship, nor are child and parent usually; nor car owner and driver, except when the state passes a statute to create the relationship.

Comparative Negligence

While malpractice or professional negligence law was originally made by case law, it has been modified to some extent by statute in all states. To read the details of the state malpractice law statutes, the nurse can look in the index of state statutes in the local or central library under such headings as Malpractice or Professional Negligence or Tort.

The theory of comparative negligence is particularly of interest to nurses because it is relatively more favorable to the plaintiff/patient. In states with that system the nurse could be considered at fault, even if there is some negligence on the part of the plaintiff. The percentage of each party's fault would be decided, damages established, and judgment given accordingly. Under the original contributory negligence principle above, a patient who was at all negligent would lose.

As an example of a judgment under comparative negligence: Assume the nurse failed to instruct the patient properly about his medication, but the patient was also negligent in not reporting that he had a reaction. His total damages were set at $20,000; nurse and patient were each found 50 percent at fault. Nurse pays $10,000. The significant change here is that under traditional case law, if the patient was negligent at all (contributory negligence), he lost everything.

Such a change in the law may have been made by state statute, in which case the statute can be found in the statute index. Or the change from contributory to comparative negligence may have been made by the court (judges) in the state; in which case the section on History in the statutes on malpractice will refer to and describe the case and decision establishing comparative negligence in the state. Any lawyer consulted in the state in which the nurse practices, should know if the state has a system of comparative negligence.

MALPRACTICE INSURANCE

To assess whether they need personal malpractice insurance, the nurse should ask the employee's risk manager if the agency has malpractice insurance that covers nurses and (1) whether the policy covers employees as individuals, (2) whether the insurance is "occurrence or claims made," and (3) limits of coverage.

Lawsuits against nurses are unlikely, but insurance may be warranted if the nurse's individual economic situation warrants protecting large assets, or if buying it will increase the nurse's comfort level.

Occurrence policies (preferred) cover for any *occurrence* during the time the policy was in force. Claims-made policies cover for any "claims made" during the time the insurance is in force.

Nurses who buy malpractice insurance may increase the odds of suit against them, if the plaintiff's lawyer knows of the insurance.

Insurance coverage exists only as long as the insurance company stays in business.

Insurance usually will not cover the punitive damage part of a liability judgment since such damages are meant to punish the wrongdoer and insurance would prevent that punishment.

Insurance does not cover fines levied for criminal acts, for the same reason; so, malpractice insurance generally does not cover costs of defending an action taken against the nurse's license by the board of nursing.

Some ethical argument may be made for carrying malpractice insurance, to compensate a patient unavoidably harmed by a nurse's mistake.

Nurses frequently ask if they need malpractice insurance and, if so, what kind and how much. First the nurse should ask the employer's risk manager if the agency has malpractice insurance that covers nurses in the event that they are sued. Nurses need to know if the policy covers employees, not only the agency. Nurses also need to know whether the insurance is "occurrence or claims-made" (the difference is explained below), and the dollar amount of the coverage.[15]

The policy should cover employees, whether the agency is sued *with* the employee, or the employee is sued and the agency is not. Policies usually do, but the nurse should ask and request the answer in writing.

The agency's policy should cover nurses individually. It needn't name the nurse personally, unless there is some question about whether the nurse is an employee or an independent contractor. If the policy is "claims-made" and not "occurrence" insurance, it should cover employees *after* they leave the employer, for acts done *while* an employee.

If the nurse employer's policy does this, then the nurse may not need a personal malpractice insurance policy. The data show that nurses are rarely sued, even more rarely found liable, and the average damages are very low. The employer's malpractice insurance would almost invariably cover the nurse adequately.

Few errors rise to the level of malpractice. Errors injure patients relatively rarely, injuries even more rarely result in a lawsuit, and rarest of all do malpractice suits result in a judgment against the nurse. If nurses can't stand words like "rarely" and want the confidence that insurance coverage brings (and don't mind spending money on something that is marginally useful), they should buy the insurance. Nurse insurance is still cheap relative to the cost other professionals pay, and the premium may be worth the "peace of mind" from the small danger.[16]

Nurses should examine their own economic situation; if they have considerable assets to protect, they may want to buy insurance. (If they have large assets, they also have more money to spend on insurance.) If not, they have little that will tempt lawsuit and little money to lose in the event of an adverse judgment. For the nurse who decides to spend the money for malpractice insurance, there are two different kinds of policies, occurrence and claims-made.

Occurrence policies are preferred. They cover the nurse for any *occurrence* during the time the policy was in force. If the occurrence happened in 1981 and the nurse had a policy that year, the nurse would be covered even if not sued until 2002. (Such a scenario could happen in a pediatrics case in some states.) Nurses will be covered, that is, if the insurance company is still in business.

Claims-made policies are cheaper; they are the only kind of malpractice insurance that some professions can get. Claims-made policies cover nurses for any "claims made" during the time the insurance is in force. If the policy is in force during 1981 (the nurse has paid the premium) and the claim (lawsuit) is made during 1981, the nurse is covered. If the claim is made at any time after the insurance is no longer in force (premium paid), the nurse is not covered.

The biggest worry is not the liability (rarely found and usually small). The more likely event (but still uncommon) is that the nurse would have to hire a lawyer to defend a suit that has no merit, filed because other nurses have bought liability insurance and the perception was created that nurses have deep pockets.

Nurses buying malpractice insurance increase the expectation of plaintiff's lawyers that all nurses have their own insurance in addition to that of the hospital; nurses are thereby converted into "deep pockets." As more nurses obtain insurance, the possibility is increased that nurses will be sued individually in addition to their employer's being sued.[17]

The advantage to having one's own policy of malpractice insurance is that the insurance will pay for an attorney if a suit is brought. If the nurse is covered only by the hospital's insurance, the attorney hired by that insurance company may be less interested in the nurse's particular liability.

In extreme cases, the hospital's insurance might find it helpful to their case to characterize the nurse's actions as illegal, thus freeing the hospital of responsibility. In such situations they have an obligation to notify that there's a conflict of interest and that the nurse should have separate representation.

The insurance company's lawyer, whether hired through the hospital's policy or the nurse's own insurance, is paid by the insurance company, not by the nurse or by the hospital. Some doctors hire their own attorney and pay privately, in order to protect their own (not the insurance company) interest.[18] The insurance company will choose the attorney, unless the nurse pays out of pocket.

If the nurse or agency have claims-made insurance, it is necessary to have coverage continue *after* the nurse stops working there or retires. "Tail" insurance, as it is called, covers claims made after the nurse leaves, on occurrences that happened while still working. A new problem is that agencies go out of business; the risk manager should know if the agency policy covers the employees after the agency closes, or what arrangements are made for that eventuality. If a hospital goes bankrupt, injured patients might have no one to recover from except the individual nurse or doctor.

Nurses need "tail" coverage only for the time period of the statute of limitations in the state. After that, a patient alleging negligence cannot sue successfully. Some kinds of practice (surgery, pediatrics) might require a longer tail. "Tail" coverage is proportionately cheaper than for coverage of current risks.

As an alternative to buying extra malpractice insurance: If the employer already covers the nurse, the nurse can spend the money for an "umbrella" coverage policy for self, family, home, and car liability. Check with the agent; such a policy usually doesn't cover the nurse at work, but it needn't if the employer's policy does.

In general, the nurse must be aware that personal coverage (as well as that through the employer) is exactly as reliable as the insurance company is.

Punitive Damages Usually Not Insured

Punitive damages are a way to punish; they enforce the value, Doing No Harm by providing a penalty for people who *do* harm with a large degree of recklessness or even intent. Insurance usually will not cover the punitive damage part of a liability judgment. Punitive damages are not related to the injury of the patient (in some states they are called exemplary damages); they are levied by the jury and judge to punish or make an example, in order to deter really awful behavior.

There is an ethical reason for the legal and contractual policy of not covering punitive damages by insurance: If insurance covered the "punishment," the individual or agency wouldn't really feel any pain. Such damages are not for unintentional behavior, and are rarely if ever merited in negligence actions.

People are not usually deliberately bad, but if the nurse committed an accidental medication error and then *intentionally* did not inform in order to cover it up, her action would be classed as intentional. If serious damage resulted, the jury or court could be provoked to award punitive damages.

It is argued that unlimited damages could violate a defendant's Fourteenth Amendment due process rights. In that argument it is asserted that, in an action by the government (for example, in enforcement of a lawsuit), damages could be enforced that were completely arbitrary and unrelated to behavior punished. In 1991 the U.S. Supreme Court was asked to put some limits on unlimited discretion to decide punitive damages, and declined.[19]

Insurance Doesn't Cover Criminal Acts

Rarely will insurance cover for fines that must be paid as result of a crime—a crime is usually deemed to be intentional. The insurance company covers only for "accidents" (negligence), not for something done deliberately. Crimes of "strict liability" don't require intent, but they're usually about acts like selling liquor to minors.

Most importantly and more likely than being charged with another crime is the situation in which the nurse is threatened with discipline by the licensure board. Since this is not a malpractice action in civil court, the malpractice insurance policy will not cover costs or attorney fees unless the coverage is specifically written into the policy (rare). The nurse who must respond to the board of nursing in the state must hire an attorney and bear costs personally.

Most nurses need little if any malpractice insurance as protection, but there is an ethical question as to whether they and other professionals (doctors, in particular) have a duty to carry insurance or have enough assets to protect patients they might harm. Every patient of a nurse is at some risk; every nurse risks doing harm to the patient in the course of practice.

Since nurses are human and humans make mistakes, there is no way to prevent some degree of malpractice. People who accidentally hurt others are not evil, but in this society they are held responsible for their actions. Can a case can be made that the ethical nurse buys malpractice insurance, not to protect herself, but to reimburse the patient against the risk of causing harm?

General Tort Law

VICARIOUS LIABILITY

> Vicarious liability enforces responsibility for the actions of another; one example in nursing is the liability of the employer agency for the actions of the employee nurse—*respondeat superior*.

Supervisors or staff nurses are not liable for the negligence of staff under their direction, unless they are negligently supervising (failing to act as a reasonable and prudent supervisor would act in similar circumstances).

Nurse and supervisor are liable for any malpractice they personally commit, regardless of staff unavailable. All levels of nursing are responsible for communicating dangerous conditions to management, including unsafe staffing numbers.

The agency is responsible for damage to patients from unsafe staffing since the burden for unsafe staffing will not be shifted as a risk to the patient.

The agency is liable for nurses who appear to have authority to act for the agency (ostensible agency theory).

Vicarious liability is another way of saying "those who benefit bear responsibility" or "the deep pocket loses." Vicarious liability enforces responsibility for the actions of another; in nursing, it is liability of the employer agency for the actions of the employee nurse. The Latin is *respondeat superior*—the superior responds (pays). This does not mean that the supervisor nurse is responsible for the acts of all employees under supervision. The supervisor is liable under this doctrine only if the nurse is actually the employer (pays salary, hires and fires, and reaps profit).

Under the theory of negligent supervision (a different theory of liability), a supervisor *may* be liable for the acts of negligently supervised workers if the supervision is negligent. For example, the supervisor may be liable for negligently assigning an LPN to care for a patient on a ventilator, *if* the supervisor knows or should know the LPN never had training or experience with such patients.

Supervisors or staff nurses are *not* automatically liable under the law for all the acts of all the people under their supervision. (This is a version of the "Captain of the Ship" theory, formerly used to get to the *doctor's* pocket for nursing negligence—necessary in the days when hospitals were charitable institutions and were immune from liability.) Nurses may *feel* responsible if someone under their supervision is negligent, and management may hold the nurse responsible, but the law will only find negligence, and hold the nurse responsible for *damages*, if the nurse has been negligent in supervision in some way. The standard is: How a reasonable and prudent supervisor would act in similar circumstances. Reasonable and prudent supervisors do not stand over people, nor do all their work for them. Reasonable and prudent supervisors do assign people work they can do, and make checks on the quality of the work done.

Supervisors are liable for making assignments—assigning enough staff to do the job; competent staff, able to care for those particular patients, and with adequate time allowed.

When alerted to a problem, supervisors must respond (very important in sexual harassment incidents). The supervisor must teach and inform appropriately, ascertain that staff complied generally with policies and procedures, verify that the staff's training was adequate, report conditions that could injure patients (including staffing levels) to senior management, and provide for student supervision. Supervisors have more than enough responsibility for negligent supervision, without being responsible for any and all damages of any staff action.

Responsibility for Staffing—Too Few or Untrained

Neither staff nurses nor supervisors are held responsible for poor staffing (there being either too few trained staff, or adequate numbers with deficient training)—*if* the harm to the patient is not due to the nurse's own negligence or the supervisor's decision to assign inadequate staff. The staff nurse and supervisor *are* liable for any malpractice they themselves commit, regardless of staff unavailable. As noted above, it is not the patient's problem that nurses have too many patients or unskilled assistance; it is not the patient's problem that the agency has too few nurses or hires unskilled people.

Nurses are responsible for meeting the objective standard of the practice of the "reasonable prudent nurse." The standard is not subjective—it is not the standard of the "reasonable prudent nurse with too many patients" or the "reasonable prudent supervisor with too few skilled nurses." If there is a danger to patients, the nurse/supervisor's duty is to communicate that to whatever level of management can deal with the problem. Staff nurses must tell supervisors that staffing is inadequate—every time it happens, and in writing. The supervisor must do something with that information; investigate, assess, and if needed, either supply more staffing (if within authority) or inform the next level of management (if not).

The agency is responsible for damage to patients from unsafe staffing; this responsibility is levied because the agency represents to patients that they will provide safe nursing care in return for payment. Agencies take the money, and then must deliver or face liability. If the nurses and managers involved communicate their concerns properly, they as individuals should be protected. Whether nurses cease to work for such an agency is an ethical issue for them, possibly a higher duty than the minimum ethic imposed by law. The law will hold the agency liable if the patient is injured and sues, under the theory of corporate liability.

Vicarious liability can be applied to find the *employer* liable for the nurse employee's negligence, even if the employer had hired supervisors doing a reasonable job of supervising. All that is necessary is to find the nurse liable, and the employer is automatically liable for that negligence, too. In addition, the employer can be found liable for negligence on a theory of negligent hiring (failure to check out skills, references, and licenses, at the time of hire) and on their own negligent supervision of nurses.

These theories are used also if there is difficulty in proving that the nurse was an employee; they have been used successfully in suing hospitals, even for the acts of doctors and nurses who are considered independent contractors.

If a nurse appears to act on behalf of the agency, the agency may be liable whether or not the nurse actually has authority to act; this theory is called ostensible or apparent agency. The agency is liable for permitting the nurse to *appear* to have authority whether the authority is actual or not. For example, the hospital may be held liable for the acts of a temporary nurse who does not work for the hospital, because the temporary *apparently* (to the patient) has the authority of an employee of the hospital.

STRICT LIABILITY (Assumption of Risk, Product Liability)

Strict liability torts (not based on negligence) create liability for procedures so inherently dangerous that they cannot be made safe; the ethical value underlying them is to protect people from unavoidable harm (doing no harm, doing good).

Assumption of the risk is a defense to strict liability, and a defense to a suit for malpractice (professional negligence) that alleges negligent informed consent.

To assert that the patient assumed the risk of danger, the defendant must prove that the plaintiff/patient knew of the risk, and voluntarily proceeded.

In strict liability law, risk may be assumed by express agreement. Express agreement is precisely what is obtained with a specific and detailed consent form listing "all" risks.

Products liability tort law uses strict liability analysis; but nurses provide services, not products (blood transfusions are considered a service).

Strict liability is a theory of recovery *not* based on negligence. Some procedures are so inherently dangerous that the doer cannot make them safe, even if very careful and not negligent. The ethical policy that people must be protected, causes laws to be constructed that enforce that ethic. An absolute duty to make the activity safe is placed on people who are engaging in ultrahazardous activity, such as causing explosions during excavations. In reality the activity cannot be made 100 percent safe, so the people doing the activity must assume, as a cost of doing business, the damage that is caused. Someone injured by such activity need not prove the defendant was negligent, only that the act was done and injury resulted.

Ultrahazardous activity is that which (1) presents a risk of serious harm to persons or property, (2) can't be made safe, and (3) is not a common activity (so, flying is not classed as an ultrahazardous activity). The last qualification is also probably why surgeries or other procedures don't fall under strict liability law; they're commonly done. Also, such inclusion would mean that every surgery that went wrong would leave the surgeon, nurses, and hospital strictly liable for damage, regardless of their use of extreme care; few practitioners operating would be the result. Note the resolution of the question in favor of the ethic of doing good for the patient (promoting surgery) over the ethic of doing no harm (compensating for any injury regardless of negligence).

One example of strict liability is having dangerous animals: The snake handler doesn't have to be negligent if a snake bit someone; the only proof needed in a suit is that he had snakes and that one of them bit the plaintiff. In contrast, having a nondangerous animal doesn't qualify for strict liability until the animal exhibits dangerous tendencies—the dog gets the first bite "free."

Contributory negligence is a defense to a case brought in strict liability, but only if the plaintiff knew of the danger of an action and engaged in activity that harmed her (it amounts to an assumption of the risk defense).

Assumption of Risk

Assumption of the risk is a defense to strict liability. More pertinent to nursing practice, this theory is a largely unacknowledged, but real defense to a suit for malpractice (professional negligence) based on failure to obtain informed consent. A consent form that lists all the possible risks of a procedure to the patient contains much "assumption of the risk" language.

To defend against a lawsuit by asserting that the plaintiff assumed the risk of danger, the defendant must prove two things:

1. *The plaintiff/patient knew of the risk.* The knowledge of the danger is implied where the risk is one that average persons would clearly appreciate. However, average persons would not clearly appreciate the specific risks in most medical procedures; hence the need for a long list of warnings of possible side effects and complications in the consent form, so they'll know the risk.
2. *The plaintiff/patient assumed the risk by voluntarily proceeding despite the risk.* But the patient is not deemed to have assumed all the risk of proceeding voluntarily *if there is no available alternative* to proceeding. If the only alternative offered for his condition is surgery, the patient might not have assumed all the risks.

If the patient had other options and chose surgery, the case would be stronger that he had assumed the risk. This defense cannot be used in strict liability cases (or in malpractice for failure of informed consent) if there is evidence of fraud (lying to the patient), force (obviously not voluntary consent), or emergency (no alternative, therefore not voluntary). These are exceptions to the use of the "assumption of the risk" defense in cases using a theory of strict liability. They can be seen also as exceptions in cases proceeding under an allegation of negligent failure to obtain informed consent.

In speaking about the strict liability defense, the law says that risk may be assumed by express agreement. The usual consent form reads like that express agreement, perhaps encouraging the patient to believe he's agreed to assume the risks.

A suit for failure to inform is different from a suit for malpractice. By signing the consent form, the patient agrees that he knew of the risk (so the signature can be used by the defense to prove that the patient *did* have enough information to consent). But signing such a consent, with many risks listed, does not mean the patient agrees to *assume* the risks listed—it merely shows he *knew* of them.

Products Liability

Products liability is an area of tort law in which strict liability is one of the theories used. In a product liability suit, the plaintiff can allege either negligence or strict liability (if the seller of the product is in business and the consumer gets the product unchanged through the seller from the manufacturer). In addition, buyers of bad products can sue for damages caused by the product's failing to do what it was sold to do; this is breach of an implied warranty of merchantability. The law implies (assumes) that the seller is guaranteeing that the product will do what it is sold to do.

The major "product" sold in illness care is a service (in legal terms), not goods; so, the service is not subject to suit under product liability. Blood and blood products have been ruled to be a "service" and not a product, so patients harmed by blood have to prove that the provider was in some way negligent. Strict liability (liability without proof of negligence) won't be imposed on the provider of the blood—a decision based on the value and need to do good for the public (maintain the blood supply), in preference to a need to punish harm (compensate for damage) to the individual.

Satisfaction and Release. In common law (before so much statute law was written), to release or dismiss one defendant meant all defendants were released from the suit. This rule, satisfaction and release, has been changed by statute in most states so that one defendant can settle with the plaintiff and be released from the suit while other defendants continue to trial.

Survival of Lawsuits

Torts for property and personal injury "survive" the death of the plaintiff because they are for past harm; the malpractice action continues. Suits for defamation, invasion of privacy, and malicious prosecution can only be pursued by a living person, the ethical principle being that the reputation died with the person (at least the emotional feeling about it).

Living people have many rights, including the right to sue for remedy of wrongs done to them. Many lawsuits survive a patient's death; they will be prosecuted in the name of the plaintiff, by the estate (the administrator or executor). They may be initiated after the patient's death by the estate, which can happen when the estate is sued for an outstanding hospital or doctor bill.

Not all torts "survive" the death of the plaintiff, however. Torts for property and personal injury do, so the malpractice action can continue; but suits for defamation, invasion of privacy, and malicious prosecution of a lawsuit do not. These wrongs are personal to the living person's dignity, not to his body or material goods. The ethics (value) behind such law is: No living person, no (or at least less) dignity.

Lawsuits can be brought after the patient's death, to compensate survivors of the patient wronged by the death. Wrongful death lawsuits, generally established and defined by statute, allow recovery for damages to the family or dependents (usually spouse and next of kin) of the dead person. Creditors who lose money by the death can't sue—and note the value judgment implicit in this legal distinction: The economic interests of families are more important than the economic interests of businesses. Wrongful death suits are likely when the patient has alleged malpractice and then dies from the condition caused by the alleged negligence. Wrongful death suits are the *civil* (not *criminal*) punishment for causing someone's death, either negligently or intentionally.

IMMUNITIES

Immunities from suit for family members, charities, and governments (to the extent they exist) enforce the ethic that protecting the potential defendant (for some reason) is more important than holding the responsible party liable.

Governmental (sovereign) immunity has been abolished or limited in application, but may protect nurses who work for federal, state, or local governments to some extent.

All immunities are in some way designed to protect people, who may indeed be liable, from the effects of their liability. Immunities protect "guilty" people from punishment, because some other principle with an ethical base is considered more important than holding the responsible person liable. Some of the immunities from lawsuit and their resulting liabilities are discussed below.

Intrafamily Immunity

Intrafamily immunity enforces the policy that family relationships (value) are more important than punishing a wrongdoer within that family. Many jurisdictions do not allow one family member to sue another.

In some states, exceptions to the immunity for family members are made—another way of saying that intrafamily immunity does not always apply. The immunity does not apply in some states, for example, if family members sue each other for property damage, intentional torts, or negligence while the defendant is not a member of the family (such as, after divorce). Such immunity from suit by another family member extends only to husbands, wives, parents, and little children.

Charitable Immunity

Charitable immunity once protected agencies that performed "charity work" from lawsuit (they're now called not-for-profits); such immunity has been eliminated in most states.

Much of what charities used to do is now done by government. The immunity from suit of charitable hospitals was a reason for the development of the "Captain of the Ship" doctrine (mentioned above, under Vicarious Liability). Under that theory, the doctor was liable for negligence of all "hands" on the watch; the plaintiff could recover from the doctor for the negligence of a nurse even though the nurse was not the doctor's employee. Today, plaintiffs can sue hospitals (either no or much less charitable immunity), so the need for and use of the "Captain" doctrine has practically disappeared. If payment for care by government decreases, the need for charity care will increase and some form of immunity from suit for charity care will again be needed.

Sovereign Immunity

The nurse who works for the government may be protected from lawsuit, to some extent. In the days of kings and queens, the sovereign could not be sued; the sovereign was thought to be ordained by God, Who could do no wrong, so neither the sovereign nor God was responsible for wrong. As a practical matter, enforcing a judgment against the sovereign was difficult (and good policy from the government's point of view). That viewpoint continued as kingdoms developed into democracies, evolving into governmental immunity. In recent decades the policy of governmental immunity, too, has been abolished or limited in application, but governmental immunity can still have meaning for nurses who work for agencies run by local, state, or federal governments.

In many states nurses who work for the state or local government have limited liability for malpractice; the agency's liability is limited, too. Some state employees may be covered by a liability insurance pool, information that can be obtained from an agency's risk manager.

Nurses who work for the federal government (for instance, Department of Veteran's Affairs) have immunity from lawsuit for any negligence (but they can be sued for wrongs done intentionally).

The Federal Tort Claims Act applies to all federal agencies; for example, war veterans as patients harmed can sue the Veterans Administration (VA) for negligence and for intentional torts. This protection from liability probably has some effect on doctors and nurses who enjoy it; but it might be studied whether immunity reduces responsibility, whether immunity from suit reduces the practice of (and cost of) defensive medicine, or whether the immunity improves practice, worsens it, or has any effect at all.

Sovereign immunity/governmental immunity may protect government workers and officials for "discretionary" but not "ministerial" acts; this means that managers and officials are immune from the effects of most of their policy decisions. However, the employees who carry out automatic functions of the job (ministerial acts) may not be immune, if they are negligent. Sometimes an act that can only could be done by government (such as police work) is immune, but government functions that are "proprietary" are not; proprietary functions are those that could be farmed out to private business (like trash collection).

The nurse who works for a governmental (taxpayer-financed) agency should check with the risk manager or management as to whether the agency and/or nurse are protected from suit by governmental immunity in state law. The nurse can in addition find the statutes in the local library, using the index under Immunities.

JOINT AND SEVERAL LIABILITY

Joint and several liability holds that all "tortfeasors" (wrong-makers) are held equally liable; if the other defendants don't pay their share, the one who *can* pay must.

Contribution theory means codefendants have a claim against each other if one paid more than a correct share of the judgment.

Indemnity refers to the ability of a defendant to get reimbursement (indemnification) from another person who actually caused the damage that the defendant was held liable for—it is rarely done in nurse liability. Indemnity seeks to shift the entire liability to another (not just a share as in *contribution*).

This legal concept of joint and several liability (now modified in several states) holds that all "tortfeasors" (wrong-makers) are held equally liable. Each is liable for the whole of the patient's damages, if the other defendants don't pay their share.

Scene. A nurse, doctor, and hospital were all sued individually.

The hospital is liable on *respondeat superior* grounds for the nurse employee's negligence, or under apparent agency or another corporate liability theory.

The patient is awarded $100,000 total for all damages—medical expenses, loss of earnings, and pain and suffering (to the defense lawyer, noneconomic damages). The doctor's assets are in the spouse or children's trust or in a trust in an offshore island, and the hospital has filed for bankruptcy.

It could happen; and it does.

Under the theory of joint liability, all three defendants in the above scenario were jointly liable; each owed one-third of the judgment (assume no percentage of fault was assigned to the patient or that this was not in a state with comparative negligence). But assume the other two codefendants are "judgment proof" (lawyer talk meaning a judgment against them can't be enforced—the money can't be gotten from them). The nurse is now severally (*severably*) liable. The other defendants are "severed" and the nurse is liable alone, owing the plaintiff the whole $100,000.

If the nurse doesn't have insurance, enforcing the judgment may *not* take all the money, the oldest child, and her 50 percent of all earnings from now on. In the scenario, the hospital's bankruptcy trustee may allow some of the judgment to be paid out of the hospital's frozen assets; and the doctor likely has money in U.S. accounts. If neither of those is true, the nurse's lawyer may advise the plaintiff's lawyer that, unless there's agreement reached for less money, the nurse might take bankruptcy.

The plaintiff's lawyer may then offer to settle because, depending on the nurse's financial status and state limits in bankruptcy, the plaintiff might not get much unless the lawyer makes a deal with the nurse for what is affordable. The nurse who declared bankruptcy (depending on the state's law) might be able to keep a car, the equity in her house, personal things, pensions, some bank account, and be free of debt (including the $100,000 malpractice judgment). Bankruptcy is a last resort, but useful if the worst happens.

Nurses do not lose a lot of money in lawsuits, and airline mechanics are not the main target when the plane crashes for the same reasons.

States with comparative negligence may ask the jury to assess each defendant's degree of fault, in case any single defendant is not liable for the whole judgment. The nurse is only liable for the percentage of the judgment that the jury assessed individually.

Variations of joint and several liability laws have been enacted by creative state legislatures. For example, in Texas, nurses will not be joint and severally liable if their percentage of liability is less than ten percent, *and* if that amount is less than the percentage of liability assigned to the patient. Such formulas are hard to remember, even for lawyers, and they are not worth worrying about until verdict time in a malpractice case (and Texas changed the rule in 1995!). If that very unlikely event happens, by then the nurse-defendant will be an expert.

Contribution and Indemnity

These concepts are related to joint and several liability and to insurance law.

The concept of contribution means codefendants have a claim against each other if one paid more than the correct share of the judgment. (This rule may be changed in states with comparative negligence; there, the loss may not be joint and several, but instead is exactly the percentage determined by the jury.) Codefendants who commit intentional torts cannot get each other to contribute. The ethic/value underlying that law: Don't worry about fairness, between people who intentionally do acts that injure others.

If the patient sues the hospital for nurse malpractice and the hospital is held liable under a vicarious liability theory, the hospital theoretically can then sue the nurse to *indemnify* them for any loss suffered as a result of the nurse's action. In contrast to contribution, indemnity shifts the *entire* loss (not just a share). This is rarely done because (1) nurses don't have much money; (2) the hospital's own liability company (who also insures the nurse under the agency policy) would probably have to pay itself; and (3) it's not good public relations for recruiting nurses and patients.

STATUTES OF LIMITATION

A statute of limitations limits the length of time in which the injured person can bring a lawsuit.

The statute may say the time limit for suit starts (1) at the time of the injury, or (2) at the time of the *discovery* of the injury, or (3) at the date when treatment ceased (or any other variation the legislature devised).

Concealing injury or complication from the patient may "toll" (suspend) the running of the statute. Plaintiffs may be required to give defendants notice of intent to sue before filing a lawsuit.

In the past, most malpractice law was made by the courts (case law). More recently, much malpractice law has been made by legislators (statutes). A "statute of limitations" limits the length of time the injured person has, to bring a lawsuit.

If the patient waits longer to sue than the time specified in the statute, the case is lost automatically. Such statutes are written so that people who intend to file a lawsuit will do so relatively quickly, while evidence is fresh and available. The statute also limits the time that potential defendants live under the threat of lawsuit for their past acts.

Most states have set the time limit to sue for professional negligence (malpractice) at from two to five years. In a particular state's statute, this limitation of time to sue may be shorter for suits against illness care workers than for suits against other people. Depending on what the state statute says, a person injured in a car wreck might be able to wait almost five years to sue the other driver, while a person injured by an operation may have only two years to sue the doctor or nurse.

The statute may say the time limit for suit starts (1) at the time of the injury, (2) at the time of the *discovery* of the injury, or (3) at the date when treatment ceased—or some other variation the state legislature devised. Two years from the date of discovery to sue, may be a long time to bring suit; the patient may not discover the injury for many years, and has two more years from that date of discovery to sue. (The patient with a retained sponge or hemostat may not discover the injury until years later, at a subsequent surgery.)

If the injury is concealed from the patient (for example, if the nurse fails to inform of complication), the time available to sue will not start until the patient actually makes the discovery of the injury. That concept is *"tolling the statute"* (delaying the start of the running of the time available to sue). Deliberately concealing the possible existence of malpractice is called fraudulent concealment, which carries penalties of its own—not least of which, that juries tend to punish practitioners who engage in such behavior, even if not they are not actually negligent.

Many state statutes provide that plaintiffs give defendants notice of intent to sue before filing the lawsuit. That notice tolls (suspends) the running of the statute.

The statute also usually specifies how long a minor has to sue. In traditional case law, the minor could (or even had to) wait until no longer a minor (21 years old; later lowered to age 18), and then sue. Some states have changed this case law by statute.

If the patient cannot point to any one incident that is the particular malpractice, then the end of a course of treatment (the treatment that is the basis of the malpractice) may become the starting point for the running of the time of limitations. Patients with chronic diseases, in which complications can be prevented by careful early treatment, may not know of malpractice until complications develop. One example is the patient with diabetes; it is now known that complications can be greatly reduced by early and aggressive control.[20] The doctor or nurse who sees the patient, and who says not to worry about the blood sugar—"200 and below is fine"—might face liability in ten years if the patient loses eyesight. A two-year statute of limitations will probably not begin to run until the patient discovers the complication. Practitioners could develop an "informed consent" for patients who are educated but continue to be noncompliant with treatment suggestions.

Good Samaritan Laws

> Good Samaritan statutes change the standard of care to which volunteers in emergency are held, from liability for ordinary negligence to liability for gross negligence.

Good Samaritan statutes, which excuse negligence on the part of rescuers in emergency, are of interest to nurses but rarely of use. The term Good Samaritan refers to a person who voluntarily helps another in need.

THE STORY BEHIND THE NAME

The story from the New Testament is about the poor fellow who had been mugged on the road to Jericho. Lying there bleeding, he was bypassed by a judge—symbol of a formal legal system that should help such people. He was also ignored by a priest—symbol of the formal ethic/religious system that should help such people.

Finally, he was aided by a member of a rival gang, the Samaritans—symbol of the private, informal, voluntary, instinctive, human response to do good for another person. It was not the Samaritan's job to help anyone (much less a member of another gang) but he did. Hence the term "Good Samaritan" (as opposed to the usual Bad Samaritan), for one who stops to aid a stranger, enemy or not.

The story illustrates that one needn't be an ethicist or a lawyer (*or a paramedic*) to help out on the road.

As part of a general fear of lawsuits, nurses and other practitioners express concern about stopping to aid at accidents. They say they fear the person aided will sue them. Such suits happen no more often than when nurses are at work (they are far less common). But the fear remains. Despite that, one writer says that nurses may have a moral (not legal) duty to act when faced with emergency situations, and that fear of legal recourse may be no excuse for failing to provide first-aid care.[21]

Many practitioners stop to help in emergency, regardless of the fear of lawsuits. (The fear voiced by some, might be an excuse for doing something the ordinary Samaritan doesn't want to do anyway.) And, in response to the fear of suit, state legislatures have modified the case law on malpractice in many states to insulate practitioners from extremely rare lawsuits by the rescued. Instead of being held to a standard of ordinary negligence like the rest of the public, the nurse or doctor *can* be ordinarily negligent in a volunteer emergency situation. But they still may be liable if grossly negligent.

If there is a state statute on Good Samaritan protection, the general rule is that nurses *will* be held liable for gross (great) negligence. Nurses will *not* be held liable if not at all negligent (as is usual), nor be held liable if ordinarily negligent. In the hospital, nurses who are negligent (not a reasonable and prudent nurse) lose the lawsuit. If they are similarly negligent at the side of the road, they won't lose the unlikely suit (because of the Good Samaritan statute protection).

Nurses should stop at accidents if they feel ethically bound to do so; they're very unlikely to be sued, and even more unlikely to lose the suit. Nurses should not stop at the accident if they don't want to. (There's no legal duty to stop, except in a handful of states in which laws mandate *anyone* to rescue persons in danger; these statutes—in Vermont, Minnesota, Wisconsin, Wyoming, and Quebec—run counter to centuries of legal tradition and are likely to be unenforceable). If nurses decide to stop, they can't rely on the Good Samaritan statute to totally immunize them from suit; they simply shouldn't do procedures they don't know how to do, and should rely on good nursing judgment and common sense as always. Good practice is good ethics is good law.

TORT REFORM

> Tort reform statutes, passed by state legislatures and contemplated by the Congress, seek to limit lawsuits and/or awards to plaintiffs by limiting access to the courts, limiting amounts of damages, changing methods of resolving conflict, limiting lawyers' fees, limiting availability/amount of punitive damages, and presuming no breach of the standard if guidelines are met.

In addition to passing Good Samaritan and duty-to-rescue laws, state legislatures for the last two decades have been writing tort reform statutes. (The federal government is also writing similar laws.) These laws are in response to what at various times are called "malpractice crises." Changes in the law include capping noneconomic damages available for pain and suffering, limiting attorney fees, and penalizing frivolous suits.

These changes are of interest to nurses, too; any changes in malpractice law for doctors always is applied to nurses as well. Nurses, however, have far less to worry about than doctors; the nurse lawsuits are far less frequent than suits against doctors.[22]

Many varieties of tort reform were tried in the 1970s (when malpractice insurance for doctors became very expensive). In some systems the patient-plaintiff had to submit the case to a panel of doctors and others before going to court. Some reforms put a cap on damages, especially noneconomic damages (pain and suffering). Many states have required various "proofs" of the legitimacy of a lawsuit for malpractice, before the court will allow the suit to be filed or go to trial.[23] (Some of those legislative solutions were found contrary to the U.S. or state constitutions, as limits on the citizen's right of access to the courts.)

The Seventh Amendment to the U.S. Constitution limits tort reforms:

In suits at common law where the value in controversy shall exceed twenty dollars, the right of trial by jury shall be preserved. . . .

State constitutions have such guarantees too; the text of the state constitution can usually be found in the front or back of the set of state statutes at the library.

Attorney Fee Reform

Some proposed reforms of tort law limit lawyer contingency fees (some lawyers charge 40 percent for cases that go to trial, and up to 50 percent for cases that are appealed, because of the expense of prosecuting such cases). Some doctors push for a maximum fee to the lawyer of 15 percent. But Rand Corporation studies in 1993 have found that restraints on lawyer fees don't reduce the number of suits filed.[24]

In 1987 Oregon repealed its 33 percent cap on contingency fees, when that state found the cap didn't make any difference in the numbers of suits. Studies have shown that shorter statutes of limitation and ceilings on damage for pain and suffering *do* reduce the number and size of awards.

The downside of such reforms is that it becomes hard for poor patients to get to court, say consumer advocates.

Reform Using Guidelines

Another reform: Maine tries to limit liability for doctors who use and adhere to guidelines. If practitioners follow the established guideline (checklist, protocol, critical pathway), then the injured plaintiff has to prove that the doctor unreasonably deviated from the guidelines, in order to win.

Maine is conducting a five-year experiment in reform through guidelines in four specialties: obstetrics/gynecology, radiology, emergency medicine, and anesthesiology. Over 80 percent of eligible doctors signed on to the program. Now, using the guidelines, 50 percent of patients suffering falls and car wrecks get neck x-ray—compared to 95 percent receiving such tests before.

But obstetrics/gynecology doctors all now do an extra test before hysterectomy for bleeding. Further, there are 11 requirements for transferring patients, mirroring the federal regulations that prohibit "dumping" of patients. The doctor completes the list and attaches it to the patient's chart. In legal terms, completing the list creates a rebuttable presumption that the care was correct. The plaintiff can introduce evidence to rebut (refute) that presumption—such as showing that procedures were charted but not done. The law says that the guidelines can't be used as a sword against the practitioner (that the plaintiff can't show *non*compliance with guidelines as evidence for negligence). Theoretically that prohibits *failure* to follow the guidelines being used as evidence of negligence.

Lawyers who defend practitioners warn that such lists may do more harm than good to them. Such lists make it hard to explain to juries why the practitioner deviated from the list.

Other states watch to see the outcome of Maine's attempt: Several considering guidelines as part of reform plans. If Maine's plan works, other states (and possibly the federal government) might adopt it as well.

Malpractice insurance rates won't go down until test cases of the reform laws are made, years in the future, so that insurers can see if doctors are indeed protected by the guidelines. The rate of cesarean sections—an indicator of defensive medicine to some—continues to rise. Checklists require extra tests that some doctors do not do in all cases.[25]

OUTCOME OF USING CHECKLISTS TO AVOID LAWSUIT

The bottom line: Dr. Christopher Clark, Emergency Room doctor, says, "I feel better that the parameters are there . . . I feel safer."
Could that be the real outcome desired, that doctors "feel safer"?

Enterprise Liability

One proposed reform of malpractice law would be to substitute for personal responsibility of the doctor and nurse, responsibility of the agency, known as *enterprise liability*. This exists to a degree in the Veterans Administration system, and under corporate negligence doctrines.

Some believe making the institution liable, as in enterprise liability reform, would cause the institution to find its own errors and correct them, such errors being seen as largely preventable.

Very important to consider—when evaluating enterprise liability reform in which individuals sue large institutions instead of doctors and nurses—is the public's attitude toward different types of defendants. "In a dispute between an individual and a large corporation, the individual's version is more likely to be believable" (70 percent). Further, "to a big company, being forced to pay $1 million in a legal dispute is just a slap on the hand" (60 percent).[26] Such a concept when applied to the reform of malpractice law, is a substitute for personal responsibility (in which the doctor and nurse *are* liable for their actions). Such reform creates a new enterprise liability, in which the "enterprise," the hospital or other employer, is liable for any negligence. The enterprise is already vicariously liable for the acts of its employees under the theory of *respondeat superior*, and also individually liable under the theories of negligent hiring, supervision, admission to staff, and others.[27]

The difference in this new approach would relieve the professionals, nurse and doctor, from liability and put all risk on the employer.

The wish is that doctors would stop wasting money by ordering tests and treatments as defenses to potential lawsuits. But some studies indicate that this "defensive medicine" factor represents only a tiny contribution to the cost of illness care, and that physicians mainly use the specter of lawsuits to justify the ordering of tests and procedures, which they would order anyway. (It's asserted that they learned to practice medicine the "defensive" way and that the real inflation in costs is caused by the belief of doctor and patient alike that the care is "free," since the costs are paid for with money from the taxpayers or premium-payers.)

Existing Enterprise Liability

Enterprise liability—at least liability for the institution, in addition to the doctor or nurse—is already an informal reality, because of market trends and court rulings. The liability will fall on whomever has the ultimate authority and accountability for the delivery of care. Since HMOs control more of the market and employ more doctors than ever before, HMOs are more often sued.

More than half of 640,000 doctors in United States have affiliated with HMOs. About 11 percent formally employ the doctors. In these situations, there is automatic vicarious liability for the employee's act (although the employee is still liable, too) under the theory of *respondeat superior*. If the doctor is affiliated with the HMO by independent contract, the contract probably says that the HMO furnishes malpractice insurance or pays legal costs and damages. Nurse practitioners are in this situation even more often, since fewer NPs are solo practitioners.

At least two dozen state court decisions have found the insurance plan and hospital liable, even if the practitioner is not their employee, nor their independent contractor. The HMO is responsible for negligence when patients believe its doctors act as agents (ostensible agency), and the HMO so advertises.

The courts will let the practitioner have liability for personal actions as well. In one case, the doctor who was designated "on call" for a Humana prepaid plan, and who was consulted by the emergency room doctor, was found to have potential liability. The court said the case could go forward to trial; there was no automatic lack of duty and there was potentially a doctor-patient relationship, despite the fact that the defendant doctor never saw nor spoke to the patient.[28]

The courts say that HMOs must be held to high standards because, if the HMO is not held liable, it would be able to cut costs by buying cheap (less competent) practitioners. California courts have held the insurer liable, demonstrating that, increasingly, the insurer is the HMO and vice versa. The insurer's decision not to pay for earlier treatment was found to have caused injury.

Practitioners are still named as codefendants in these cases, a difference from a formal enterprise liability program. But the employer/institution has more money and will always be sought or held responsible. It is harder for such defendants to win even when justified; patients will not refrain from suing an agency. Patients have no feeling of restraint, which they might have against the practitioner, and juries see deep pockets.[29]

Enterprise liability would further increase supervision and intervention into practitioner practice by HMOs—one reason some practitioners oppose any enterprise liability plan.

Although some practitioners might welcome any proposal that exculpates them from liability, there remains an ethical problem: To relieve professionals from responsibility for their actions strikes at the very heart of "professionalism." Nurses who would be autonomous must be responsible. If they want authority, they must also have the duty. To remove their responsibility for their actions would itself produce harm. It would destroy the assumption that the doctor or nurse is an adult professional responsible for her actions.

> "We must never make our professions immune to suit for damages we cause by our negligent acts for two reasons. If we cause harm we must pay, and the fear of a suit serves as a deterrent to negligence and causes us to strive toward at least the standard of the reasonable nurse under the circumstances."[30]

Demystifying Lawsuits

MYTHS DEMYSTIFIED

Lawsuits are usually won by *defendants*; poor people are *less* likely to sue for malpractice; frivolous suits are *usually* dismissed; and median awards are *much lower* than the highest would indicate.

A Silly Suit? A Texas lawsuit was filed (everyone's right), dismissed by the judge, appealed by the plaintiff (again, a right). The plaintiff's contention was that injuries caused by an elderly bad driver were the responsibility of General Motors: General Motors should have warned the driver, or instructed the dealer, about dangers presented by elderly, impaired drivers.[31] The dismissal was upheld by the appellate court.

Despite the publicity they get, silly suits are usually dismissed by the court. Plaintiffs don't always win; in fact, they *usually* don't. Of all malpractice suits filed in North Carolina from 1984 to 1987 (1,195 cases in all), only 117 cases actually went to trial. All others were settled. In almost 500 cases, the plaintiff got nothing. The median award—the point at which half the awards were above and half below (not the average, which gets skewed upwards by the big awards)—was $36,500. This study showed 15 claims filed per year for every 100 doctors (a small percentage of claims go to trial, a fraction of those get awards, and a very few get big money).[32]

Contrary to practitioner belief, one study shows that poor people injured by malpractice are only 10 percent as likely to sue as wealthier people with similar injuries. ("Poor" was defined in the study as having a household income below $10,610 using 1984 data.) Earlier studies showed that the poor were more likely than the non-poor to be injured by medical negligence, and the poor do file other kinds of personal injury suits more often than the non-poor. But they often have trouble finding lawyers willing to represent them on medical malpractice, because such cases are so expensive to litigate.[33]

Unjustified payments to injured patients, whether by settlement or jury verdict, are said to be uncommon. Data reported show that the severity of patient injury has little bearing on whether a physician loses a case (something defense lawyers dispute).[34] The amount of payment does correlate with the severity of injury, whether through settlement or jury verdict. Physicians usually win cases in which care is deemed to meet community standards. Defense lawyers say that small numbers of wins for plaintiffs in jury cases don't help reduce the fears of doctors, nor their practice of defensive medicine. They say the jury awards set the pattern for settlements and fault the system for the time required to get a settlement of the suit (as long as five years). Justice delayed is justice denied, for plaintiff or defendant.

Less than 25 percent of the money spent for malpractice insurance premiums actually goes to patients, argue the defense lawyers. They believe, along with some plaintiff lawyers, that insurance money is not a contractual bet, which one party or the other wins (the reality). They obviously consider the insurance to be an escrow account, held for the benefit of people the doctors injure.

Malpractice plaintiffs succeed 20 to 43 percent of the time, depending on geographic area of the country. Other kinds of plaintiffs succeed 50 to 64 percent of the time, depending on location. Awards average $58,000 to

$255,000 per lawsuit, also depending on area of the country.[35] (This amount is an average, combining very large amounts with very small. The median award—half the awards higher and half lower—would be less.)

Problems with the Malpractice System

Suits for malpractice are considered unsatisfactory for addressing the problems; it is estimated only one in ten of the people injured by malpractice sue, and some people who sue (estimated as one-third of them) are not injured.

Alternative Dispute Resolution (ADR) has been tried with some success as a substitute for malpractice suits; ADR includes mediation, in which parties voluntarily try to settle with a helper (outcome not binding), and arbitration, in which parties agree to binding decision by judge-like decider.

It is said that malpractice suits don't deter accidents. Researchers found that only eight of 280 patients who experienced adverse events caused by care, filed malpractice claims. Malpractice suits don't compensate for most injuries, because most malpractice is never sued on. It has been asserted that fewer than ten percent of people who are negligently injured sue. But of people who did sue, one-third were not actually injured (according to the researchers' assessment). At most, one in ten of the people injured by malpractice are compensated, but some people who sue and are compensated actually were not injured.[36]

Is there a better way?

Alternative Dispute Resolution

Punishing malpractice—thus enforcing the duty of beneficence owed to the patient—is done under law by malpractice suits against nurses and doctors and agencies. Alternatives to that system of punishment have been proposed and used with limited success; these are grouped generally under the heading of Alternative Dispute Resolution (ADR). The ADR process is either through arbitration or mediation, in which groups provide either decision makers (arbitrators) or facilitators (mediators), from outside the court system.

In *mediation*, the parties have a mediator or go-between who helps them compromise among themselves without going to court. In *arbitration*, the parties submit their arguments to an arbitrator, who functions much like a judge to make a decision for the parties—but without the cost, time, and formalities of the legal system. Some research indicates, however, that the cost of arbitration to the defendant is not lower than going to court.

The arbitration panels are not easier on doctors and nurses than courts are. A 1980 study showed that panels found for the plaintiff 36 percent of the time, about the same as court cases that went to trial or were settled. The settlements in arbitration were higher. A 1992 study[37] found that panels found for the plaintiff even more often, 52 percent of the time, as compared to a malpractice suit finding for the plaintiff only 33 percent of the time.

Almost 90 percent of cases were settled prior to a hearing in both systems. Arbitration is faster, with hearing time two to four days, while a malpractice trial could last several weeks (but *rarely* does). And in arbitration, time from filing to resolution of the claim averages 19 months, compared with 33 months for a lawsuit.

Arbitration is sometimes agreed to in the patient's HMO contract. The issue there is whether the patient's agreement to arbitrate is freely chosen, since the patient cannot join the HMO in some cases without agreeing to arbitrate malpractice instead of suing. This is the same issue faced by buyers of stock: The contract with the broker may provide that any dispute must be resolved by arbitration.

As well as being used in health care conflicts, arbitration can be used in other kinds of disputes, such as divorce and child custody cases.

Another alternative to using malpractice law to enforce the minimum of the value, Doing Good, would be to use contracts between patients and practitioners; this is the mechanism that HMOs use to get patients to agree to arbitration. Patients could even write contracts with physicians guaranteeing certain standards of care; violation of the contract to be remedied under the law of contract, not the law of negligence. This would have the advantage of specifying what care was acceptable and what was not.

Suggested reforms of the malpractice system include processes for resolving malpractice suits out of court, first in mediation panels; if that fails, then the patient can sue. But mediation panels have already tried and failed in over 30 states. The costs are not decreased but increased, along with delays in trials, so six states have repealed those reforms. Mediation panels are still used in 25 states.[38]

The AMA advocates a system of "malpractice hearing officers" who would give decisions on patient claims, which would not have to allege malpractice. Their decisions would be appealable to an administrative board—like worker's compensation claims. They assert that more patients would receive compensation.

Avoiding Lawsuits

The most common areas for malpractice suits overall are medication errors, poor history or nursing assessment, poor physical exam, failure to consult a specialist or the doctor when appropriate, faulty diagnosis, anesthesia problems, failure to provide any care, complications of cesarean sections, and manual delivery of infants—all, in some way, are failures to maintain a minimum standard of practice. All demonstrate the thesis: Good practice is good ethics is good law.

From 1985 to 1991, according to Walsh, the ten most common reasons for malpractice suits were as listed above. (Note especially the last two: The obstetrician can't win by adopting an "all-cesarean" *nor* an "all-vaginal" policy.) All of the ten are in some way failures to maintain a standard of practice. There can there be no better demonstration of this book's thesis: Good practice is good ethics is good law.

Commonly, lawsuits that arise in the operating suite are for retained sponges and surgical instruments. Techniques to avoid these problems include computerized counts and standardization of sets of instruments. Such cases rarely go to trial; liability is practically automatic, so they are difficult to defend. The nurse counts, so she's liable, her employer is liable, and the doctor, too, if she participated in or signed off on the count, or just because she's there.

In general, if fewer than ten percent of injured patients actually sue, lawsuits are not prompted merely by committing malpractice. Nurses can create a climate that can lead to a lawsuit if the patient has any reason to suspect malpractice; nurses may make the patient want to sue by performing or mis-performing, as listed below (adapted from Walsh).[39]

THE NURSE WHO WANTS TO INSPIRE MALPRACTICE SUITS

Is not personable and informal and friendly. Reads the chart and does only the work—doesn't smile at patients.

Acts uninterested, doesn't make eye contact.

Uses superior body language. Never sits down by a patient; towers over when possible.

Doesn't listen; interrupts.

Doesn't encourage patient talking; asks only for yes or no responses.

Makes a mistake(?). Covers it up.

Doesn't explain anything to patients; when necessary, uses jargon.

Disregards any specific interest in treatment. If pressed, becomes hostile.

Dis-respects the patient; calls the patient by first name always; makes derogatory entries in the chart.

Doesn't treat the patient as an individual; treats all alike—or better, as a body part (the gallbladder in Room 220).

Following are suggestions to prevent lawsuit—in addition to the obvious good practice mandate:

Establish rapport.

Don't get mad.

Don't argue in front of the patient.

Get consent (assumes *informed*).

Document (see below).

Don't promise/guarantee results.

Don't chart to "get" people.

The commonest nurse malpractice suits: Medication and treatment errors, lack of observation and timely report on the patient, defective technology or equipment, infections caused or worsened by poor nursing care, poor communication of important information, failure to intervene to protect the patient from poor medical care—all are legal problems that can be avoided by practicing average nursing and adhering to minimum ethics.

The best way to win a lawsuit is never to be sued. The most likely examples of negligence in nurse lawsuits:

1. Medication and treatment errors. The five "rights" work: right patient, right medication, right dosage, right route of administration, right time.
2. Lack of observation and timely reporting on the patient.
3. Defective technology or equipment. This *is* the nurse's fault, too, if it's not reported and such equipment is kept in use.
4. Infections caused or worsened by poor nursing care. Infections are usually the result of poor nursing technique; and the most important basic nursing technique is frequent handwashing.
5. Poor communication of important information.
6. Failure to intervene to protect the patient from poor medical care.

Lawsuits that arise from negligence can be avoided by merely *average* practice; nurses know better than to do *bad* practice.

Nurses learn everything they need to know about avoiding malpractice in nursing school.

Give medications to the right patient—the right med, right dose, right time, right route. Observe and report on patients as taught in nursing school. Don't use equipment that is working incorrectly; use it according to its instruction manual. Don't use equipment if it appears defective in any way. Use sterile technique on wounds; move patients away from other infected patients, turn cough and deep-breath patients after surgery, and *wash hands* as taught.

Communicate about the patient to the person who needs the information and who can help the patient—also learned in nursing school (and just common sense).

Nurses should not carry out orders that are not understand, or that they believe will be bad for the patient. Disagreement about choice of antibiotic is not a reason to decline an order, but serious, real danger to the patient is. Don't give known overdoses of medication, even if the doctor repeats the order and insists; if given, of course, the doctor will be liable *and so will the nurse*. Don't keep reporting and documenting that the patient is going downhill, while accepting ineffectual orders and "just watching the patient." The nurse has a moral responsibility as both a human and a nurse to do good, not to harm the patient. This is so, regardless of who has ordered what. If nurses don't adhere to a minimum moral responsibility, the law may impose on them a legal responsibility.

MANAGING LAWSUITS

If sued, one expert has this advice:

Contact the insurance company immediately—the nurse's own and/or the employer's.

2. Realize that the nurse personally, not the insurance company or their attorney, is being sued.

Don't call the opposing attorney, who may be a wonderful person, but not the nurse's friend in this case.

Check out the assigned attorney. All attorneys are not born equal.

Start a file.

Get copies of all records to the attorney.

Teach the attorney medicine and nursing.

Research the literature personally.

Suggest expert witnesses.

Read depositions and comment on them to the attorney.

See number 2, above, again.

Prepare for deposition (this will make or break the case—remember that 90%+ are settled before trial).

Provide questions to the attorney, to ask of the opposing expert.

See number 2 again.

Ask about a settlement (in some cases it's not in the defense attorney's interest to expedite the process—more hours worked, more fee).

Prepare for trial, if that's a reality.

Sit through the whole trial—let the jury know someone cares.[40]

If that's the nurse's job—or, if the nurse wants to work in risk management—there are specialty journals dedicated to preventing malpractice, such as *Medical Malpractice Prevention*,[41] and they should be consulted.

Witnessing in Court

Advice on testifying as a defendant or witness: Talk to the lawyer, practice Q&A, tell the truth, read all statements, understand the questions, think before answering (say "I don't know" if you don't), don't accept the other lawyer's statement as fact, don't argue, don't volunteer anything, look at the judge and jury, be courteous, be cooperative, take time, correct mistakes, don't guess, don't assume, don't chew gum or candy, don't smoke during deposition, dress neatly and conservatively, in a blue suit.[42]

Testifying as a witness is a happier time to be in court than is testifying as a defendant in a malpractice case (or as a plaintiff). The nurse might be a plaintiff if injured by malpractice, or if the nurse sues an employer in a job-related suit. Or the nurse might be hired as an expert by the plaintiff or defendant, or may be required to testify to facts known about the case or the patient (fact witness).

In general, spend a lot of time with the lawyer, going over what will be asked by lawyers on both sides. Practice. If asked on the stand whether testimony was discussed with the lawyer, the answer is of course yes—it's the truth and it's expected that witnesses will discuss testimony before testifying.

The most important rule: Tell the Truth. The nurse who is found lying has done worse than if not testifying, and might go to jail for perjury.

Look over all documents and statements made or signed, especially if questions were answered earlier in a deposition.

The witness should be sure to understand a question; if not, the witness can ask to have the question repeated. If the question is still not understood, say so. It's not a test; it's the attorney's job to make the question clear. Nurses are not required to know everything. Think before answering; if not sure of the answer, say, "I'm not sure" or "I don't know" or "I don't remember"—whatever is the truth. It is better to look uncertain or even dumb, rather than to give an untruthful answer.

Don't accept the other lawyer's statement as fact just because it is stated. Don't try to figure out the lawyer's strategy. Don't argue. Don't worry if the opposing lawyer harasses you—the jury or judge will be more sympathetic to you.

Every question is important; think carefully before each answer. *Don't volunteer anything*. The nurse's lawyer will bring out what should be said that may have been left out, on cross-examination. Look at the jury (if it's a judge-tried case, look at the judge). The nurse, not the attorney, is the person on trial (or being judged as a witness). The jury will judge the nurse, not the attorney.

Be courteous, be cooperative; take time; correct mistakes as soon as realized. Testify to what is known from personal knowledge about the situation, not to what has been heard from someone else about it. Give reasonable estimates about data, if they can be made, but realize that guessing is not required. If assumptions are made in the question and in the answer, state them aloud; for example, "Yes, the nurse should have answered the patient's signal *if she saw the light*."

Don't chew gum or candy. Don't smoke during a deposition. Dress neatly and conservatively. Blue suits are always safe.[43]

Documentation

> Documentation is (1) required by law (state licensure statutes and malpractice standards), (2) necessary for reimbursement and accreditation, and (3) needed for the continuity of care of the patient.
>
> It is not true to say "not documented, not done," but a lack of documentation may create a *presumption* that the care was not done.
>
> Lists of "do's and don'ts" of documenting are all based on the standard for documentation: an accurate record of the patient's condition and care.
>
> New kinds of documentation (for example, computerized, voice-activated, negative-only, flow sheet) will all be accepted as "legal" if they meet the standard of an accurate record of condition and care.

Documentation is discussed under Doing Good since it is often the issue in malpractice, and "lawsuit" is the reason often given for documenting. Documentation is more than that, however: (1) it is required by law (state licensure statutes and malpractice standards),[44] (2) it is necessary for reimbursement and accreditation, and (3) it is needed for the continuity of care of the patient.

> *The standard for documentation:* The record should correctly inform about the patient's condition and care.

Licensure Law Requires Documentation

Documentation is enforced in licensure statutes and regulations, as well as by malpractice law. For example, the Texas Administrative Code—regulations made by the Board of Nursing—in defining unprofessional or dishonorable conduct, includes:

> 5) failing to make entries, destroying entries, and/or making false entries in records pertaining to care of clients.[45]

Can nurses buy malpractice insurance and forget documentation? No. Insurance companies go out of business, and in many states a malpractice case will be reported to the nurse licensure agency. If the malpractice suit alleges action that is also a grounds for licensure loss, the nurse may be disciplined by a board of nursing regardless of what happens in the malpractice suit. Some state licensure regulations for nurses specifically mention observation and documentation as standards nurses must meet, or face loss of licensure (see above). Those regulations are also used by plaintiffs to establish a standard of care in an attempt to prove that the nurse breached the standard.

Malpractice Law Requires Documentation

Malpractice (case law) enforces the duty to document. Underlying the duty to document is the professional duty to do good for the patient. Good documentation is good nursing practice; the law does not create a new or different obligation, but merely enforces that fundamental responsibility. Malpractice cases often hinge on documentation.

To some, the most important purpose of documentation of good care is that written evidence is a great aid to spoken testimony in court. The maxim, "if it wasn't charted it wasn't done," is not strictly true; but a nurse who testifies that the side rails were up when she left the room, and who also has charted it, is in a better position than if it weren't documented.

A juror assumes that the testifying nurse is tempted to remember the most favorable version of events; it's human nature. If the nurse's version is charted, too, the jury will assume that the nurse had no reason to lie in the chart since the chart note was made prior to the lawsuit (and prior to the incident/accident).

LACK OF DOCUMENTATION
EQUATED WITH LACK OF CARE

Example: No observation was charted for seven hours, of the toes of a patient whose leg was casted. The first note after seven hours was that the toes were noted to be "dusky and cold"—this allowed a jury to conclude that failure to document indicated failure to observe, which breach of the standard of nursing care led to liability for amputation.[46]

Vital signs were ordered hourly on a post-operative patient—they were not recorded hourly. Instead, they were recorded every six hours. The patient's temperature rose in one period from 101.4° to 105.2° with resulting brain damage. The failure of the record resulted in a judgment that reasonable post-op care was not given.[47]

Worse for the nurse who documents poorly is that some cases draw the inference that poor record keeping is itself an indicator of poor nursing care. (Some nurse-experts for the patient-plaintiff have so testified; whether true or not, that's the expert testimony, and that's the inference.) The reasoning is that, if notes are sloppy, probably so is the care. Nurse-expert witnesses for the patient-plaintiff may use poorly kept nurse's notes as support for a conclusion that the patient is poorly monitored by nursing staff.[48]

The common saying, "not documented, not done," is *not* true; nurses can testify as to what was done.[49] But lack of documentation may create a *presumption* that the care was not done. A blank flow sheet in a chart for a whole shift, or a shift without any notations about the patient's condition, looks as though the patient got no assessment or care. The presumption can be overcome, but overcoming it will require testimony. The nurse who does not document appropriately must be able to remember and to testify to what she did this morning—even five years from now.

Document for Continuity of Care

The number one reason to document is the number one reason nurses do all practice: for the good of the patient. Continuity of care is an essential part of good practice. Good care demands that the next shift, the next nurse, the next doctor know what has gone on before, with the patient.

Document for Reimbursement and Accreditation

Documentation has other purposes, too. The first is reimbursement by a third-party payor, so that the agency and then the nurse will get paid. Only the patient knows that the nurse did the work, unless it's documented. When patients pay for care directly (and if they do again in future), the patient will base payment on direct knowledge and not on documentation; but indirect pay for care requires documentation now.

Another purpose of documentation is the accreditation and/or licensure of the agency, to prove the nurse is doing the good work described in policies.

Do's and Don'ts Commonly Noted

DO DOCUMENT . . .

Legibly—"legibly" means so that other people can read it. The patient-plaintiff's nurse-expert who, examining the record in the suit, can't read the handwriting, may advise filing suit because she can't tell whether the nurse was negligent or not.

In ink—usually in black.

Date with every page and time with every new entry.

Every blank—draw a line in those not used.

Corrections to errors with a single line, signing initials and date and time.

With signature after all entries, lining through empty spaces.

Using standard abbreviations.

Without defaming anyone—patient, doctor, another nurse.

Efforts to protect the patient.

Responses to intervention.

The patient's symptoms in the patient's own words, with nurse observations.

What has been done—not what *didn't* get done.

The nurse's own personal notes, but NOT in the chart if the information is not pertinent to the patient's condition or care.

The nurse's own narrative of any worrisome event, signing and dating it, to be used in court later if needed. The legal terms are Present Recollection Refreshed, or Prior Recollection Recorded; the notes are not in the chart, but in the nurse's own files at home.

Late entries, as needed, but dated and timed at the time actually written.

DON'T . . .

Retaliate in the chart.

Destroy and rewrite, or erase, white out, or write a late entry dating it as though it were made earlier.

Add to a printed document unless the patient initials next to the addition.

Add *anything* after the patient signs. If needed write a new document and get another signature.

New kinds of documentation are being developed. Computerized, voice-activated, negative-only, flow sheet, and other kinds of charting will all be accepted as "legal" if they meet the standard as an accurate record of the patient's condition and care given. Some experts recommend using the SOAPIE method (Subjective Objective Assessment Plan Intervention Evaluation) of assessment and planning; any accurate, consistently used method will work, however. Straight time documentation, flow sheets, checklists, and computerized records are all acceptable.

Computer documentation carries its own hazards: For example, an error entered in some fields will be carried forward forever, automatically. Some systems will document everything—which may carry a hazard to the practitioner too: Surgery computers will read out and document the patient's vital signs every 15 seconds, together with medications given (click the mouse on the drug and dose). The nurse who is poor at computer technology may inadvertently create a record she will have to disavow in testimony.

Regardless of form, all documentation has in common the following rules:

1. Document only what is personally known.
2. Sign only what one is responsible for.
3. Make the record as clear as possible.
4. *Never, ever destroy a record, and substitute a new one.*
5. Sign each entry. Late entries are a good idea if needed.
6. Clearly document changes in orders.
7. Precisely document phone orders.
8. Don't use the chart just to "get" other people.

Document only what is personally known. Never assume that something has been done.

Sign only to things the nurse is responsible for. If asked to sign on an LPN's or helper's records, the nurse should make sure they sign first. Additionally, the nurse should document the reason for her own signature before signing, to clarify that the entry is *not* a record of her own observations and work (for example, that the nurse has reviewed the chart or assessed the patient or whatever the reason for signing).

Make the record as clear as possible. Be sure there's a date on every page. Don't skip lines. Line out errors, and write "error" above; don't white out, erase, or mark out so that what is underneath can't be read; people reviewing such an entry may suspect someone is trying to hide something.

NEVER destroy a record and substitute a new one. The malpractice case will be lost before it goes to trial. The defense lawyer would rather settle for maximum money than face a jury sure that some evil was hidden. An altered medical record may mean automatic liability for whatever happened to the patient. ("Altered" does not include correcting errors by lining one line through, writing "error" with initials, date, and time.) A real alteration (white-out, rewriting, destroying) immediately establishes a suspicion of a cover-up, fraud, lies, . . . evil. Here the value of telling the truth (detailed in Chapter Six) is enforced by the laws against perjury. Short of that crime, the jury in a malpractice case sometimes will exact its own "legal punishment."

PUNISHMENT FOR ASSUMED COVER-UP

Examples: Expert testimony was that the record of temperature, before a seven-year-old's minor surgery, showed correction and erasure; the original notation could not be read.

The child arrested in surgery with severe brain damage. The jury decided the operation should have been postponed and returned a $4 million verdict. They assumed (even if wrongly) that the record had been changed to protect someone.[50]

One nurse had used liquid paper to cover an error. So suspicious or interested were the parties that x-rays were done to see what was underneath.[51]

Juries who hear that nurses have changed a part of the record will believe that the records may be erroneous in other respects; they will fail to trust any of the records, and the nurses' testimony. The reasoning: the nurse who will "lie" in the record will probably lie on the witness stand.

Sign each entry, since someone else may make another entry before the end of shift. Late entries are a good idea, if needed; but, note the current time they are made, and clarify that the note is about an earlier event (enter the time of the earlier event).

Document clearly all changes in orders—calls to doctors and supervisors, patient's change in condition, efforts to clarify orders and to alert regarding changes in condition.

Document phone orders precisely. Spoken phone orders should be repeated. Do not accept relayed orders unless the situation is an emergency (in which case, act according to protocol or policy); there is usually time to get a direct order, or for the relayor to carry out the order himself.

Don't use the chart just to "get" the doctor, another shift, another nurse, or the patient. Any trouble for them will "get" the nurse, too. The chart is not the place for working out working conditions. Revenge charting does nothing for the patient, looks bad in lawsuits, and does nothing to solve the problem that the nurse is having with someone.

Incident Reports

Incident reports are made to help analyze problems and solve them, so that errors are not repeated. They may or may not be discoverable in a lawsuit, depending on the state's law at any given time.

Nurses should keep work sheets made during the shift, recording patient condition and assignments, as an aid to memory or even evidence of an incident in a future lawsuit or licensure action.

If an incident seems likely to result in legal action, the nurse should make a detailed personal record of the situation, and sign and date it; it will aid memory and might be used as evidence.

The purpose of incident reports is to analyze problems and solve them so that the same thing or worse doesn't happen again. The filing of an incident report needn't be mentioned in the chart (it's not related to the patient's condition). The plaintiff's attorney may assume there was an incident report and seek to "discover" it (get a copy to look at). The incident report may be considered a self-serving document, made by a "defensive" practioner, and the defense may not be allowed to introduce it into evidence at trial.

Some states protect these reports as part of the attorney-client privilege since they may be communicated directly to the agency attorney. (A "privilege" means the communication can be kept confidential.) A doctor-patient privilege means the patient can keep that communication confidential; the doctor can't testify to the privileged statement. Nurse-patient privilege is rarely written into state statutes. Even in a state with such a privilege, there are so many exceptions to this rule that it is better to assume that any communication to anyone—*except* an attorney in the context of a court case—can be obtained (discovered) for a lawsuit. There will be no privilege for confidential communication in a criminal trial, nor in a lawsuit for malpractice brought by a patient.

Nurse Notes Not in the Chart

Nurses should keep the work sheets they use to get report on the patient's condition, whatever notes were made to report to the nurse following, and notes used to make assignments (this information is possibly all on the same sheet). Much information not in the patient's chart is in the notes. Examples are what the nurse was told about the patient (and what was not mentioned), what notes the nurse made, concurrent with care and assessment, and the context in which the care was given. Such information—how many patients the nurse was assigned, how many and which patients the helpers were assigned, which patients were in which room—may not be in the chart, but it will be available in the work notes.

Whether as defendant or witness, the nurse in a malpractice case may perhaps not testify until years after the occurrence; any information kept will help preserve the memory of what happened. Such documents may be admissible in court as past recollection recorded or as present recollection refreshed.[52]

If the nurse is involved in a troubling incident or one that seems likely to produce litigation, the nurse should also write one more thing: In addition to reporting and recommending needed changes, charting in the patient record, and doing incident report documentation for risk management, the nurse should also make a detailed personal record about the incident, and sign and date it. This record, too, can be used as past recollection recorded, if the nurse can't remember the information, even after reviewing the notes. The nurse who can remember the information after reviewing such a personal record, may testify to it as present recollection refreshed (the opposing lawyer in such an instance will be allowed to see the notes so used).

ENDNOTES

1. Emanuel, E.J., and Emanuel, L.L., "Four models of the physician–patient relationship," *Journal of the American Medical Association*, 1992; 267(16):2221–2226.
2. Amundson, R., "Liability in the physician in classical Greek legal theory and practice, *Journal of the History of Medicine*, 1977; 32:172–203.
   Harrison, L., "The development of the principles of medical malpractice in the United States," *Perspectives in Biology and Medicine*, 1985; 29(1):41–72.
3. *Ibid.*
4. *Ritchey v. West*, 23 Ill. 329 [Orig. 385] (1860).
5. Popp, P.W., "Experts in malpractice litigation—What about nurses?" *Legal Medicine*, 1992:165–178.
6. See, for example, Audet, A.-M., *et al.*, "Medical practice guidelines: Current activities and future directions," *Annals of Internal Medicine*, 1990; 113:709–714.
7. Lumsdon, K., and Hagland, M., "Mapping care," *Hospitals and Health Networks*, 20 October 1993, pp. 34–40.
8. Murphy, S., "Legal issues for nurses: IV conscious sedation," *Texas Nursing*, January 1993, pp. 8–15.
9. 1991 Joint Commission, *Accreditation Manual for Hospitals: Vol. 1. Standards*, Oakbrook Terrace, IL: The Commission, 1990.

10. Woolfe, S.H., "Practice guidelines: A new reality in medicine: III. Impact on patient care," *Archives of Internal Medicine*, 1993; 153:2646–2655.
11. *Thompson v. Nason Hosp.*, 527 Pa, 388, 591 A2d 783 (Pa. 1991), citing *The Poor Sisters of St. Francis Search of the Perpetual Adoration, Inc. v. Sharon Catron*, 435 NE2d 305 (Ind. Ct. App. 1982).
12. "Headlines," *American Journal of Nursing*, 1993; 93(12):9.
13. See, *e.g.*, Fiesta, J., "Legal update for nurses—1992, Part I," *Nursing Management*, 1993; 24(1):16–17.
    Fiesta, J., "Legal aspects—Standards of care: Part II," *Nursing Management*, 1993; 24(8):16–17; and "Legal update for nurses—1992: Part III," *Nursing Management*, 1993; 24(3):16–17.
14. Doerhoff, D.C., "Supreme court adopts 'but for' causation rule," *Journal of the Missouri Bar*, January–February 1994, p. 5.
15. Lippman, H., "Malpractice protection—How much is enough?" *RN*, May 1993, pp. 61–67.
16. Kolodner, D.E., "Are you considering professional liability insurance?" *MEDSURG Nursing*, 1993; 2(3):213–214.
17. Hall, J.K., "Malpractice insurance and case law," *Nursing Outlook*, May/June 1990, p. 119.
18. Marks, A.R., "Where is the *real* conflict of interest," *American Bar Association Journal*, February 1993, p. 112.
19. *Pacific Mutual Life Insurance Co. v. Haslip*, 59 U.S. 4157 (1991).
20. Personal conversation with Endocrinologist Harold V. Werner, M.D., regarding the Diabetes Control and Complications Trial.
21. Castledine, G., "Ethical implications of first aid," *British Journal of Nursing*, 1993; 2(4):239–241.
22. Birkholz, G., "Malpractice data from the National Practitioner Data Bank," *Nurse Practitioner*, 1995; 20(3):32–35.
23. For example: Grant, J.A., "Florida's presuit requirements for medical malpractice actions," *Florida Bar Journal*, February 1994, pp. 12–19.
24. Danzon, P., head economist, Wharton School, *Wall Street Journal*, 12 October 1993, B8.
25. Felsenthal, E., "Cookbook Care: Maine Limits Liability for Doctors Who Meet Treatment Guidelines," *Wall Street Journal*, 3 May 1993, A1,A9.
26. Metricus National Juror Opinion Survey, Rupert Howard.
27. Crane, M., "The malpractice reform idea that won't go away," *Medical Economics*, 1993; 70(14):27–34.
28. *Hand v. Tavera*, 864 SW2d 678 (Tex. App. San Ant. 1993).
29. "Medical Plans Take on Greater Liability," *Wall Street Journal*, 18 October 1993.
30. Cazalas, M.W., *Nursing and the Law*, Germantown, MD: Aspen, 1978, p. viii.
31. *Salinas v. General Motors Corp.*, 857 SW2d 944 (Tex. App. Houston, 1993).
32. Kilpatrick, J., "Plaintiffs Don't Always Win," *Amarillo Globe*, 31 January 1993.
33. Burstin, H.R., *et al.*, "Do the poor sue more? A case control study of malpractice claims and socioeconomic status," *Journal of the American Medical Association*, 1993; 270(14):1697–1701.
34. Hirsch, B., "Flawed malpractice study finds unjustified payments are uncommon," *Texas Medicine*, 1993; 89(6):50–51.
35. *Ibid*.
36. Localio, A.R., Lawthers, A.G., and Brennan, T.A., "Relation between malpractice claims and adverse events due to negligence," *New England Journal of Medicine*, 1991; 325(4):245–251.
37. U.S. General Accounting Office, *Medical Malpractice—Alternative to Litigation*, Washington, DC: 1992.
    Felsenthal, E., "What Happens When Patients Arbitrate Rather Than Litigate," *Wall Street Journal*, 4 February 1994; B1,B11.
38. Felsenthal, E., "Clinton's plan for malpractice has failed tests," *Wall Street Journal*, 1 August 1993; B1,B4.
39. Walsh, L., "Communication Averts Malpractice Suits, Doctors Told," *Arkansas Democrat Gazette*, Little Rock, 13 January 1993, 6B.
40. Materials for conference by Kip Poe, Office of General Counsel, Texas Tech University Health Sciences Center, Lubbock, Texas, 23 January 1993.

41. *Medical Malpractice Prevention*, published monthly by World Medical Communications Organization, 7 Ridgedale Ave., Cedar Knolls, NJ 07927.
42. From Fitzgerald, W.B., "Checklist for the witness," *For the Defense*, July 1992; 18–23.
43. *Ibid*.
44. Blackwell, M., "Documentation serves as invaluable defense tool," *American Nurse*, July/August 1993, pp. 40,41.
45. Tex. Admin. Code. 22 §217.13(5) (1995).
46. *Collins v. Westlake Community Hospital*, 12 N.E.2d 614 (Ill. 1974).
47. *Robert v. Chodoff*, 393 A. 2d 853 (Pa. Super. 1978).
48. *Maslonka v. Hermann*, 414 A.2d 1350 (N.J.App. 1980).
49. Hall, J.K., "No substitute for good practice," *Nursing 1994*; 24(12):4.
50. *Quintal v. Laurel Grove Hospital*, 397 P.2d 161 (1965).
51. *Ahrens v. Katz*, 595 F.Supp. 1108 (D.Ga. 1984).
52. Hall, J.K., "Cheap insurance," *American Journal of Nursing*, 1990; 90(8:20), p. 20.

THREE

Ethics and Law of
Doing No Harm
(Non-maleficence)

TOPICS COVERED

Ethical basis of the law enforcing the value, Doing No Harm (Non-maleficence)

Laws enforcing the value, Doing No Harm

Intentional torts

BATTERY • ASSAULT • FALSE IMPRISONMENT • INTENTIONAL INFLICTION OF EMOTIONAL DISTRESS, OTHERS • DEFENSES TO INTENTIONAL TORTS

Quasi-intentional torts—injury to economics and dignity

DEFAMATION • INVASION OF PRIVACY, AND OTHERS • DEFENSES

Statues prohibiting maltreatment

PROHIBITING ABUSE • REQUIRING REPORT • ANTIDUMPING

Research protections against harm

Licensure

PURPOSE AND EFFECT • CREDENTIALING • COMMON PROVISIONS • CONTESTING BOARD DECISIONS • LICENSURE LIABILITIES • NATIONAL PRACTITIONER DATA BANK • ETHICS AND LAW OF NURSE EDUCATION • MANDATORY CONTINUING EDUCATION • COMPETENCE • ALTERNATIVES TO LICENSURE

Non-Maleficence:
The Value As Basis for the Law

$\triangledown$

"I never wonder to see men [and women] wicked, but I often wonder to see them not ashamed." [BRACKETS ADDED].
—JONATHAN SWIFT, *Thoughts on Various Subjects*

$\triangle$

> The duty not to harm others is mandated of all people, not just nurses (different from the duty to do good to others, only mandated of nurses and others who voluntarily assume the duty).
>
> The ethical duty to do no harm is the base of all criminal law, and the civil law also enforces the value through liability for wrongs (torts) done intentionally.
>
> The ethical values of doing good (beneficence) and doing no harm (non-maleficence) are enforced in laws that mandate the practitioner to provide competent care.

Every member of a society is under a duty not to harm others (to leave other people alone). More people are subject to the ethical and legal mandate to do no harm than are subject to the mandate to do good (beneficence).

To distinguish the value of non-maleficence from the value of beneficence: Only people who assume a duty to do good are punished when they fail. Doctors and nurses undertake to do good for patients, and they are punished—by licensure law or a malpractice suit—when they fail to meet that standard of care.

This duty not to harm (essentially a negative duty) is the base of all criminal law. Murder, theft, rape, assault, and battery (all crimes) are violations of this basic human value enforced in criminal law. Particular crimes that nurses are more likely to encounter, such as child and adult abuse, are discussed later in this section.

The civil law also enforces the value, Doing No Harm, through liability for all the wrongs (torts) that are totally or partly intended by the actor. These are different from the failure to do good (to be beneficent), punished as detailed in the preceding chapter by malpractice suits. Those acts of negligence/malpractice are considered to be *un*intentional (more or less accidental or "negligent").

The Latin term for the simple Anglo-Saxon value of Doing No Harm is *non-maleficence, non* meaning "not," *mal* meaning "bad," and *ficence*, to "do or make." The value is easy for nurses to understand: Nurses help patients if they can, but at least they avoid making them worse. The things nurses and doctors can do to people, however, make this easier said than done.

Considering the iatrogenic (provider-caused) illness that is possible, just coming into the hospital or being a patient in another setting is a risky business. Another Latin term, *primum non nocere* (pronounced "preemum non no-cherry"), is the nurse's mandate to *"first, do no harm."*

The self-interest nurses have in doing no harm is the same interest they have in doing good (beneficence); they feel good, are seen as good, and adhere to professional values. Not harming enhances the individual's self-esteem as a valued member of society. If nurses don't hurt others, they are less likely to be hurt by others in turn. Nurses who don't harm others avoid breaking laws made to punish people who hurt (either intentionally or negligently). If nurses do hurt other people, criminal prosecution could cost liberty and even life, and civil lawsuits could cost psychic pain and money.

From both values, of doing good to people (beneficence) and doing no harm to people (non-maleficence), come the mandates for the practitioner to provide competent care. Professionals are mandated to keep their skills and practice competently; these standards arise from the values of doing good for the patient, as well as doing no harm. Most of the codes for professionals hold competent practice as an ethical value, a value of competency based on the principles of doing good for, and doing no harm to, the patient.

The malpractice suit is a result of the values (of doing good and doing no harm) *not* being adhered to. The people as a society want to compensate the patient if the practitioner fails to do good. The people, through lawsuits, may also punish the practitioner who "intentionally" does harm (specific torts are explained below).

It would seem unnecessary to say that the value of nursing is "don't harm the patient," since nurses have an even higher duty than the negative "don't harm"—they have a duty to do good. The law that enforces the value of doing no harm is more developed for people in general who don't have the additional higher duty to do good. Such *general* "don't harm" law applies also to nurses. As always, adhering to the value of not harming makes the nurse's practice ethical, thus legal.

In a lawsuit for strict liability, people who engage in what is considered ultrahazardous activity are automatically liable when someone is harmed. These acts are so inherently dangerous that they cannot be made safe. The person sued needn't be negligent to be liable, but is liable merely for harm done by performing the act (even very safely). The mandate not to harm is so strong that, in those situations, even if no negligence is present, having someone harmed produces automatic liability. There is some analogy here to surgery—some medical procedures may be so inherently dangerous that they cannot be made safe. Then why don't we hold nurses and doctors automatically liable for a bad result? Does the difference depend on who may benefit from the dangerous activity?

Laws Enforcing the Value, Doing No Harm

INTENTIONAL TORTS

Intent to injure is not needed for liability under the civil law; only general intent to perform an *act*, knowing the result with substantial certainty, is necessary.

To convict of some crimes may require specific intent (that the actor intended the *result*, not merely the act).

General intent can be presumed from an act, together with advance knowledge of the result of the act, since the law can never know with certainty what is in another's mind.

Motive and intent distinguished: Intent is *what* the person meant to do; motive is *why* the person did the act.

Children (the age depends on state law) and incompetents can have the requisite intentional will to commit intentional torts (civil law), not usually crimes (criminal law).

The word *tort* means "wrong" in Old French (the early language of law in England, the basis for American case law). Insurance for malpractice (negligence) may not cover the intentional torts defined here. But if the "intentional" tort arises in the course of the nurse's work (for example, a suit for lack of consent/battery/an intentional tort), the individual policy may cover it.

That a nurse would ever *intend* to injure a patient is not acceptable, but there is evidence that some nurses have done exactly that—for example, in Germany under the National Socialist government.[1]

Usually the nurse did not intend to injure; intent to injure is not needed for liability under the civil law. The only intent needed is intent to perform an *act*. An intentional tort occurs when the nurse acts in a certain way that causes injury. The law does not assume that the nurse intended *injury*, but law does assume the nurse intended the deliberately done *act*; the nurse may be held liable for the injury that results from the act.

Intent in criminal law may be classed as general or specific. Some crimes (not "intentional" torts) that nurses may commit make the specific/general intent distinction. For example, the crime of assisting suicide requires specific intent: "*intentionally* causes or aids another to commit suicide."

Mere general intent means the actor knows with substantial certainty that specific result will happen. General intent is found merely from doing the act (for example, writing a prescription) together with knowing with substantial certainty that the act will cause or contribute to a result. In the situation of assisted suicide, the prescriber *knows* that writing the prescription may contribute to the result of death by suicide, and may or may not intend the result.

If the law requires specific intent, as in assisted suicide, the prosecution must prove that the actor's *goal* in acting is to bring about specific consequences. It is not enough to prove just that the writer *knew* with substantial certainty that the act would cause or contribute to the result. To find specific intent requires, in addition to knowing of the result, that the result be intended.

General Intent: Intend act → know of injury

Specific Intent: Intend injury → cause injury

Transferred intent means to intend to cause specific consequences to one person, but to end up with consequences to another. In criminal law, one can be guilty of transferred intent crimes only if charges are for assault, battery, false imprisonment, and trespass to land and chattels.

Anglo-Saxon law is clear on the role of intent in defining crime. In the case of assisted suicide, the court will never actually know the prescriber's intent ("prescriber" is used since nurses may be able to prescribe lethal doses to assist suicide under laws contemplated). Since the law can never know with certainty what is in another's mind, intent is presumed from the act, together with advance knowledge of the result of the act.

If the *only* result of a prescription can be its use by the patient to cause death, the prescriber's intent to assist suicide is presumed. If there is another *possible* result of the act of prescribing (to cause sleep, to relieve pain), the law need not inquire into the prescriber's subconscious intentions. If someone prescribes poison or a dosage that has no other purpose than to kill the patient, the intent to aid suicide will be presumed from the act of prescribing together with the knowledge of the certain result of the act.

Meaning of motive *and* intent *distinguished.* Motive is *why* the person did the crime, and intent is *what* the person meant to do. Motive may be relevant to the degree of the crime and to punishment, but not to whether the crime was done. Some writers have suggested the recognition of "partial intent," at least in the area of assisted suicide.[2] To recognize "partial intent" might be psychologically helpful to the prescriber, but the law does not recognize such distinctions.

Infants (children under varied ages, depending on state law) and incompetents can have the requisite intentional will to commit intentional acts— torts, under civil law, not usually crimes, under criminal law. They can be held liable for damages they have caused under the civil law, but not usually for crimes that will result in punishment that is not monetary.

Intentional torts are different from negligent torts in several ways. First, the nurse must have *intended* the act sued upon. (This is not true in negligence cases.) Second, depending on the kind of tort, the patient may not have to prove specific injury (damages), as is necessary in a suit based on negligence. The law is generally harder on someone who does something intentionally than if the act was accidental. Torts can be classed according to how much intent was involved in the act that produced the injury.

TORT LAW SCALE OF INTENTION

↓	↓	↓
Negligence Torts (M)	Quasi-intentional Torts (D, I/P)	Intentional Torts (B, A, FI)

M = Malpractice
D = Defamation
I/P = Invasion of privacy
B = Battery
A = Assault
FI = False imprisonment

Battery

The usual lawsuit for battery, in the context of illness care, arises when surgery or some other procedure is done on a patient who has not consented specifically to that procedure.

Battery is harmful or offensive contact to plaintiff's person, with intent, and caused by the defendant.

Consent is a good defense to battery lawsuit.

The most common intentional tort in illness care is battery. In common usage today, the word *batter* means physical beating, such as results in an abused spouse. But the Old English word for battery in law means only "offensive touching without consent"—merely touching someone without consent is to batter. Though the patient may not have to prove specific injury (damages) to win the case, a court will be unlikely to award damages unless some injury results from the unconsented touching.

The lawsuit for battery in the context of illness care arises when surgery or some other procedure is done on a patient who has not consented specifically to that procedure. (Consent is a good defense to battery; if the person consents to touching, there's no battery.) Consent can take many forms. Patients are assumed (*implied*) to have given consent for a lot of touching when they voluntarily come in for treatment.

Battery is formally defined as harmful or offensive contact to plaintiff's person, with intent, and caused by the defendant. The contact can be direct or indirect—for example, setting up a machine that will hit the patient—and the contact can be with merely clothes, purse, or bed. Plaintiff needn't know of contact, nor need prove special damages. The more direct and harmful the contact, the more damages.

Assault

> Assault is "fear of immediate harm from a battery" (one step short of a battery).
>   Unlike battery, the plaintiff suing only for assault must be aware of the assault.
>   Immediate threat to the person is required (not threat of future harm, or violence to another).

Nurses rarely are sued for assault on a patient; the legal definition is "fear of immediate harm from a battery." Assault is one step short of a battery; if the nurse threatens to hit the patient, and acts so that the patient has reason to believe a battery is imminent, the patient could sue for assault. Usually the two torts, assault and battery, are committed and sued on together.

The formal definition is apprehension of immediate harmful or offensive contact to the person, together with intent to cause the apprehension, by the defendant. The apprehension must be reasonable; it needn't be actually possible to cause injury, but must be apparent to a reasonable person.

Unlike battery, the plaintiff suing only for assault must be aware of the assault. The plaintiff doesn't necessarily have to know that the *defendant* is causing the apprehension of battery. Mere words aren't enough, but words together with an overt act are. The appropriate words can turn an innocent gesture into an assault; and, vice versa, kind words can soften an apparent threatening gesture. An immediate threat to the person is required; it is not sufficient to be apprehensive of future harm, or only of violence to another.

Like battery, proving damages is not necessary with the intentional tort of assault. But also like battery, assault without special damages may not provide enough potential judgment to make it worth suing.

All nurses would agree that it is unethical to strike a patient unless in extreme self-defense. No nurse anticipates doing so. But the stress of work and handling combative patients, particularly those who must be restrained, can provoke a situation in which it can happen. In the midst of a crisis, nurses might try to envision how the situation could look to a jury (legal) or to a respected peer (ethical and possibly legal). Rarely should a patient need to be physically subdued. Care of such a patient is not a contest for control; time and careful observation will allow many such patients to calm themselves. If immediate restraint is necessary to protect a patient or staff, the people who are trained in using physical force should do so. Restraining carries with it the possibility of liability for false imprisonment.

False Imprisonment

> False imprisonment is defined as confining a person to a bound area by force (including threat of force to the person or property, and acts or words reasonably implying force).

False imprisonment includes failure to provide a means of escape when the defendant has the means to do so and includes situations when the plaintiff is under the defendant's control or can't leave without the defendant's help.

Moral pressure or *future* threats to detain are not sufficient to produce liability.

Lawsuits about the use of restraints on incompetent patients will probably allege negligence instead of false imprisonment.

Psychiatric and emergency nurses can follow the ethic that the patient should not be harmed (restrained without reason). The law enforces the ethic by punishing one who intentionally imprisons *without good reason*.

The "good reason" to restrain is for the safety of people who are a danger to themselves or others, but only to the extent necessary.

Consent is one defense to false imprisonment, and necessity (need to protect the patient) is another.

Two nursing situations that may produce liability for false imprisonment are:

1. Restraining a patient who is in no danger to self or others against the patient's will in order to provide "protection," and
2. Keeping a patient from leaving by forbidding the patient to leave.

Unwarranted physical restraint is sufficient for false imprisonment, but a suit can be successful even without physical restraint. The patient who believes leaving is impossible also can allege false imprisonment.

The formal definition of the tort is confining a person to a bound area by force. That force can also include threat of force to the person or property, and acts or words reasonably implying force. The definition includes failure to provide a means to leave when the defendant has the means to do so (for example, a wheelchair). The tort also includes situations when the plaintiff is under the defendant's control or can't leave without the defendant's help; for example, the nurse who says, "No, I won't get a wheelchair for you so you can leave the hospital."

Police have special rules that prohibit them from invalidly using their legal authority to imprison. Private citizens can arrest others if a felony was actually committed and the citizen has reason to believe the detained person did the felony. A merchant who has reasonable grounds to believe a customer has shoplifted is protected from lawsuit liability if the customer is detained "reasonably" to investigate the circumstances.

Moral pressure and *future* threats made to detain someone are not enough to produce liability. But the plaintiff needn't resist a forceful imprisonment (analogous to victims of rape). The duration of time the person is confined relates only to how much damages are given, not to the issue of whether the person was actually confined. The plaintiff must have known of the confinement, unless it causes injury. For example, a patient who is confined without cause in a mental hospital, but who is drugged and un-aware of the confinement, would have to find some injury it caused (which may not be difficult).

No confinement occurred if the plaintiff was aware of any reasonable means of escape. Like the other intentional torts, there is usually no require-ment of special damages in order to make the case, but recovery is certainly better if damages can be shown.

> *Examples of false imprisonment*: The patient is competent and wishes to leave (against medical or nursing advice) and the nurse says the patient may not leave. The patient who is ready for discharge is told that leaving is not permitted without paying the agency's bill.

Lawsuits about the use of restraints on incompetent patients will prob-ably allege negligence instead of false imprisonment (assuming the patient's incompetence is not at issue). It may be appropriate to restrain the patient for her or his own protection (from walking out of the agency into the street), a motive that would be a defense to false imprisonment; then, the issue on malpractice is whether the physical restraints were appropriately used or negligently done.

Special laws govern the actions of nurses who work in emergency rooms and psychiatric settings, with people who are made patients involuntarily. The ethic is clear: The patient should not be harmed and his freedom should be protected as much as possible. The ethic is enforced by laws that punish intentionally imprisoning someone *without good reason* (the "false" in false imprisonment).

The laws enforcing the ethic of doing no harm are state statutes that set out in detail the procedure to follow in order to care for people who are a danger to themselves or others, without their consent. Following the ethic will also result in compliance with the law. Nurses who work in areas where people are made patients against their will may want to read the state statute, which can be found in the local or central library, or from the agency's management. The statute will say that the person can be forced to accept care without consent only if a danger to self or to others. This assessment of "dangerousness" is a judgment call, like all else in nursing and in life.

If the statute allowed involuntary commitment under any other situation, the law would probably be unconstitutional under the U.S. Constitution or state constitution. Constitutions mandate that no person may be denied lib-erty without due process (the law enforces the values Doing No Harm and Freedom here). In this case, due process means the patient can't be restrained (committed) past the time of immediate danger to self or others—unless there is some substantial reason for it (*substantive due process*). And a procedure to allow the facts to be ascertained—procedural due process—must be followed to allow the patient to have a say. (Due process is described in Chapter One, Values in Ethics and Law, and in Chapter Five, Ethics and Law of Fairness.)

Defense to False Imprisonment

Consent of the patient is one defense to a lawsuit alleging false imprisonment; necessity (need to protect the patient) is another. The nurse can defend by establishing that the action was reasonable to protect the patient from danger to self, and that another reasonable prudent nurse in the same situation would have done the same. If the patient is incompetent, in the hospital, and in danger of falling when getting out of bed without help, false imprisonment is not the question. The patient needs to be prevented from harm; how this is done and whether restraints are necessary, and safely applied, are malpractice questions of negligence law, not questions rising to the level of the intentional tort of false imprisonment. (Some authorities now say beds should be low and *without* rails.)

The nurse has a duty to reasonably protect the patient from falls but is liable for damage from improperly used restraints. Answers are (as always) determined case by case, using good nursing judgment and documentation. First, the nurse should "restrain" self while assessing whether some other solution will work. The process should be documented; restraints should not be used unless determined to be necessary, and then done according to agency policy.

Intentional and Negligent Infliction of Emotional Distress

Intentional infliction of emotional distress (outrageous conduct that makes the plaintiff experience severe emotional distress) does not require that the nurse intend the *result* that the patient actually be distressed; general intent suffices (to intentionally do the act with knowledge that such an act could cause the distress).

Negligent infliction of emotional distress is a nonintentional tort treated under the rules of negligence malpractice and is more likely to arise in nursing situations than the intentional tort.

Rarely would the nurse be sued for intentional infliction of emotional distress, since few nurses will intentionally harm patients physically *or* emotionally. An action that might lead to such a suit is the following: A nurse knows that the patient is very worried about a pending HIV lab result and deliberately tells the patient the test is positive (when it is not). Note that the nurse does not have to intend the *result* that the patient actually be distressed, only to intentionally *act* with the knowledge that such an act could cause the distress. In legal terms, general (not specific) intent suffices in this tort as in all the civil torts. As noted above, some crimes require specific intent—that the nurse intend the *result*, not merely the *act*. The nurse cannot defend by saying that there was no intent to make the patient distressed; intent to do the act is enough (in this example, intent to give a false result) with knowledge that the patient could be distressed.

The legal definition of this tort is outrageous conduct that makes the plaintiff experience severe emotional distress. Contrary to some other intentional torts, the person pleading intentional infliction of emotional distress is required to prove damages; because the causation of the damages is more difficult to see than with an obvious battery.

There is a problem with *transferred intent* in these cases. If a second person sees outrageous conduct (words rarely suffice) and suffers as a result, the second person can win a lawsuit only if (1) present for the conduct, (2) related to the person intended to be harmed, and (3) the second person's presence and relationship was known by the defendant.

The *negligent* infliction of emotional distress is a nonintentional tort treated under the rules of negligence like malpractice (plaintiff must show duty, breach, causation, and damages). Negligent infliction is more likely to arise in nursing than the intentional infliction of emotional distress. Such a suit might arise in a number of ways, including inappropriate handling of dead bodies witnessed by the family, or a relative's witnessing of negligent care given to a loved one (generally unsuccessful suits). Suits for emotional distress without any resulting physical injury are not favored by the courts in states east of California.

Other Intentional Torts

Other intentional torts include trespass to land, trespass to chattels, and conversion; they are enforcement of the value placed on private property (the result of labor).

Other intentional torts are not often encountered in nursing practice, but they may be important to nurses in their private lives. Almost all of these torts reflect theories of law that in some fashion protect property or punish harm to it; in that sense, they enforce the value, Doing No Harm, since harming one's property harms the person (the person's ability to survive). Other intentional torts include *trespass to land*—entering property without permission—land occupying a special place in law and human thinking because it was and is (though dimly realized) the source of food and thus the means of survival.

Trespass to chattels includes any action done to another's personal property (anything movable) without permission. The origin of the word *chattel* is cattle; the word was later applied to slaves. Chattel is in general all personal property which is not land.

Conversion is another intentional tort. Conversion is defined as acting to exercise dominion and control, as though an owner, over another's chattel. This tort is the civil equivalent of the crime of theft.

Instead of the police prosecuting the thief, the owner of the property can sue the thief in court to recover the property. Nurses rarely will need to know about these torts in the context of practice. If a situation involving one of these torts arises in private life, the nurse should seek legal advice.

Defenses to Intentional Torts

> Defenses to the intentional torts include consent (express: written or spoken; and implied: apparent or implied by law), self-defense, defense of another, defense of property, and necessity.

Consent (to the action that is alleged to be the wrong) is always a defense to an intentional tort. If the patient alleges the intentional tort of battery (that no consent was given before a procedure was done), the defense is the written consent and/or testimony that the patient indeed did consent to the procedure.

Consent can be express (written or spoken) or implied (apparent or implied by law). People without capacity—incompetent, inebriated or drugged, and children—are considered to be unable to consent.

One cannot consent to a *criminal* act, although it may look also like a *civil* intentional tort (which one *can* consent to). If the action is bad enough to be considered a crime, letting the act go unpunished is considered to harm the general public, not only to the individual actually harmed. To say that the person consented to being beaten is not a good defense to a criminal charge of battery.

Consent can be exceeded; for instance, a consent for a pelvic exam does not extend to consent to pelvic surgery. The law of consent reflects and enforces the value placed on the freedom of the individual (power over the body). (Consent law is fully discussed in Chapter Four, on laws enforcing the value, Freedom.)

Self-defense can be used as a defense to an intentional tort, as well as a defense to criminal charges. Defense of self can excuse an act that would otherwise produce liability for battery and assault. To be excused for the act that is otherwise wrong, the person who asserts self-defense must have had a reasonable belief that attack was imminent. There is no need to run, but no retaliation after an attack is excused.

The self-defense exculpation may be allowed even if the defender injures a third person while defending from the attacker. Defense of another person is justifiable if the defended personally had a reasonable belief that an attack on him was imminent.

Defense of property has different rules from defense of self or another person. To defend property and have a valid defense for the action if sued later, the defender must first ask the person to stop bothering the property before taking any action. The defender of property may use only reasonable force to effect the defense of the property. Deadly force to defend property will not be excused, unless also defending life or preventing forcible entry into the home.

Related to the idea of self-defense is necessity; necessity is a general defense to intentional tort liability. As noted, defense to a suit for false imprisonment of a patient is that the act was *necessary* (in that case, to protect the patient). The person defending on necessity grounds will allege the act was needed to do either a public good or a private good. Even if excused from liability because the action was necessary, the damage done in accomplishing the public or private good still must be paid for. The classic example is the defense against trespassing on (tying the boat to) a private dock if a storm makes it necessary: The boat owner still has to pay for damage to the dock, if any.

The necessity defense has arisen in the context of illness care and ethics. Some anti-abortion demonstrators, charged with trespass on private property of abortion clinics, have sought to defend on grounds of necessity (to save fetal lives). Statues that make such trespass a federal crime may obviate that defense.

QUASI-INTENTIONAL TORTS— INJURY TO ECONOMICS AND DIGNITY

Quasi-intentional torts (also called "injury to economics and dignity") are a middle ground between intentional torts and nonintentional torts (negligence).

Defamation is an injury to the person's reputation, resulting from an untrue statement made to a third person ("publication" of the defamation).

Written defamation is called libel (damages automatic); spoken defamation is called slander (if slander *per se*, damages are automatic).

Quasi-intentional, or half-intentional, torts are a middle ground between the intentional torts (battery, assault, false imprisonment) and the nonintentional torts, principally negligence. The designation "injury to economics and dignity" has been applied also, possibly because it is logical to treat intent as an all-or-none quality: Either one intends an act or one does not intend it; under this logic, there can be no "half-intent." Whether the designation persists will be seen with time.

Defamation

This area of tort law also clearly enforces the ethical value of doing no harm (non-maleficence). The ethic is more easily relevant to nurses when stated,

"Don't harm other professionals." More likely than suits by patients are suits by doctors and nurses against each other, or sometimes employers, for defamation.

Defamation is an injury to the person's reputation, resulting from an untrue statement to a third person; the making of the statement is called "publication" (for example, writing a defamatory remark in the patient's chart). If the statement is true, it is not defamation. Making the statement only to the person spoken about isn't "publishing" the defamation (but it is published if the writer of a letter knows the secretary will see it, too).

Written defamation is called libel; spoken defamation is called slander. And there are degrees of offense (and degrees of defenses). Damages depend on how widespread the publication and how clearly the statement is damaging. The statement may not clearly damage on its face; but it may be damaging in the whole context in which it was made—in which case, it is termed *innuendo*.

The statement may not directly identify the plaintiff; but the person may be recognizable in the context of the situation—known as *colloquium*. The plaintiff who is a public figure will have a harder time recovering (winning); public figures are presumed to tolerate some notoriety as a payment for their advantages.

A defendant news organization is less likely to lose than other defendants. The laws that protect the freedom of the press reflect the value placed on truth in the society. Punishing every misstatement of the media might result in self-censorship of the press (and result in less information to the people); that policy consideration outweighs the need to protect individuals from defamation in some cases.

Libel law in Britain makes it much easier for the plaintiffs to win; the law is tougher on the media there. For example, the defendant publisher has the burden to prove that a statement is true. In the United States, the plaintiff has the burden of proving the statement is false. The British legal system makes the loser of a lawsuit pay the other side's legal fees, which means that many potential plaintiffs who might sue for defamation are reluctant to sue, even if they deserve to win, for fear they can't afford to lose.

In the United States, damages for defamation are automatic if defamation is proved. (Automatic does not necessarily mean large damages, however.) No proof of actual injury is necessary if the defamation is made in writing (libel). Damages are also automatic if the spoken defamation is any one of the following four lies (in legal terms, slander *per se*—slander all by itself):

1. The person has a loathsome disease. (This used to include leprosy; now HIV positive may be sufficient.)
2. The person is guilty of a felony.
3. The person's reputation in a profession or business is injured (as in, "She's a terrible nurse. I have seen her hit patients").
4. A woman is "unchaste." (This is seldom sued upon any more, since a reputation for being "unchaste" is not as injurious to women as in the days when virginity and fidelity were considered more important.)

The third item above is a prime area of interest for nurses: First, due to intemperate statements, nurses could be defendants in a lawsuit by a colleague or patient. Second, nurses could be potential plaintiffs if their reputation in their profession is damaged by some untrue statement. Here the ethical mandate, "first, do no harm," means not to harm patients *or* coworkers. Employees are increasingly likely to bring lawsuits against employers for alleged defamation made in the context of discharge, discussed in Chapter Five, Fairness.

Defense to Defamation

> Truth is an absolute defense to a charge of defamation; so is proving that the statement was opinion and not allegation of fact. The plaintiff must prove the statement was false.

Truth is an absolute defense to a charge of defamation. The plaintiff has the burden of proving (presenting evidence) that the statement is false; the defendant will probably seek to prove that it's true. In addition, people are allowed to express *opinion* without fear of lawsuit. The difference between defamation and opinion can be close but, in general, an action for defamation will have to establish that the defendant made some statement of fact. To say, "I don't think she's a very good doctor," or "I don't like her at all," is a statement of opinion. To say "she's not a good doctor" is a statement of fact, especially if supplemented with another allegation "because she snorts cocaine during surgery."

Patient charts are accessible to third parties, so writing in the chart would be considered "publication"—which proves one element of the tort. That's another reason to chart only what is observed and only what is pertinent to the patient's care; and, that's also a good reason not to "fight" with doctors or other nurses in the patient's record.

Invasion of Privacy

> Suits and violation of statutes for invasion of privacy that are most likely to affect nurses are from the classification "disclosure of private facts."
> Truth is not a defense to invasion of privacy, but consent and necessity are.

The quasi-intentional tort invasion of privacy is another area of law that enforces the ethical value of doing no harm. In addition, a lawsuit for invasion of privacy enforces the ethical value of keeping secrets (confidentiality) through case law made by the courts.

There are several classifications of this tort, invasion of privacy, including the use without permission of one's face or name for advertising. The classification most applicable to nurses and their patients is styled as "disclosure of private facts."

Damages need not be proven in order to recover in a lawsuit based on this tort as is also true in other intentional torts (but, as always, if there is no injury apparent, the recovery will be small). For purposes of a lawsuit, disclosure of the patient's diagnosis, treatment, prognosis, or just about any fact known to the nurse because of the special relationship to the patient, could be considered a private fact.

The fact disclosed must be one a reasonable person would find private. The patient's address, while not generally known, is probably not a "private" fact. Disclosure of the fact that the patient has delivered a baby and is not married has been successfully sued upon. As in other areas, changing morals might make disclosure of some "private facts" less actionable if the society in general doesn't find them private.

Defense to Invasion of Privacy

Truth is not a defense to invasion of privacy. Even if true that the patient is HIV-positive, the patient can sue for the nurse's breach of confidentiality. Neither are defenses available of negligence (unintended breach of confidentiality), good faith of the nurse, nor lack of malice on the nurse's part. In that respect this tort is more like one of a strict liability analysis. Plaintiff need not prove the nurse was negligent but merely that something was revealed that should not have been revealed through the nurse's action.

As always, consent is a defense. When the person becomes a patient, some implied and written consent is given for limited disclosure to others (which disclosure is necessary to care). Revealing confidences necessary to the next nurse or next unit or the consultant *are* necessary to care. Patients should be asked to give consent or sign a release (consent) before their information is shared with others who request it (even other doctors or agencies).

The nurse might have the privilege of disclosing private facts about a patient in the patient's best interest (to protect the patient from harm). A qualified privilege to reveal information might be asserted, when revealing is in the interest of one who might be harmed without the information (such as the sexual partner of a patient tested positive for HIV).

Before acting to disclose private facts about a patient, nurses should take extreme care to be sure the action is ethically justified under the value, Doing No Harm. If the action is right, it will probably be legal; but the circumstances must be that keeping the confidence will surely harm the patient or someone else, in order to justify violating that confidence.

In this area the nurse's ethical judgment may be enhanced by knowing the specific state law and regulations (especially in the HIV situation). The statute can be found through the statute index in the local or central library, or from agency management/policy.

Statutes on Invasion of Privacy

Some states have statutes that protect patient confidentiality in legislative law (statutes) as well as the case law (common law) outlined above. Often that statute will allow a lawsuit for release of confidential information. Even without a statute this lawsuit is allowed, but the statute is usually more specific. The statute may provide that a patient can even get an injunction from the court, ordering a physician or other provider not to release information.[3] (An injunction is an order by the court to a person, *not* to do something; this remedy is not always available without a statute.) If the statute did not grant the power to enjoin the other party, the plaintiff would have to wait until the damage was done and then sue.

> Other quasi-intentional torts are malicious prosecution, and intentional misrepresentation. (Negligent misrepresentation follows the legal rules for negligence—duty, breach, causation, and damages).

Malicious Prosecution

This quasi-intentional tort usually is alleged by a physician or nurse who says that a patient sued without any basis, "maliciously." (Note the root word, *malice*, of malicious.) To succeed in the suit, the doctor or nurse must:

1. Win the lawsuit the patient filed in the first place,
2. Prove the patient had no reasonable basis for bringing the suit, *and*
3. Show malice on the part of the patient (that the patient wanted to "get" the defendant).

It is difficult to meet the second criterion—usually there's *some* reasonable basis for the patient's suit, other than malice.

Intentional Misrepresentation (Fraud, Deceit)

This tort has been rarely used in medical/nursing law, but it may become more prevalent in the future.

> #### A SUIT FOR MISREPRESENTATION
>
> A medical technician in California sued the patient for not revealing that the patient was positive for HIV. A jury gave the technician $102,500 in damages for the mental anguish of worrying whether HIV had been contracted from the patient. A judge upheld the award at the trial court level, saying that the patient has no obligation to tell the provider his HIV status—but if he doesn't volunteer it, and the worker suffers harm thereby, he may be liable.[4]

Elements of the tort of intentional misrepresentation, in a scenario like the case above, include these:

1. False representation of material fact (asserting "I'm not HIV positive"), and
2. Scienter (guilty knowledge)—knowledge that the fact is false ("In reality, I know I am HIV positive"), and
3. Intent to induce plaintiff (provider) to act or not in reliance on misrepresentation (take care of him), and
4. Justifiable reliance (the provider reasonably relies on patient's word and thus exposes self to HIV), and
5. Causation (the effect of the misrepresentation eventually caused anxiety), and
6. Damage (in California, courts award damages for worry).

The plaintiff can't justifiably rely on *opinion* ("I don't think I have HIV"). Nor can the plaintiff rely on a statement of the value or quality of something ("This house is worth $100,000"), unless the statement of value is made by an expert. For purposes of a suit for misrepresentation, one can "rely" on the legal opinion of a lawyer to a layperson, or a statement of future intent if the maker of the statement has control over the event ("I'm going to fix that weak floor before you move in").

There's usually no duty on the part of the defendant to reveal a material fact (one doesn't have to announce one has HIV), but if one deceives about the material fact (says "I don't"), there is then a duty to set the plaintiff straight. One can't actively conceal a material fact (one that matters or on which the plaintiff will act); for example, secretly removing the HIV-positive result from one's own chart on the way to outpatient surgery.

Negligent misrepresentation is also actionable, but the defendant is only liable if the reliance by that particular plaintiff was foreseeable. For example, if a nurse didn't know the results of the patient's HIV test but negligently allowed the patient to think the result was negative, it can be foreseen that the patient would rely on that information.

STATUTES PROHIBITING MALTREATMENT

Nurses are included in the general mandate not to harm (enforced by many criminal statutes). Nurses are also specifically mandated to report harm they know about.

Without knowing specific laws, nurses can assume that the ethic, Doing No Harm, will be enforced in criminal law and civil lawsuits that prohibit (and will punish) people who abuse people unable to defend themselves; and that the law will require that nurses report known or suspected abuse of dependent persons.

The duty of the nurse to nondependent adults who appear to have been intentionally injured is to ascertain the cause of the injury, treat, and offer referral for the underlying etiology. (Reporting without the patient's consent may not be mandated and may be prohibited).

The case law outlined above allows lawsuits for the various harms that people do to one another. In addition, legislatures have added many statutes that seek to prevent or punish harm. All of criminal law ultimately enforces the value of doing no harm. Much of the criminal law once was case law, but the modern tendency is to put all criminal law into statues; sometimes these are called penal codes (*penal* meaning "punish," originating in "pain").

The assumption that laws will cure problems results in many state and federal statutes written to prevent harm to innocent people, and to punish harm when it is done. Some of the laws that mandate people not to harm specifically address nurses. Nurses are included in the general mandate not to harm, and nurses are also specifically mandated to report harm they know about, a higher burden on nurses than on the general public.

Prohibiting Abuse

All states have statutes prohibiting abuse of children and dependent adults. The statutes usually provide a criminal penalty for abusing patients, and they may make neglect illegal (of particular concern in nursing home and home health practice). Some statutes make failure to report abuse or neglect a crime.

Child Abuse

All people, not just nurses, are under a mandate not to harm children. One U.S. law that enforces the ethical value of non-maleficence is the federal Child Abuse Prevention and Treatment Act of 1974, which gave incentives to states to set up programs for child abuse research and programs for identification, prosecution, and treatment of offenders. The law was expanded several times, increasing federal funds allocated to states. To qualify, states had to pass legislation to provide immunity for all people reporting child abuse (for example, nurses), and to provide by statute criminal penalties (fines and/or prison) for failure to report by professionals (including nurses). All 50 states and the District of Columbia have passed such legislation.

Every nurse knows the ethic that underlies another law, the Child Abuse Amendments of 1984; the ethics, Doing Good and Doing No Harm, are enforced in that law, passed after the "Baby Doe" case. A Down's syndrome baby with esophageal atresia was not operated on (a mentally average baby would have been) and was allowed to dehydrate/starve to death at the request of the parents. As a result, the federal law was passed to mandate that states must "establish programs and procedures in child protection services systems to respond to reports of medical neglect."

MEDICAL NEGLECT DEFINED:

". . . withholding of medically indicated treatment from a disabled infant with a life-threatening condition." That definition was elaborated as being a "failure to respond to the infant's life threatening conditions by providing treatment (including appropriate nutrition, hydration, and medication) which in the treating physician's medical judgment, will be most likely to be effective in ameliorating or correcting all such conditions, EXCEPT if the infant is chronically and irreversibly comatose; if treatment would merely prolong dying, not correct all life threatening conditions, or otherwise be futile in terms of survival; or treatment would be virtually futile in terms of survival and treatment would be inhumane. . . ."[5]

The short answer for nurses (incorporating the ethical principles and enforcing law) is: Don't dehydrate to death infants who have a treatable condition. The hospital will have a policy and possibly a copy of the law; a hotline number should be available for nurses' use if they believe the law is being violated. In some borderline cases, the ethics committee of the agency may be consulted. The 1984 law established Infant Care Review committees to watchdog in each institution,[6] and they too can assist nurses with concern.

NEGLECT AS ABUSE

Abuse laws can be carried somewhat further than the lawmakers may have foreseen. Refusal to immunize a child has been charged as neglect in one state, even though the father asserted that he was exempt from the law because of strong religious convictions against vaccinations. The judge found the father's convictions based more on beliefs about medicine, than on religion. Though the judge found the child officially "neglected," the measles emergency had passed and he did not order the child vaccinated.[7]

Abusing Dependent People

As a general rule, nurses can assume that the ethic, Doing No Harm, will be enforced in laws that prohibit (and will punish) people who abuse those unable to defend themselves, such as the young, the very old, and the disabled. The laws almost always provide immunity from harm for the reporter of abuse (some make failure to report itself a crime).

In addition to the crime of abuse, the civil law through a lawsuit can enforce the ethic of doing no harm (and also the ethic that it's right to report harm). If a child is injured by an abusive parent, and if a nurse has reason to know the child is abused (through an emergency room visit, perhaps) and does not report, the child can sue the nurse for subsequent injuries. Likewise, the nurse who fails to report a situation in which the patient is unjustifiably dehydrated, could face a criminal charge of failure to report neglect, along with the doctor and agency.

Applicable abuse statutes may be indexed in statute books under Abuse—Children, Adults, Minors, Disabled or Challenged (whatever euphemism the state uses). The nurse can find read the statute, or can assume that abuse of dependent patients is a crime and that reporting it is mandatory.

The nurse will not err in reporting abuse of a dependent patient to people who can help, if there is a reason to believe the dependent patient has been abused. A legal label for that ethical behavior is that nurses have a qualified immunity from liability when acting to protect the patient. Even if there is no statute requiring a report, the nurse's failure to report reasonably suspected abuse might be considered negligence for the purpose of a malpractice suit.

When the statute refers to some penalty for a crime such as abuse or failure to report abuse, it will say what "class" of felony or misdemeanor is the penalty. Searching an index of statutes, under Felony, will lead to the statute that specifies amount of jail time and/or fine imposed.

Intentionally Injured Adults

*Non*dependent adults who have been intentionally injured present less clear duties to the nurse. (The phrase "intentionally injured" is more specific than "abuse," which has been defined as loosely as "ignoring your feelings.")[8]

Patients who from history and physical exam appear to have been intentionally injured, should be questioned about the cause of the injury, treated, and offered referral (this is standard diagnosis, therapy, and prevention). Writings that suggest *all* patients be screened for intentional injuries may be inviting legal risks to the nurse or doctor by establishing an unnecessary standard.[9] Doctors and nurses should be aware of the statements, but as with any other recommendations from political entities, each must decide if there is evidence warranting a change in standard approach to diagnosis.

Some states require all "abuse" of adults be reported, including people intentionally injured. But in other states, involuntary reporting is considered to cause more danger to the injured. The nursing supervisor and nursing management, especially the emergency room department, should know the status of the state law (it changes year-to-year)—and the patient *must* be consulted.

Extreme caution should be used if the law requires reporting this injury without the patient's permission. In all cases, doctors and nurses should rigorously protect the patient's confidence and thoroughly document their actions.

Reporting Disease

> State statutes may require reporting of certain diseases, injuries, and crimes; in general, the rule is that any condition of the patient that could harm public safety needs reporting and probably is mandated by law.
>
> The professional (and legal) duty to protect the patient's confidentiality is a *qualified* duty; the patient's condition may be reported, only to the proper authorities, only as necessary to protect the public or the patient.

Other statutes also require reporting of certain diseases, injuries, and crimes. Specifics of the law may be available from agency management; the actual wording of statutes can be found from an index of the state statutes (possibly under the heading, Report Required).

Without specific knowledge of the law—but only with practice of the ethic that the public is served by doing no harm—nurses can assume the rule: Any condition of the patient that would be important to public safety should be reported to the proper authority. That rule might require reporting communicable disease (for instance, tuberculosis or AIDS); results of tests required by the state (phenylketonuria [PKU] in newborns); and evidence of crime (gunshot wounds, injuries from violence).

The professional (and legal) duty to protect the patient's confidentiality is a *qualified* duty; this means the patient's right to confidentiality is not absolute. The nurse may have a duty to report the condition, to the extent that is necessary to protect the public. The nurse has a qualified immunity from lawsuit or prosecution for revealing the patient's condition—but only to the proper authorities, and only as necessary to protect the public or the patient.

> *CAVEAT (Warning) About Reporting*: A practitioner may be sued for reporting to the *police* a child believed to be abused. The statute may require (and only protect) reporting to the *social welfare* or some other specific agency. Nurses who work in areas where suspected abuse is often encountered should get specifics on their state's statute from management or from the library's set of statutes.

ANTI-DUMPING

> The ethic of not harming patients is enforced by federal statute, which requires a hospital with an emergency department to stabilize the patient before transfer.

"Anti-dumping" is an inelegant name for good ethics: Don't harm patients who present to a hospital, by transferring them out to another hospital without stabilizing their condition. The resulting law which enforces the ethic, has had some unintended consequences, however. The federal Emergency Medical Transfer and Active Labor Act (EMTALA),[10] says that hospitals must:

1. Have policies that comply with the Act,
2. Maintain records for five years, of patients transferred out of the emergency department, and
3. Keep a list of physicians on call to provide treatment needed to stabilize emergency patients.

If the hospital has an Emergency Department (ED), it must provide an appropriate screening exam to see if a medical condition exists that needs stabilization. Regulations have been written to flesh out the requirements of the statute.

Regarding EMTALA, some questions have arisen:

When is the patient "in" the ED for purposes of the law? When in contact by car phone, or in the ambulance by radio contact? No.—If the patient is on the property, in the vehicle, the patient is "in" the ED.

What's a screening exam? A substandard result of the exam will produce liability.[11] In addition, maternal patients in labor also must be stabilized before transfer. The ED must either provide an exam and treat to stabilize, or transfer the patient.

If patient wants to leave, must the hospital still do the paperwork required in the law? The patient can go if the patient desires; refusal of treatment is valid if informed. The ED should get a signed written "informed refusal of treatment."

The patient can refuse to be transferred if the hospital offers transfer *and* explains the risks and benefits; nurses should document such a situation thoroughly.

The motive for "dumping" was once thought to be motivated by the patient's inability to pay; the EMTALA law would seek to remedy that harm. But the "dumping" does not have to be motivated by the patient's inability to pay, meaning that a charge of "dumping" can't be defended by explaining that the transfer wasn't because of the patient's insurance status.

Federal law may preempt state tort law (which requires negligence before a patient can recover). If so, a strict liability tort has been so created if the following evidence applies:

1. The patient went to the ER, *and*
2. The patient had an emergency condition, *and*
3. The patient did not get an adequate screen, *and*
4. the patient was discharged before stabilized, *and*
5. thereby damaged.

The possible *negligence* in that scenario is the failure of "adequate screen." and discharge before stabilization.

The EMTALA provides remedies (rights exist only where there are remedies for wrongs):

> *The patient can sue for tort in federal court.* This remedy may give rise to a new federal cause of action, beyond medical malpractice. The patient can also sue for medical malpractice under state law if negligence exists.
>
> *The government can assess fines against the providers,* up to $50,000 per violation. The hospital and doctor (and nurse) can be excluded from future Medicare and Medicaid payments. The hospital can lose federal building funds, and its tax-exempt status, because it is "not providing community benefit."

In its attempt to prevent harm to patients, this law presents potential danger to nurses. The nurses in the ER and Obstetrics (OB) departments should first remember the ethic that the law enforces: Doing No Harm to the patient by transferring without first stabilizing.[12]

More "Doing No Harm" Statutes

> Federal law enforces the value of doing no harm by encouraging practitioners to report information about medical devices that harm patients.

The Safe Medical Devices Act of 1990 is an effort in law to enforce the value, Doing No Harm by encouraging practitioners to report information about medical devices that harm patients. If a medical device caused or contributed to a patient's death, serious injury, or serious illness, the Food and Drug Administration (FDA) or its manufacturer should be notified. If providers (doctor and nurse) disagree about reporting, there are no *legal* penalties for not reporting, as of this writing. The *ethical* penalty for not reporting rests with the nurse, personally.

The FDA's regulation of the medical devices industry means that patients can't sue alleging failure to warn of possible injuries from medical devices. This is an example of federal law that is interpreted by the courts to be the only remedy in a field of law. Such law completely supplants state laws' remedies.

The FDA has been criticized as lax in enforcement, but its oversight sometimes shields companies that comply with the act from lawsuits based on state product liability grounds.

Laws about adult and child abuse, along with laws that mandate reporting, enforce two values: Being True (as Veracity) and Doing No Harm (Non-maleficence). Such statutes enforce both those values, just as a lawsuit for invasion of privacy enforces both those values (Confidentiality, not Veracity, in that case). (More discussion about the mechanism for reporting "serious adverse effects" due to drug and medical devices is included in Chapter Six, on laws enforcing the value, Being True.)

NON-MALEFICENCE IN RESEARCH

> In addition to the ethical values of doing no harm to the patient/subject, nursing and other scientific research upholds the value, Being True (Telling Truth above all).

Nursing research (and all scientific research) carries within it its own ethical values, in addition to the usual "first, do no harm" to the patient/subject. The researchers must first have sought the *truth*. To have validity, research must continually challenge whatever is the presently-believed knowledge. Greek pre-Socratics started the Western world's long chain of seeking truth, even at the cost of destroying their own and others' dearly-held dogma.

Challenging the status quo is the basis for furthering all science, including nursing science. Nursing science and nursing ethics do not progress (or even survive) if no position is ever taken that is adversary to the current knowledge and wisdom. Consensus in science, as in ethics or politics, represents a failure of leadership. In science, consensus is dead dogma.

The great philosopher of science, Karl Popper, asserted that humans can never *know* the truth. The idea of an absolute perfect truth is a mirage; any idea can be improved upon. The most that can be known is that a hypothesis can't *yet* be falsified. Instead of truth, scientists must settle for hypotheses that challenge, refine, falsify, and destroy the old truth.[13]

Research Concerns

> The values most important when dealing with subjects of research are doing no harm (non-maleficence) and telling the truth (veracity).
>
> U.S. federal law and regulations establish Institutional Review Boards (IRBs) to oversee research with federal funding; the review board's responsibility for oversight is to look at the purpose of the research in relation to protecting the subjects, and balance those interests.
>
> The terrible example of Germany's National Socialist government saw physicians and nurses freely participating in often horrible experiments on people who had not "consented," to say the least.
>
> Despite laws and ethical guidelines, the ultimate responsibility for ensuring ethical research practice rests with the individual investigator and the people who work in research.

Research practitioners know that the interests of subjects must be protected. The values of doing no harm (non-maleficence) and telling the truth (veracity) are paramount; don't harm the subject, if possible, and tell the subject the truth.

A U.S. syphilis research study, begun in the early 1930s, was not made public until the 1970s. Some patients in the study remained untreated for decades after penicillin was available to cure the disease. The failure to prevent harm to research subjects is the topic of the *Belmont Report*, which sets out ethical guidelines for research.[14] Currently, a federal law mandates that all experiments be reviewed by IRBs (discussed in Chapter One).

The review board's job is to look at the purpose of the research and to balance those purposes against protection of the subjects. Individual nurses involved in research also must balance interests: They must consider their own interest in participation in the research, and weigh it against their patient's interest in being protected from harm and in getting good care.

Awful examples of failure to protect subjects of research come from the era of the National Socialists in Germany (1930s to 1945). (Details of Nazi medical "research" is beyond this book's space, but much writing on the subject is readily available.) The rationale for Nazi practices was: Research is more important than subjects. Nurses should be aware that, under the National Socialist government, not only physicians but also nurses freely participated in horrible experiments on people whose consent was not sought. Such practices can never happen again—if people continue to remember that atrocities did happen, and that ordinary people became the perpetrators. It will never happen again if people determine that they as individuals will not allow such things to happen in their lifetimes.

Nurses, even those who are not involved in research, should know that the ethics of not harming subjects is reflected in the law. Making ethical decisions related to the protection of human participants in research can be complex—it is an art and not a science, fraught with uncertainty and conflict.[15]

To make ethical decisions about subjects of research, three thoughts provide a useful framework:

1. The value underlying all subject protection measures is doing no harm to the subject.
2. The basic principles outlined in the *Belmont Report* are about protecting the subject.
3. Federal regulations reflect the ethic of not harming.

The ultimate responsibility for ensuring ethical research practices rests with the individual investigator and the people who work with that person.

The main responsibility of the IRB is to protect the subject; to actually enforce, legally, the value of not harming. In most protocol review, that responsibility translates into making sure that the subject is informed and voluntarily consents to participate in the research. Consent by and for children and incompetents remains an ethical problem.

Consent to Research

> Consent to research involves the same principles as consent to treatment; the autonomy of the subject, along with freely-given, informed consent.
>
> Voluntary consent is the base of ethical research; if individuals cannot legally consent (children or incompetents), utmost care should be used both to protect the individual *and* their assent should be obtained when at all possible.
>
> The IRB and the researcher who adhere to the ethical mandate not to harm ensure that people at risk of coercion or undue influence are *in fact* not harmed.

Consent issues in research are generally the same as those related to treatment; however, they may be more complex because research may involve procedures not therapeutically necessary. And research participant-subjects may have less freedom of choice (autonomy). Some subjects are in the position of having only a choice between *experimental* therapy and *no* therapy.

Consent for research usually is better scrutinized than consent for treatment (for example, consent for surgery). The research consent process for each experimental program is reviewed by the IRB in advance of the procedure. In contrast, consent for usual treatment may never be reviewed, unless a malpractice action later is filed.

Often the researcher receives a fee for each patient enrolled in the research. Patients are usually unaware of how much the researcher will receive for their participation. (Whether patients should be told this information is an ongoing question.)

Sometimes patients receive a fee for participation, or parents receive a fee for allowing their child to participate—a questionable practice as it could be speculated then that the parent might not have the best interest of the child completely at heart. In addition to the parents' consent, the child's consent to research should be obtained, if at all possible. If the child is too young to understand what is happening, the investigator should explain those circumstances to the IRB. A suggested form would have, in simple language, "I Consent" and spaces for the child's signature (or mark, if the child can't write yet) and the parents' signature (or mark). The form should also allow space for the investigator to explain why the child's consent was not obtained, if that is the case.

As always, nurses should remember that the consent is a process in the mind; the paper form is merely evidence of the consent. Discussion of the use of children as research subjects is itself the subject of ongoing debate. Below is a suggested form for a child's consent to research, as modified from some in use in research protocols. This consent would be obtained in addition to the consent of the adult responsible for the child.

CHILD'S PERMISSION

"I understand why this research study is being done. I understand how it may help me or other children and what discomforts it may cause me. My questions have been answered. I want to take part in this study and I know that I can quit at any time."

Patient signature _____

The investigator (researcher) should sign the following:

"I have reviewed the contents of the Informed Consent Statement with _____ at a level appropriate to the level of his/her understanding, and I feel he/she understands these matters and their implications."

Investigator signature _____

The requirement for assent of the child is waived, because:

_____ The child is not capable of understanding an explanation.

_____ The procedure is important to the health and well-being of the child.

IRB Chairperson signature _____

(Required if assent of the child is waived)

Date _____

Incompetent Patient's Permission

If future research is done on bodies of persons in the "persistent vegetative state" and/or anencephalic babies, the permission of the next of kin may still be needed, just as permission to use cadavers is needed now.

All the major statements on research ethics stress the importance of the patient giving voluntary, fully informed consent (of course consent is not valid unless it *is* informed). Occasionally a guardian is allowed to give consent to do research on the incompetent. This is at least *in*consistent with the ethical standard of informed consent, but if the research protocol will benefit the guardian's ward, it may be acceptable.

Regulations outlining IRB procedures say that consent to research can be sought from the prospective subject *or* the subject's legally authorized representative. However, some written consents to treatment protocols allow signature by a "responsible person" who may or may not have any legal standing. If the research is minimally harmful, or there is anticipated benefit to the subject, this too may be acceptable; but the IRB must oversee the process.

The IRB and, in every case, the researcher must employ the ethical mandate not to harm, to ensure that people who are at risk of coercion or undue influence are in fact not harmed.

The principles outlined for children should also operate for people considered to be "like children" (insofar as they are dependent). Whatever their legal incapacity, such people can consent or refuse consent to the degree that they are able.[16]

Proposals are being made to use the bodies of persons in "persistent vegetative state" (PVS) for research; if so, their surrogate decision makers might be able to "volunteer" them for such use. Under such proposals, if anencephalic babies are also deemed "dead," their bodies might be used for research before cessation of pulse and respiration. If such proposals go forward, and people in PVS are declared dead, some recommend that consent might still be needed, just as consent from the next of kin is now required for organ retrieval.

Women in Research Studies

> Federal law and regulations require that women be "appropriately" represented in medical studies; research protocols that automatically exclude pregnant women may be in violation of such law.

As part of the National Institutes of Health Revitalization Act, signed into law in June 1993, the National Institutes of Health (NIH) requires that women be "appropriately" represented in the medical studies they fund and all study results must be analyzed by "gender." In addition, the act established a new agency to enforce the law. (Further information about the NIH Revitalization Act can be obtained from the Office of Research on Women's Health, National Institutes of Health, Building 1, Room 201, Bethesda, MD 20892.)

Pregnant Women in Research

Many research protocols automatically exclude pregnant women, whether or not the protocol is thought to be harmful to the fetus (teratogenic). This automatic exclusion may be considered discrimination on the basis of sex, since only women may become pregnant.

The beneficent rationale for such exclusion is to protect the fetus; but in application the exclusion of pregnant women from protocols may in fact be destructive to the fetus. A potential subject, informed that she cannot go on a protocol because she is pregnant, may choose to abort or choose to continue the pregnancy to term, delivering a baby whose mother is then at greater risk of death. Neither outcome is beneficent for the fetus/baby.

Allowing the pregnant woman on the protocol may indeed put the fetus at risk, but possibly at less risk than either of the two scenarios above. Not all treatments on protocols are teratogenic. Some would argue that a fetus and parent are better off if the fetus is aborted, better than being born with a defect. Such reasoning, however, substitutes for the values of both the parent and the potentially disabled (but alive) child. Researchers have no right and no legal authority to make such value choices for research subjects. The IRB has a general obligation to prevent researchers from engaging in discrimination and imposition of personal values on potential subjects.

The law does not require pregnant women to be excluded from research protocols that are potentially teratogenic; in fact, the law may require that women *not* be arbitrarily excluded on the basis of their sex/pregnancy.[17]

Should Quality Assurance Projects Be Reviewed by IRBs?

Some have suggested that Quality Assurance (QA) projects (projects likened to research in that patients' rights/confidentiality may be at risk) should be examined regularly by IRBs, just as they oversee research protocols to protect the rights of human subjects. They believe that all prospective QA projects should go to an IRB, just as all scientific clinical research projects do. IRBs are also urged to develop faster and better review of programs.[18]

The data gathered by QA projects are tempting sources of raw material for scientific analysis and investigation by researchers. It is asserted that proposals to access that data should be examined in advance by IRBs to protect the subjects' rights, to prevent the investigator from doing harm rather than good, and to enhance the ethical credibility of the projects. In addition, having IRB approval for access to data might help protect the investigator from possible lawsuit.

Ownership of Tissue

John Moore, surveyor on the Alaskan Pipeline, sought medical treatment for leukemia from an oncologist at UCLA. His spleen, which had grown from one-half pound to 14 pounds, was removed, and Moore's health improved.

Moore's doctor isolated and cultured a cell line from the spleen, a line that could produce several products. The doctor patented the cell line in 1984. The issue arising from the Moore case[19] is whether the removed spleen is considered as useless garbage or as still belonging to Moore, with rights to the profits from the cells. The question is: What should the doctor get for the work, without which the spleen would have been worthless?

Controversy continues over who owns the products of research. Mr. Moore had consented to research but said he had checked "no" in the box on the form that asked whether he granted ownership of the cells. The Moore case gave potential compensation and some interest in the profits to the man whose tissue was used in the research.

The case is a good example of the need to beware of total reliance on consent forms. As part of the consent process, patients should be informed if their tissue will be used and whether they will have rights to share in profits from the use—and this should be reflected on the consent form.

Finders' Fees for Research Subjects

Another controversy is about the payment of finders' fees for residents or other practitioners who identify and refer patients to researchers. Such fees range from $50 to $350. Researchers say the fees are justified by the difficulty of finding suitable patients for protocols. Some believe the use of such fees will influence "finders" to persuade patients to enroll in research projects regardless of the value to the patient.[20] A related question is whether patients should be told how much the researcher is being compensated for each patient enrolled in a study.

Animal Research

> Research and experiments using animals raise issues and reflect values we hold and apply also to people labeled less than human.

Research using animals is controversial, too (beyond the scope of this book); those interested in the range of controversy can easily find information elsewhere.[21] Some of the issues raised in research using animals reflect values that may be applied to people less "human" (more "vegetable"). Thus, animal research issues are more than interesting—they become directly relevant to humans. Nurses should be, and probably are aware that different parties have differing interests.

The interests of humans are in having research that produces the best drugs, techniques, and illness care for humans.[22] (Some of the research benefits animals, too.) Animals have "interests" in life and being free of pain. Controversy arises as to whether and how humans value (or don't value) animals, and whether humans have the right to dominate other species.

Research in animal behavior itself reveals more intelligence and "feeling" than was previously suspected—and perhaps more than some wanted to know. Humans can impose their will on other living creatures. The question is whether the power makes the right. Do humans have only a responsibility to other humans, to use whatever resources they have to promote only the human species' survival and well-being?[23]

The more "intelligent" the animal, like dolphins, the more they seem like humans. That "human-ness" makes any "use" of them worse, to some. Intelligence (brain function) is a valued condition, in animals and in humans. "Cute-ness" and rarity are also valued conditions or traits—baby seals being saved as often because they're cute as because they're endangered.

However, *if* they were as common as rabbits, and more of a "pest," would it be OK to kill them? Some humans worry more about the living conditions of veal calves than the dying conditions of old cows.

Rabbits are considered vermin in Australia—to say the least, their "rights" to life in Australia are suspect, along with many other "non-native" species. Whether dingoes are "native" has yet to be decided, and even the aboriginal *people* are not indigenous to Australia, having arrived about 40,000 years ago.

When it comes to some animals, however, a visitor from a foreign planet might believe the human species values some other animal species more than its own—the visitor might perceive a subtle form of self-hatred at work. Indeed, if it concentrated on some human laws, might the alien visitor conclude that humans value baby seals more than baby humans?

Environmental Ethics

Further ethical issues arise when the environment is threatened in order to provide illness treatment. Related issues are apparent when a threat to the environment is seen to cause illness. An obvious example is the use of the bark of a rare species of yew tree to extract an anti-cancer drug. The lives of women with breast cancer are weighed against the killing of all the yew trees; the lives of yew trees might be preserved at the cost of women's lives. Will the search for ethical compromise yield a ratio, say X number of trees per life saved?

A utilitarian argument is implicit in the yew tree issue: that it is OK to lose some individuals (trees or women) for the greater good. But such an all-or-nothing argument is rarely useful (ironically, *not* utilitarian). The "good news" for women and yew trees is that technology (a dreaded concept to some) has produced a taxol analog to the yew extract that can be produced without killing trees.

Health risks to and within the environment are major issues. Is the value, Autonomy (the individual's Freedom), to be compromised for a small decrease in risk to many (the good of many citizens)? Is it ethical to prohibit all smoking, when smoking causes health risk to a relative few?

LICENSURE

Licensure, the most important state statute for nurses, enforces the value of doing no harm and punishes failure to uphold the value of doing good, by seeking to assure that only capable people perform tasks that might harm.

State government has the power to license (the power to regulate practice was not granted to the federal government in the Constitution; the power was reserved to the states by the Tenth Amendment).

Licensure creates a monopoly (granted and maintained by government), which restricts the supply of services only to the group of people licensed.

The monopoly is justified if the safety (prevention of harm) of the public is valued as more important than the freedom of the unlicensed person to nurse or the patient's freedom to choose an unlicensed nurse.

> Licensure supplants the information-gathering function for the individual, in that the state functions as a "market," inquiring as to the education and ability of the practitioner.

The licensure statute in any state has enormous importance for nurses. The statute enforces the value emphasized in this chapter, Doing No Harm, as well as punishing failure to uphold the value and mandate of nurses' Doing Good for patients. Licensure law proposes to assure that only capable people perform acts that could potentially harm patients.

> ### CONTACTING THE STATE LICENSURE AUTHORITY
> To contact the state board for nursing, nurses may call information at the state capital or larger cities and ask for the number; that office will have the name of the executive director and the address. Nurses can ask for an annotated copy of the nursing law and regulations during the call, or they may write to the state board for nursing, at the address obtained.

Nursing education is addressed under Doing No Harm also, since licensure law enforces educational minimums and, in some states, continuing education requirements as well. The law of licensure enforces a minimum ethic, not to harm.[24] Because of their potential to harm patients (and to do good for them as well), nurses must be licensed, in all 50 states. Other illness workers, such as x-ray technicians, are not licensed in all states (although almost all technician groups seek licensure status). Each state has a somewhat different nurse licensure law, but all the laws have similar provisions.

Purpose of Licensure

The general purpose of licensure laws is to protect the public from harm (as much as can be) by ensuring that practitioners are qualified to do good and not harm the patient. That purpose, however, is limited: The laws are not written to protect the people in the licensed occupation from competition, or to limit the practice of nurses, or to advance the profession of nursing. The legislatures, not the profession, decide what laws are necessary to protect the people. The legislatures' purpose is to protect the people, not the profession.

Licensure law promotes the values of doing good and doing no harm, by protecting the public. The licensure law enforces a minimum ethic; it establishes minimum standards for practice, and probably can do no more. Although permitting only those who can pass a test to practice may prevent some harm, as in all law "enforcement," licensure law cannot safeguard the public from *all* harm; the law acts to punish after harm has been done (to remove from practice a person who has harmed).

Effect of Licensure

Licensure in the United States is regulated by state governments as one of those powers reserved to the states by the Tenth Amendment of the U.S. Constitution. Who is to be licensed, how, with what qualifications, to practice what—all are determined by state law, not federal law, because the power regulate practice was not granted to the federal government.

Licensure creates a monopoly that restricts the supply of services to those licensed; the monopoly is granted and maintained by the state government. Economists assert that a monopoly can persist only if it is maintained by force (by government power)—a monopoly in the private sector will sooner or later be destroyed by competition, but the state can use its enforcement power to maintain the monopoly as long as wanted.

In the case of licensure, a person who practices nursing will compete with other people also practicing. If a person has the knowledge and the ability to nurse, but not the required license (the monopoly permit), the government can prevent that person's work—by physical force, if necessary. Some nursing licensure statues, for example, provide misdemeanor or felony penalties for people who violate the law. Conviction could mean jail time or fines, so the monopoly is preserved through threat or actual force of the state (the en*force*ment of the statute).

In general, licensure law restricts the freedom of the person to work and restricts the freedom of the patient freely to hire a caregiver. The freedom of individuals to make contracts with each other is diminished, since a citizen cannot hire an *un*licensed person to be a nurse (even a person known from experience to be educated and competent).

The premise of licensure is that the hirer is unable to judge nurse expertise in practice. A consequence of the law is that a person who is educated and competent to nurse cannot contract to do nursing without the proper license.

The reason given for enforcing the monopoly is the safety (good) of the public. The value of doing good, in that instance is more important than the freedom of the unlicensed person to nurse, and more important than the patient's freedom to choose an unlicensed nurse.

Such state paternalism is justified if it is assumed that the public cannot know, from the usual marketplace sources, whether or not the practitioner *is* safe. With licensure, the state government takes over the information-gathering function for the individual. Thus, the state functions as a market, inquiring as to the education and ability of the practitioner.

The state then prohibits practice by any person not meeting the standards of education and ability, by not licensing that person to practice in the monoply. And the the state's agents prosecute unlicensed practice when found. But prosecution specifically for "nursing without a license" is very unlikely, unless the practitioner labels her or himself by the title "Registered" or "Practical Nurse."

INTENDED AND UNINTENDED CONSEQUENCES OF LICENSURE

Licensing of sheltered-care facilities is intended to protect people who live there; but it also creates problems of bureaucracy and a welter of regulations. In Illinois, for example, an elderly couple living in such a facility must get permission from the Department of Public Health to sleep in same bed.

Requiring licensure of such board-and-care facilities is said to prevent people from getting needed service. Unlicensed providers assert that they charge less than the amount charged by licensed facilities and could save the people/taxpayers money, while offering a homelike setting for patients. The state nurses association opposes relaxing licensure standards on safety grounds.

Some economists say that state monopoly of licensure keeps care expensive by preventing competition by less expensive caregivers, which would ultimately lower cost to the customer. As concern for the high cost of care rises, this aspect of licensure will receive more attention.

Doctors and nurses wish to delegate actions only when it is economically advantageous to them; maintaining a state-enforced monopoly to give certain kinds of care, keeps the numbers of competitors to a minimum. Nurses seek to protect patients, and to limit competition, when they resist practice by physician's assistants, LPNs, technicians, and paramedics. Use of statutes to prevent competition is expensive and state manipulation of the market encourages doctors and nurses to seek to define practice through law, not through scientific innovation and experimentation.

The effect of state-granted monopoly like licensure increases cost to the public, decreases access to the service, and thus increases the money for nurses. The intended consequence of licensure was protection of the public (enforcing Doing No Harm).

There is evidence that licensure fails to accomplish its *intended* consequence, to prevent harm and to punish harm done to patients.

EXAMPLE OF FAILURE TO PREVENT HARM

A nursing home in Texas has had a second round of deaths of medically handicapped children in its care.

Two years previous, the nursing home nearly lost its Medicaid funding after the suspicious deaths of 12 disabled children. (Many of them had not been resuscitated after going into respiratory arrest.)

At that time, the government agency charged with protecting the children by licensing the home, required the home to "train its staff, buy emergency life-saving equipment and rewrite its policies."

Two years later, two more children died after a nurse admitted turning off the alarm of the respiratory monitor. Again, the home was to "lose its Medicaid funds if it does not impose new safety measures." The home was found responsible for the nurse's actions, and may be fined up to $5,000.

Despite the presence of licensure law covering the nurses and nursing home, and many inspections and warnings, these children died.[25]

In addition to or in place of licensure, other forces may protect the public from unqualified practitioners. One force, educating people to the differences between practitioners, would allow the public access to people who will do the work, regardless of credentials. The pressure of an educated and informed public will enforce practitioner quality. Another force, the fear of malpractice, also helps keep abuses to a minimum; in situations in which caregivers are not licensed, no more harm has been documented than where licenses are mandated.

Voluntary standards, such as those of the JCAHO and insurance companies, are also a means of maintaining quality of care. The agencies in which doctors and nurses practice also require credentials and proof of quality work (references, experience, education) before they admit doctors to their staff or nurses to their employment. These forces may offer protection and guarantee patient safety more than licensure.

Credentialing

Legal credentialing is the broad term for credentialing mandated by law; nonlegal credentialing is voluntary.

The law of licensure protects the practice; the law of registration protects the title.

All 50 states require licensure (not merely registration), but from past practice, licensed nurses are still called *registered* nurses. Practical nurses are correctly designated as licensed.

The broad term for licensure and other versions of legal monopoly is "legal credentialing." Nonlegal credentialing is voluntary (not mandated by law). When doctors obtain credentials as specialists (as board-certified), they do not go through a legal process but a private one, regulated by private organizations. This is also true of nurses who get additional certification.

Licensure is different from certification by a private association or agency, but confusing the issue is the action by some licensure boards to use certification by private associations as a requirement for *licensure* as a nurse specialist. When a state agency allows a private group, such as the ANA or the nurse practitioner association, to certify, the agency lends state authority and responsibility for credentialing to a nonpublic entity. This is true of the use of any test not made by the state, even the NCLEX (the acronym for the basic licensure test for nurses used in all states).

Legally enforced credentialing is generally called licensure or, perhaps, registration. Laws that register or title practitioners designate only that the title be protected—that certain people, with certain education *or* (in some cases) competence, are registered or certified and have a protected title. The practice of what they *do* is not prohibited to anyone else, only the use of the title.

The purpose of a registration law, from the public's view, is to inform the public that this person has certain qualifications. The purpose, from the nurse's view, is an economic one: that people will choose the titled over nontitled. Even in "mandatory" licensure laws for nurses, the title is the thing protected (since licensure boards rarely prosecute for practicing nursing without a license, unless the individual has also used the title).

Titling and registration laws are considered the first step to restrictive mandatory licensure. Registration laws are permissive credentialing—one *may* be registered, but not mandated to be registered, to do the work. The next, more restrictive step is mandatory credentialing—licensure—meaning that one must be licensed in order to practice. No one, other than the person licensed, is permitted that particular practice.

Sometimes an incorrect distinction is made between "mandatory" and "permissive" licensure; using the term licensure implies that it *is* mandatory. "Permissive" licensure should not really be classed as licensure, but rather, as such registration. Such distinction is a moot point in nursing—there is no "permissive licensure" for RNs. All 50 states require licensure, not merely registration. From the past, when nurses were registered (title alone protected) and not licensed (practice protected), licensed nurses still are called *registered* nurses. Practical nurses attained licensure status later; they are correctly designated as "licensed."

Common Provisions of Licensure Laws

Licensure statutes generally have provisions that involve definitions, prohibition of unlicensed practice, minimum qualifications for licensure, minimum curricula for schools of nursing, examination for licensure, exceptions from the requirement for licensure, establishment of boards of nursing, and reasons the board can discipline the license.

Licensure statutes generally include the following kinds of provisions:

1. Definitions. Definitions tell what the words in the statute mean; one of the words defined in nurse licensure statutes, for instance, is "nursing." Usually there will also be some broad explanation like "practice, for compensation, requiring education, judgment and skill based on certain sciences." The sciences may be listed (biological, physical, nursing sciences), along with a list of examples of what nursing "acts" are.

The statute may define specific types of nurses: practical, registered, nurse practitioner, nurse anesthetist, nurse midwife, clinical nurse specialist. The qualifications for those specialties may also be listed.

In nurse licensure laws the definition of nursing has changed since the 1970s, to remove requirements that nurses practice under the supervision of physicians. Ironically, as nurses perform more independently as nurse practitioners, advanced practice nurses, and nurse clinical specialists, the legal requirements for their practice usually include that they practice in collaboration with a physician. ("Collaboration," more often than not, is interpreted as "supervision.")

Further discussion of licensure for nurses in independent practice is found in Chapter Four, Freedom, since those nurses are considered more autonomous than others.

Nurses who want to make changes in their state nursing law, or want them modeled after what elected officials of the ANA suggest, can obtain the proposed language of state legislation from the ANA, in a model Nursing Practice Act, a Nursing Disciplinary Diversion Act, and a Prescriptive Authority Act.[26]

2. Prohibitions of unlicensed practice. State statute will say that anyone who hasn't been licensed may not *be* a nurse or practice a specific type of nursing. Such a prohibition against unauthorized practice is *licensure*, and it is different from *registration*. Registration merely protects a title, not an activity. (See above, under Credentialing.)

3. Minimum qualifications for licensure. Another section of the licensure statute lists the qualifications required for licensure as an RN and as an LPN (LVN in Texas). At present, all states except North Dakota use the same exam for graduates of the three different kinds of educational programs—associate degree, diploma, and BSN. (Changes have been proposed; see under Educational Entry Level for Licensure.)

4. Minimum curricula for schools of nursing. The nursing licensure statute (or regulations written under that law) may require the minimum curriculum for schools of nursing. Statutes or boards may define the minimum qualifications of school faculty, needed if a school is to be accredited by the state to prepare nurses to take the nursing licensure examination. Such specific requirements may not be written in the statute passed by the legislature but, instead, may be authorized in the statute, and actually written by an administrative body, the board of nursing. Regulations must be published in a state listing of regulations, in order to become law.

5. Examinations for licensure. Nurses in all states now take the same exam, the NCLEX. Graduates of foreign nursing schools may have to take the CGFNS (Commission on Graduates of Foreign Nursing Schools) exam before they take the NCLEX. Such uniform testing enables states to make some provision for licensure by "endorsement." Endorsement is the process of having the nurse's original state endorse the application for licensure in a new state, along with providing test scores. The nurse's original state of licensure endorses the nurse's status to a state to which she or he has moved; the nurse who graduated before the NCLEX was in use may have to prove that her original education was equivalent to that required in the new state at the time of original graduation.

The term "reciprocity" is properly used only if two states have a reciprocal agreement to honor one another's licensure; that is, if Alabama licensed Florida nurses on condition that Florida licensed Alabama nurses. This arrangement is common in lawyer licensing and other occupations, and it may be useful for new kinds of nurses like nurse practitioners, whose licensure requirements are not the same in all states.

A standard nationwide exam was pioneered by nurses; few other occupations have such a system. With a standard exam, nurses have the freedom to move from state to state and gain licensure easily, so problems of distribution of nurses are more easily met. When one area of the country has fewer nurses or more patients (supply of labor goes down), nurses can be compensated more (demand for labor goes up) and nurses will increasingly move to those areas.

6. Exemptions to licensing requirements. The licensure statute usually lists exemptions from the provisions of the law. In physician statutes, many other *licensed* occupations (such as nurses, physician assistants, pharmacists, etc.) are exempted from being required to be licensed as doctors. But in nurse statutes, often many *un*licensed people are exempted from needing a nursing license to "nurse."

Usually exempted: Nursing done by student nurses, by nurses travelling with patients, nursing done for free or in homes, or by Christian Scientists. If, however, the intent of a licensure statute really is to protect the public (with no economic effect), then the unlicensed would not be allowed to give potentially unsafe care, even for free. Although monopoly by licensure statute can affect patients, exemptions mean nursing licensure statutes aren't entirely monopolistic in practice. The many exceptions to the requirement for licensure can turn nurse *licensure* statutes into more nearly *registration* statutes: Only the person "licensed" (more like registered) can use the title, but anyone can perform the function—the practice.

7. Establishing boards of nursing. The statute will provide for a board, or some other agency, to administer the law. The board of nursing then writes regulations to implement state licensure statutes. Such boards write rules about how they'll inspect and certify schools of nursing, for example; and they may list the specific functions permitted a nurse practitioner or other nurses.

The statute may also grant other powers to the board, depending on what the statute authorizes. The licensure statute will say who will be on the board (what kind of people: LPNs, RNs, lay members) and who appoints the members of the board and how (usually the state's governor has that power).

The board will be authorized, either specifically or implicitly, to grant the nurse's license, suspend or deny renewals of the license, and perhaps give temporary licenses. The law should say what reasons the board may use to deny renewal or revocation of license; this section of the law should most concern nurses since it most directly endangers their careers.

8. Disciplining the license. Most licensure laws list "unprofessional conduct" or "professional misconduct" as one possible reason for disciplining the license. In an extreme example, a license can be lost for neglecting to file an income tax return, a crime of "moral turpitude."

A nurse in Massachusetts challenged that state's requirement appearing on the renewal application form, that nurses swear they have filed state income taxes; the Massachusetts Supreme Court ruled she had to swear to that, even if it had nothing to do with safe nursing practice.[27]

Other examples considered by nursing boards to be professional misconduct include advising a patient of a cancer treatment alternative the the patient's doctor opposed (see the *Tuma* case, below); and giving patients needed and ordered morphine from another patient's supply (the "hospice six" example, below). In a more recent case a nurse lost her license for "unprofessional conduct" because, after much deliberation, consultation, and an independent assessment, she did not report her coworker for misappropriating drugs.[28] As an example, the Texas nursing board defines "unprofessional" and says the rules they made are intended to protect clients and the public from "incompetent, unethical, or illegal" conduct of licensees. The Texas board does have authority over *illegal* conduct, and *incompetent* conduct should also be illegal; but *unethical* conduct is not necessarily incompetent or illegal. Ethics covers higher optional actions than the minimum legal safe practice.

The Texas board further says the purpose of the definition and rule making about professional conduct is to identify behaviors of the RN (Texas has a separate board for LVNs) that the board believes are likely to "deceive, defraud or injure clients or the public." Some bad behaviors are actually listed, but others *not on the list* can also be punished. Most licensure boards, for example, have the power to discipline a nurse's license because of failure to blow the whistle on a colleague.[29]

EXAMPLE OF THE EXPANSION OF BOARD POWER

The Missouri Board of Nursing sought to establish broader power to discipline nurses by "assisting the chemically dependent or recovering nurse through monitoring without the potential negative implications often associated with disciplinary measures." The board proposed to monitor the nurse beyond mere abstinence from the drug; not only the nurse's actions, but the mind of the licensee would be monitored in assessing "recovery mindedness." Further, they hoped to be able to identify the behaviors of such a "recovery minded person" in addition to abstinence from drugs (demonstrating the right attitude according to the board).[30]

"Professional misconduct" is a catchall phrase that can be used unfairly by boards. It may be useful, however, in that it covers many situations without the need of specifying them, for example: patient abuse, negligence, falsifying records, endangering patients, abandoning patients, and violating confidentiality. The more clearly a nurse's action violates expected and usual standards of professional conduct, the more likely a court is to uphold a board's discipline of the nurse's license on grounds of "professional misconduct." The practice makes the ethics, which the law enforces.

In addition to unprofessional conduct, the licensure law lists other behaviors that can cost the nurse her license to practice. Although the law varies state to state, other common reasons are: obtaining a license through fraud (lying on the application), incompetence, and addiction. Nurses can be disciplined for abusing drugs if their drug abuse endangers their patients or affects their practice.

It is not certain that private actions that do not affect the nurse's competence may be used to discipline the license. If so, such "status crimes" (for example, being a person who drinks alcohol or smokes) could be cause for discipline, even if the behavior did not affect nursing practice.

Drug abuse is the single largest reason that nurse licenses are disciplined; but discipline for drugs will be more difficult after passage of the Americans with Disabilities Act (ADA), discussed further in Chapter Five. State licensure laws all give the boards established, the power to deny licensure because of drug addiction (also described as drugs, chemicals, substances: intoxicating and illegal; substance abuse, use, dependence). The Texas statute mandates that each agency employing at least ten nurses have a nursing peer review committee that must notify the board if a nurse is impaired or likely is impaired by chemical dependency. Certain provisions of the federal Americans with Disabilities Act protect persons with disabilities, out of which may ensue conflict with the state licensure boards.

LICENSURE/ADA CONFLICT

A court might find that nursing boards can't investigate nurses who reveal past drug abuse or psychological problems; imposing extra (unnecessary) burdens on qualified individuals with disabilities would seem to be prohibited by the Americans with Disabilities Act.

Contesting the Board's Decision

The judgment of whether nurse conduct is unprofessional is necessarily subjective, but the board must act in accord with due process.[31]

Licensure board decisions can be reviewed in court; the board must have complied with the nurse's right to due process and the state's administrative procedure act.

Due process includes, at minimum, notice of charges, the right to defend against the charges, and unbiased decision makers.

Licensure board decisions can be reviewed in court (with some difficulty). The board's findings of fact (their decision and the facts that are the bases) are analogous to the initial tribunal or court in the legal system in that the findings of fact are given great weight if appealed to the courts—the reason being that the board has personally heard the live witnesses and personally seen the evidence. The appeals court can only review the case from the cold paper record.

The weight given to board decision is the same credence (belief) given to the trial courts' findings on appeal to higher courts. The appellate court will not always agree with the board, but the board starts with some advantage over the nurse who appeals a board's decision.

Full discussion of how nurses can contest administrative decisions is found in Chapter One, under Administrative Law. Such information is useful when boards go beyond enforcing the law of minimum safe practice, to enforcing "ethical behavior." In the now well-known *Tuma* case,[32] an Idaho nurse believed she should discuss with a patient a therapy that the doctor had not mentioned. The nurse was disciplined by the Idaho nursing board for unprofessional conduct.

The *Tuma* case is known only because the nurse appealed the Idaho board's discipline of her license and won. That appeal took several years, much money, anguish, and publicity. Thousands of other cases in which boards find unprofessional conduct are never appealed.

Another "unprofessional conduct" allegation: A Texas nurse who did not document drug administration on the 24-hour flow sheet—*instead of or in addition to* the medication sheet, had her license revoked (several other faults were also alleged) by the Board of Nurse Examiners. The nurse appealed that board's decision to court, and also won.[33] Good practice (here, minimum safe practice of charting drugs in only one place) was also upheld as minimally lawful.

THE "HOSPICE SIX"—NURSES WHO CONTESTED A BOARD

Six hospice nurses began to keep a stock of extra doses of narcotics, mostly morphine suppositories, donated by families of deceased patients. The nurses gave morphine only after a doctor's order—but sometimes out of their illicit stockpile, because there was no all-night pharmacy. Sometimes the stockpile was used for patients without money; once for a patient who couldn't swallow liquid morphine.

A nurse told the supervisor about the stockpile, and the supervisor reported it to the Board of Nursing in Montana (under some state law the supervisor could be disciplined had she not reported). The Board placed the six nurses on probation for unprofessional conduct, for periods ranging from three to five years.

The nurses appealed the Board's action in court.

A district court judge said the violations were "procedural, rather than substantive" and ordered the board to reduce its discipline to letters of reprimand. (The Board's appeal of the judge's decision to the Montana Supreme Court was rejected.)

The ethics and therefore the law require nurses to do good to the patient and not to harm the patient. Unless the above "stockpiling" would in some way harm, the doing good that was intended should fulfill the ethic. The law should enforce only that minimum. Although the nurses "broke the law" in the eyes of the board of nursing, eventually they were found to have committed only a technical violation, warranting only a warning. In this case the nurses did good to patients, and they did not harm patients—and both are ethical *and* substantially legal.[34]

The experiences of Florida nurses accused of violating their Nurse Practice Act (the agency found that they had probably violated the law) are revealing. The nurses had a hearing, but unlike nurses who have fought their sentences, these were eventually required to comply with some order from the board of nursing that disciplined them.

Researchers believe nurses experience a transformation of professional identity, with the five phases of the change consisting of being confronted, assuming a stance, going through it, living the consequences, and re-visioning themselves.[35] The difference from the "hospice" case and *Tuma* is that these Florida nurses were all deemed "guilty"—that they didn't (or couldn't) defend themselves and maintain their first vision of themselves as "innocent."

Nurses do have some protections against unfair use of power by boards under both state and national constitutional requirements for due process, as well as under state and federal administrative procedure acts.

Administrative Procedure Act

State law will include some kind of administrative procedure act, which specifies just how the board may investigate, prosecute, and judge a complaint filed. Decisions of administrators may be wrong, so an appeal after final board action can be made to the court system (due process).

The constitutional guarantee of due process, from both the Fifth and Fourteenth Amendments of the Bill of Rights, provides that the licensee must be treated fairly (justly)—which includes:

1. adequate notice of charges;
2. a chance to defend, including the right to a lawyer; *and*
3. a right to unbiased decision makers.

Nurses who are the subject of an investigation by the licensing board should get legal help immediately; they must not volunteer anything (records or answers or remarks), must not believe the investigators are friends, and must obtain a lawyer who specializes in administrative law, defending people in similar situations. The state nurses association at the capital, the state bar association, or the nurse's personal lawyer can help find such an expert.

Licensure investigations are serious. (Being innocent is not a guarantee of a good outcome, and malpractice insurance will not cover the cost.) The consequences could be far worse and linger for longer than a malpractice suit—beyond money, the nurse could lose a career.

Liabilities of Licensure

> State legislatures may use licensure laws for other purposes than protecting the public.

State legislatures may see an opportunity to solve money problems by using the licensure laws. The increased cost of illness care (from increasing demands caused by increased use of indirect payment) has caused legislators in some states to shift the cost of care for Medicaid by including in licensure requirements mandatory free labor in behalf of Medicaid patients. A Massachusetts law requires doctors to accept assignment for Medicare patients (to accept a minimum fee as full payment and not bill the patient more); the same has occurred in West Virginia. These laws have been upheld in court as being reasonable actions on the part of legislatures.[36]

The court's test as to whether that kind of law is fair was not based on whether the requirement is related to the safe practice by the practitioner, but whether the action of the lawmakers in any way related to the problem seen by lawmakers; the court asked the question: Does the lawmaker's action have *any* rational basis? If the answer is yes, the law stands.

EXAMPLE OF THE RATIONAL BASIS TEST

A Massachusetts nurse objected to a question on her license renewal form that asked whether she'd paid her state taxes. The appeals court said that the question was a legitimate one for the state to ask (had a rational basis). Failing to pay taxes—or, in this case, to answer questions about them—is relevant to licensure.[37]

Lawmakers can grant a benefit (the a state-enforced monopoly of services) when they license nurses. They may, however, be charging a price: One edge of the licensure sword may cut out any competition from the uneducated/unsafe/unlicensed people—the other edge of the sword may cut the licensed.[38]

Government may make of licensure law enforcement a "sword" by tying other work requirements to licensure, requirements that have nothing to do with the safety of the public or competence to practice.

Is licensure an illusion? The fundamental reason for licensure is not only to protect the safety of (prevent harm to) the public. Legislatures also know licensure to be an economic tool that can keep competition down (keep supply of practitioners low so demand stays high). Nurses may reap the economic benefit of a state-granted monopoly, but some states may ask them to pay dearly for that monopoly.

Licensure Records

Nurse managers have a work duty and usually a legal duty to maintain records of the licensure of their nurse employees. This legal responsibility would be an enforcement of the ethical duty to assure (as nearly as possible) that people hired are competent to do good to the patient (the ultimate responsibility of the nurse manager). Maintaining such records has the added benefit of reducing risk of liability in a lawsuit brought under the theory of corporate or personal liability, alleging incompetency of staff employed. Again, the underlying value enforced by malpractice law is to do good to the patient and to protect from harm. Nurse managers may use whatever technology is efficient and appropriate to meet that record-keeping duty, keeping in mind the value that the practitioner also is owed a duty: confidentiality of records.[39]

The legal enforcement of the ethical value to prevent harm to the patient, is to keep good records on the staff's education and licensure. This mandate may rise to the level of a licensure requirement for nurse managers (in Texas, standards of practice require nurse managers to set up strategies to see that staff are licensure-compliant).

National Practitioner Data Bank

> Federal law enforces the values, Doing Good and Doing No Harm, by collecting and making available information about "bad" doctors (and nurses).

The National Practitioner Data Bank is the result of a federal law, the Health Care Quality Improvement Act, that enforces the values of doing good and doing no harm to the patient in a way somewhat similar to licensure laws. The National Practitioner Data Bank seeks to collect information about "bad" doctors (and nurses), in one place, so that practitioners who harm patients can be tracked. The problem the Data Bank was created to remedy was that state boards and hospitals could not readily find out that a doctor (or nurse) had been in trouble in another state; the perceived need was for a national bank of data on these people.

Such law has negative implications for the ethics of confidentiality: In the case of the Data Bank, the secrets are mainly those of the practitioner, not the patient. In some cases, it might be the patient who wants to know the practitioner's secrets kept by the federal government. The law creates a federal repository of data on malpractice payments and adverse actions taken against the clinical privileges and licenses of *all* practitioners (nurses, too). Disciplinary banks have existed before,[40] but this one is national; and a reform proposal by the Clinton Administration would have made all the data in the bank available to the public.

The National Data Bank mandates specific reporting requirements: When, for example, any money is paid out on a malpractice action (whether settlement preceded trial, or was the result of a verdict), it is to be reported. Any discipline by the employer that affects nursing practice must also be reported (this could be a medication error that resulted in supervised medication administration). And, further, any action against the nurse by a state board must be reported.

Agencies must inquire of the Data Bank before admitting doctors or nurse practitioners to staff. If nurse specialists associate with hospitals or nursing homes as consultants, it can be foreseen that those agencies will also have to check the Data Bank before affiliation. State boards can get full reports of prior data on individual nurses who may have been subject to discipline.

Practitioners will be notified when reports are made and will be given the opportunity to correct errors, if any, in the reports.[41]

The Data Bank will also require reports from insurance companies, but only when money is paid on a claim. Many states have statutes that require insurers to report not only when money is paid, but even when a malpractice claim is *filed* against the licensee—a practice that can result in continuing investigation by the practitioner's board, even if the malpractice claim was frivolous and later dismissed.[42]

The Ethics and Law of Nurse Education

> Licensure law mandates the minimum educational level and (in some states) the minimum continuing education for nurses.
>
> The ethical values of doing good (beneficence) and doing no harm (non-maleficence) underlie the licensure laws that require educating professionals to a level of competence, and maintaining that competence.
>
> Education is used as the standard for practitioner entry into practice (instead of using competence or knowledge) because education is more easily measured.

The ethics and law of nurse education is discussed with licensure, since licensure is the law that mandates the minimum educational level and (in some states) the minimum continuing education nurses must have in order to practice.

Professionals are educated to make them good at their practice; they must to be good at their practice, for the good of their patients and in order not to harm them. Underlying the licensure laws that require educating professionals to a level of competence and that insure that they stay competent, are the ethical values, Doing Good (Beneficence) and Doing No Harm (Non-maleficence).

The value of Freedom (Autonomy) for the practitioner also touches education; freedom, liberty, power—all are seen to increase with more education. To be an illness care *profession* (or, at least, more like the professional prototype, medicine), all illness practitioner groups seek to require more education for new practitioners Whether or not more education is necessary to do the job is not always the issue. The goal is to "improve the profession" by reducing the numbers of new practitioners with certain qualifications, and by increasing their competence.

The advantage of using education as the standard for practitioner entry into practice, instead of using competence or knowledge, is that education is more easily measured: The number of hours that have been spent in chairs, listening to lectures, are easily counted. Those hours of sitting and listening are, in essence, what degrees or units of continuing education represent.

Competence and knowledge are harder to measure than education, so it is easy to understand why occupations use formal education as "standards" for entry into practice, and why they seek to "standardize" (make fixed) education for entry into practice. Formal education has the double advantage of being easier to measure and having the effect of increasing the "professionalization" of the occupation by decreasing the numbers (supply) of practitioners.

Standards—or Standardize?

> Setting standards in law requires that all practitioners prove they can achieve some standard (either in competence or knowledge).
> "Standardizing" fixes the way that practitioners are taught, so that only people educated under the standardized format can enter the occupation.

"Standardizing" education is not the same as setting standards for practitioners. Setting standards in law means that all practitioners will have to prove they can achieve the standards, either in competence or knowledge.

"Standardizing" fixes the way (even in law) that practitioners are taught, reducing the number of ways that people can enter the profession. Only people educated in the standardized format can enter the occupation, which keeps people out, cuts down the competition, increases the demand, and therefore increases the rewards for practitioners who have attained the standardized format.

Professional groups (which are, in some cases, also unions) seek more education for new practitioners as a requirement to join their group (the monopoly of licensure). Professional associations seek more education as a requirement to improve the profession and, as a consequence, the service to the patient.

Educational Entry Level for Licensure

> For many years, the goal of organized nursing was two levels of nurses: technical (two-year, junior college associate degree) and professional (four-year, baccalaureate degree).
> Licensure would mandate differences in preparation and function. LPNs would no longer be educated or licensed.

Since the late 1950s, the American Nurses Association has sought to bring nursing into what it considered the educational mainstream. Association leaders wanted all nurses to be educated in colleges, which would replace the diploma-granting schools in hospitals and the vocational-technical schools training licensed practical or vocational nurses. (Understood as part of that movement toward "differentiated practice" is deletion of the category of worker now known as LPNs.[43])

The ANA goal was to have only two levels of nurses: technical (two-year, junior college Associate Degree Nurses/ADNs) and professional (four-year, Bachelor of Science in Nursing/BSNs).

Licensure would then mandate differences in preparation, with each level's practice set in law. Nurses educated in ADN, diploma (generally three-year), and BSN programs presently all take the same examination for licensure, and no significant differences in scores on the exam can be noted in graduates of different schools. (Some associate degree schools were noted to produce graduates who did extremely and uniformly well on state board exams, but release of such data has been stopped.)

A reason given for requiring more education for entry into practice is to improve service to the patient. Unfortunately, objective data do not exist to prove that people with more years of schooling in nursing give better service. Nurses with more formal schooling give different *kinds* of service, as in management, or research, or teaching, but evidence is lacking that they give better bedside care, where the patient would see the difference.

One study looked at whether the educational level of the nurse affected what she did on the job. RNs with baccalaureate degrees were found to perform high-skill functions more often, and other studies have found that they earn more money.[44] The labor market may already distinguish between nurses with more education by assigning them different functions; if so, there would be no need to change licensure laws to provide information to the market.

Beyond differentiating between associate and baccalaureate degrees, the increasing differentiation of the nurse with the master's degree may mean that the "professional," autonomous primary care nurse is an MSN, with all others at various technical levels. This possibility is discussed further, under advanced nurse practice values, in Chapter Four, Freedom (Autonomy).

Mandatory Continuing Education Law

Mandatory Continuing Education (MCE) attempts to protect the public by preventing harm from incompetent practitioners.

No studies demonstrate that states with MCE have increases in nurse competency (no decrease in malpractice case filings, settlements, or verdicts, no fewer disciplines by state boards, no objective improved outcome measurements).

Legal challenges to mandatory CE laws have been largely unsuccessful, except when private groups are delegated to manage CE.

Mandatory Continuing Education (MCE) attempts to protect the public by preventing harm from incompetent practitioners. Unfortunately, there is little if any connection between MCE and competence.

> "Although continuing professional competence has been increasing in importance, we have not yet been able to define such competence with reasonable precision, nor measure it with adequate accuracy."[45]

Almost 30 years after the above was written, the situation has not changed.

Voluntary continuing education is not a new issue. A guild (union, association) of doctors in Florence required continuing education of their members in 1389; continuing education was voluntary since doctors were not mandated to belong to the guild, and patients could go to any doctor they liked—there was no state-enforced monopoly of licensure.

Mandated continuing education of practitioners promises safe care; moreover, it implies quality care to the public. A certain number of hours in class per year is represented as ensuring continuing competence. Mandatory CE does force changes in behavior (guaranteed attendance at courses, or payment of money for correspondence courses). But mandatory CE guarantees or measures *only* attendance; competence is hard to measure and impossible to guarantee in advance.

> "Until research efforts provide quantitative evidence concerning the relationship between benefits and costs, there should be far less emphasis on mandating CME requirements."[46]

Mandatory continuing education has not been shown to be relevant to quality of care given by providers; providers who are mandated to participate in CE cannot be shown to provide better care than those who do not. A study of doctors showed that the amount of initial *clinical training* of the doctor has the greatest influence on quality of care given, but there was no association between the amount of mandatory CME and quality of practice, nor was greater interest in CME a characteristic of the better doctor.[47] The certain cost of mandatory CME was not justified by its uncertain benefits.

The premise is that mandated CE results in a safer practitioner, but that has not been proven. No increase in competency in states with mandatory continuing education for nurses can be documented (no decrease in malpractice case filings, settlements, or verdicts, no fewer disciplines by state boards, no objective improved outcome measurements are documented in those states). One review indicated that voluntary CE for doctors could show some limited change in outcomes. Eight studies out of 18 demonstrated positive changes in more than one major measure of education (e.g., skill, memory, etc.).[48]

As of this writing, state nurse associations have established CE as mandated by law in 21 states; Louisiana mandated CE in 1994. Three of the 21 states (Washington, Oregon, and Mississippi) require MCE for nurse practitioners only. In general, CE hours required range from 15 hours every two years to 24 hours of CE per year; no scientific bases for how many hours are needed to maintain competency, have been established.[49] In most instances, credit is given only for formal programs where attendance can be verified, not for informal self-study of other kinds.

EXAMPLES OF MANDATORY CE LAWS CHALLENGED

In one case osteopaths challenged in court the 30 hours of MCE passed by the California legislature. The law was upheld, even though no requirement was made for allopathic doctors at the time.[50]

In a chiropractor challenge to MCE the court said:

> The fact that a person is once licensed does not create a vested property right in the licensee, as advancements in trade or profession may require additional conditions to be complied with if the general welfare of the public is to be protected.[51]

Pharmacist MCE was upheld in a similar case.[52]

Firing a public school teacher for failure to meet mandatory CE requirements is constitutional.[53]

In another chiropractor case, the court held invalid a legal requirement to attend programs approved by the private chiropractors association. The court said they probably would uphold requirement of attendance at state board-approved programs. The issue was unlawful delegation of the power to determine the requirements, quality, and nature of chiropractic CE to that private society.[54] One can make an analogy to the situation in which many state boards of nursing delegate their power to certify nurse practitioners to private organizations such as ANA or the academy of nurse practitioners.

Podiatrists may escape MCE if set by their professional association:

> While private, professional societies may and do act in an advisory capacity and make recommendations to the State Boards and the department of education in matters affecting their profession, they have no independent power to establish mandatory standards for professional licenses.[55]

Like other challenges to the legislature's power to make law, legal challenges to mandatory CE laws have been largely unsuccessful, except when private groups appear to benefit. The power to regulate by licensure is very broad, and whatever burdens the lawmaker chooses to impose will probably be upheld, if they are even minimally related to the license. (See the discussion of licensure disadvantages, above.[56]

Another intended consequence of such law is that the practitioner will attend courses. Such behavior is seen by some as "what good nurses do," whether or not mandatory CE increases competent practice. Merely "going" to CE seems the value here. The reasoning: Good nurses go to CE; therefore, going to CE makes one a good nurse. But going to CE does not seem to be the *cause* of good nurses; instead, it is the *result* of being a good nurse in the first place.

> "Aside from the excessive cost, the efficacy of mandatory continuing education remains doubtful. A certain number of hours at approved courses or seminars or annual meetings . . . does not demonstrate that learning has occurred. Bills for mandatory continuing education have failed to require testing of a professional's knowledge and skills. Attendance is not the equivalent of learning. Proponents of continuing mandatory education have failed to document that it will positively affect job performance. Even if competence in the classroom were to be shown, it is different from competence (in practice). . . ."[57]
>
> —Mark Alan Siegel, Chair of
> the Higher Education Committee,
> New York State Assembly

As Robert Boissoneau said:

> Has mandatory continuing education been a success or failure? On balance, the answer must be that it has failed . . . . In fact, no relationship between mandatory continuing education and improved effectiveness has been established . . . the health professions would be better advised to terminate further moves in the direction of mandatory continuing education. [Their] efforts would produce greater benefits if they were directed at revitalizing voluntary continuing education measures and, more importantly, at isolating incompetent professionals by helping either to correct deficiencies or to leave the profession.[58]

Competence

> Competence is the *advance* assessment of ability; performance is the *ongoing* assessment of ability.

Insuring competence to protect the public is the purpose of licensure law; if mandatory CE does not guarantee competence, how can it be done?

Maintaining competence does not issue directly from "going to courses." Competence is learned and maintained, not only from formal courses, but from informal experience self-sought and self-taught (the essence of true education).

Competence can be distinguished from performance; competence is the *advance* assessment of ability. It is the assessment that a nurse is able to do good or adequate work, a potential measured before the practitioner starts; the state board of nursing tests the nurse before the license is issued. One of the ways competence can be approximated (not precisely measured) is with multiple-choice tests, inexpensively administered to large numbers of candidates.

Performance or practical exams can be given, but they are used more for skilled trades, such as barbers and plumbers, than for professionals. Simulations of practice are possible, too, but separate scorers of a doctor's performance correlate on doctor competence only at the same rate as chance (computer technology may help). Chart audits can be used to measure performance, but standardized charts are needed, with standard criteria to apply to the assessment.[59]

Performance is a form of *continuing* competence, the actual doing of the work. Assessing performance is assessing the work that the practitioner has done or is doing. Performance can be ascertained with charts, peer review, or patient outcomes. State boards of nursing do a performance assessment when they investigate a complaint about a nurse. Of necessity, enforcing minimum performance is only done after the fact, and in random or very bad cases.

Minimum performance could be measured by doing chart audits on all nurses every year, but this would be very costly. Furthermore, it would still not prevent *all* harm to patients: Absolute safety is impossible to guarantee.

Minimum competency could be assured by requiring all nurses to repeat the licensing exam every year; at least, in this way, the nurse would be known to be not worse at taking the test than when she entered practice. Licensure examinations are not perfect at measuring competence either, but they are more certain than mandatory continuing education.

Law corrects harm that has already been done by punishing; and the threat of punishment will deter some people some of the time from doing harm (and thus prevent some harm). But no law will absolutely prevent harm that is yet to come. In contrast to law, ethics does seek to *prevent* harm, by encouraging people to act in ways that do not harm other people. Like law, ethics cannot prevent harm completely and, unlike law, ethics cannot punish the harmful act.

Among all the state statutes, licensure is by far the most important statute to nurses. Nurses who find and read the licensure statute for their state have done more than most other nurses (more than most lawyers) and will have read the major statute law enforcing the minimum ethic of what they do for a living—caring for, doing good for, and preventing harm to, the patient.

Licensing Alternatives

Licensing of other kinds of nurses, changing the licensure laws to license only institutions, and dispensing with licensure altogether are proposals that have been made and may be tried in the future.

Various plans have been proposed for licensing other categories of nurses. Unlicensed student nurses were early hospital caregivers, supervised by a few "graduate" nurses. Most other educated and licensed nurses worked in private practice, nursing in the home of the patient. After insurance programs started by hospitals paid for much hospitalization, people (and their nurses) moved into the hospitals for sick care. Still, not all the nursing was done by "graduate" nurses; much was done by nurse assistants (aides, helpers, technicians).

LPNs were originally a "tech nurse" plan. And the phrase now used for "aide" is Unlicensed Assistive Personnel (UAPs). (ANA supports regulating UAPs, but it is not clear if that means licensing.) ANA says the UAPs require the least restrictive form of regulation to protect the public. (Others say the very least restrictive regulation would be by the free market.) The association recommends that research be done, to compare outcomes based on skill mix: Comparisons should be done as to whether patients get better, faster, cheaper, or happier, cared for RNs, or some other mix of nurses.[60] It remains to be seen if the research shows that all-RN staffs are not as effective as mixed staffs or if all-RN staffs are of about the same effectiveness, but merely more expensive.

This issue will heat up as more hospitals cut costs by changing their nursing skills mix to rely less on RNs and more on lower-paid aides for routine tasks. In 1992 the numbers reported were: 2.2 million RNs—average 1992 income of $36,000; 950,000 LPNs—average pay of $23,000; and a virtually unlimited supply of nurse aides (UAPs)—at an average cost of $15,500. Some consulting firms specialize in downsizing the size of the licensed staff in a facility.[61] Some experts say an essential for successful change requires employees to cross departmental and disciplinary boundaries.

Institutional Licensure

Institutional licensure is a solution that has been offered at several different times in the past, to solve the problems of proliferation and restrictions of licensure. Economists, planners, and some hospital managers advocate that the state not grant licenses from the government for each kind of occupation; they recommend that institutions be licensed instead, and the qualifications of who does what be decided within the agency. In such a scenario, the monopoly of licensure would continue for agencies; but it ends the benefits of licensure (monopoly) for practitioners.

Occupations that have or seek licensure oppose this solution; the power to decide who is a safe practitioner would rest with the employer and practitioners fear that employers would not have the same interests (the professional's self-interest in professional care, in the interest of the patient, in quality of practice). Employers would certainly not have the same interest in the practitioner's economic health as the practitioner does.

Arguments for institutional licensure: Fear of malpractice is one "force" that keeps agency standards high, or at least safe (that is the case already). The pressure of competition would require agencies to employ qualified people with proper credentials (this pressure exists already, and it works).

Inspection by JCAHO would encourage agencies to employ people with specified credentials (inspections already perform this function). Insurance companies would only pay for procedures done by qualified people (already the case). The loss would be to the occupations' "professional" status—to their power as licensed people.

Since all these benefits of agency control already exist, perhaps no institutional licensure is necessary. Abolishing existing licenses (the institutions', too!) would suffice without additionally empowering agencies to formally credential people.

Note that, in a system without licensure, much control is exercised like law, but is not mandatory like licensure: For example, physicians are not licensed specifically to do chest surgery; those privileges are granted by the institutions and other groups of doctors (not a state power, but an informal, voluntary group power). People voluntarily choose to go to a hospital accredited by the JCAHO, and they choose voluntarily to get care from doctors accredited by the American Board of Medical Specialties. The market works.

If licensure were abolished altogether, the change might not be dramatic. The fear of malpractice suits, threat of loss of privileges, inability to get a job or insurance reimbursement without competence and knowledge—all could contribute protect the patient from harm.

ENDNOTES

1. Steppe, H. "Nursing in Nazi Germany," *Western Journal of Nursing Research*, 1992; 14(6):744–753.
2. Quill, T., "Occasional notes: The ambiguity of clinical intentions," *New England Journal of Medicine*, 1993; 329(14):1039–1340.
3. Tex. Rev. Civ. Stat. Ann. Art. 4495b, §5.08(l) (Vernon Supp. 1995).
4. "Law Notes," *Wall Street Journal*, 23 June 1993, p. B5.
5. Child Abuse Amendments of 1984 (P.L. 98-457) 42 U.S.C. 5101, 45 CFR 1340.14 *et seq.*
6. Also see Stevenson, D.K., *et al.*, "The 'Baby Doe' rule," *Journal of the American Medical Association, 1986; 255(14):1909–1912.*
7. *Matter of Christine M.*, Judge Gloria Dabiri, Family Court, Brooklyn, NY, in Woo, J., and Lambert, W., "Refusal to Immunize Child Called Neglect," *Wall Street Journal*, 22 February 1993.

8. Puckett, C., "Domestic Violence Batters Many Lives," *Amarillo Globe–News*, 27 December 1992; p. 2B.
9. Council on Scientific Affairs, American Medical Association, "Violence against women: Relevance for medical practitioners," *Journal of the American Medical Association*, 1992; 267(23):3184–3189, at p. 3188.
   Council on Ethical and Judicial Affairs, American Medical Association, "Physicians and domestic violence," *Journal of the American Medical Association*, 1992; 267:3190–3193, at p. 3192.
10. 42 U.S.C. 1395dd, begins at 1395cc.
11. *Cleland v. Bronson Health Care Group*, 917 F.2d 266 (6th Cir. 1990).
12. Pizza, N.F., "Patient transfers—COBRA as amended," *Health Lawyer*, 1992; 6(2):1,3–10.
13. Popper, K., *Unended Quest*, London: Fontana/Collins, 1976.
    Medawar, P.B., *Induction and Intuition in Scientific Thought*, London: Methuen, 1969.
14. National Commission for the Protection of Human Subjects of Biomedical and Behavioral Research, *The Belmont Report: Ethical Principles and Guidelines for the Protection of Human Subjects*, Washington, DC: Government Printing Office, 1983.
15. Harrison L., "Issues related to the protection of human research participants," *Journal of Neuroscience Nursing*, 1993; 25(3):187–193.
16. Candilis, P.J., *et al.*, "A survey of researchers using a consent policy for cognitively impaired human research subjects," *IRB: A Review of Human Subjects Research*, 1993; 15(6):1–4.
17. For further reading on this subject, see Hall, J.K., "Exclusion of pregnant women from research protocols: Unethical and illegal," *IRB: A Review of Human Subjects Research*, 1995; 17(2):1–3.
18. Koschnitzke, L., *et al.*, "Ethical considerations for quality assurance versus scientific research," *Western Journal of Nursing Research*, 1992; 14(3):392–396.
19. *Moore v. Regents of the U. of California et al.*, 88 Dailey Journal D.A.R. 9520 (Cal. Ct. App., 2d Dist., Div. 4, 1988).
20. Maher, E.A., "An analysis of finder's fees in medical research," *Canadian Medical Association Journal*, 1994; 150(2):252–256.
21. Two good introductions to this controversial area are: Regan, T., "The case against animal research," and McCloskey, H.J., "The moral case for experimentation on animals," in Beauchamp, T.L. and Walters, L. *Contemporary Issues in Bioethics*, 3rd ed., Belmont, CA: Wadsworth, 1989; pp. 448–458; 458–465.
22. Pardes H., West, A., and Pincus, H., "Physicians and the animal-rights movement," *New England Journal of Medicine* 1991; 324:1640–1643.
23. Another view of interest: American Medical Association Council on Scientific Affairs, "Use of animals in medical education," *Journal of the American Medical Association*, 1991; 266(6):836–837.
24. Tong, R., "The ethics of medical licensure," *Federation of State Medical Boards Bulletin*, 1991; 78:174–183.
25. Austin, A.P.: "State Agency: Nurse Acted Irresponsibly," *Amarillo, Texas, Sunday News–Globe*, 13 March 1994; p. 7A.
26. American Nurses Association Publications, Washington, DC: The Association, 1990. ANA, 600 Maryland Ave S.W., Ste 100W, Washington, DC 20024-2571.
27. Holzer, H.M., "The physician's license: An Achilles heel?" *Journal of Legal Medicine*, 1991; 12:201–220.
28. Fiesta, J., "Safeguarding your nursing license," *Nursing Management*, 1990; 21(8):20–21.
29. See *e.g.*, Tex. Admin. Code, §217.13 (Vernon Supp. 1995).
30. Tadych, R., "State board of nursing's nondisciplinary alternative for chemically impaired licensees," *The Missouri Nurse*, 1993; 62(2):22.
31. See *e.g.*, Jordan, D.R.E., "Licensing issues at the administrative hearing commission," *Journal of the Missouri Bar*, January–February 1994; pp. 23–29.
32. *Tuma v. Board of Nursing*, 100 Idaho 74, 593 P2d 711 (1979).
33. *Yeary v. Board of Nurse Examiners for the State of Texas*, 855 S.W. 2d 236 (1993 Tex. App.)
34. "Headlines," *American Journal of Nursing*, 1993; 93(3): 9.
    Conversation with Ray Linder, Director of Labor Relations, Montana Nurses Assn., 1 September 1995.
    Also see "Pain control an issue in Montana's 'Hospice Six' case," *Medical Ethics Advisor*, November 1991, pp. 136–137.

35. Hutchinson, S.A., "Nurses who violate the Nurse Practice Act: Transformation of professional identity," *Image—the Journal of Nursing Scholarship*, 1992; 24(2):133–139.
36. Holzer, H., *op. cit.*
37. *Ibid.*
38. For review of licensing issues: Kusserow, R.P., *et al.*, "An overview of state medical discipline," *Journal of the American Medical Association,* 1987; 257:820–823.
39. Sieracki, C.A., "Organizational liability prevention: Automated profiles," *Nursing Management*, 1993; 24(7):60–64.
40. Milazzo, V.L., "Disciplinary data banks are not new," *National Medical–Legal Journal*, 1990; 1(2):2.
41. Birkholz, G., "Implications of the National Practitioner Data Bank for nurse practitioners," *Nurse Practitioner*, 1991; 16(8):40, 42–43, 46.
42. *E.g.*, Mo Rev Stat 383.000 *et seq.* (1994).
43. Bollenberg, R., "Differentiated practice: Another threat to the LPN? An opinion essay," *Journal of Practical Nursing*, 1991; 41(3):36.
44. Young, W.B., *et al.*, "The effect of education on the practice of nursing," *Image—the Journal of Nursing Scholarship*, 1991; 23(2):105–108.
45. *Report of the National Advisory Commission on Health Manpower*, I. Washington, DC: U.S. Government Printing Office, 1967; pp. 41–42.
46. Egdahl, R.H., and Gertman, P.M. (Eds.), *Quality Health Care: The Role of Continuing Education*, Germantown MD: Aspen, 1977., p 126.
47. Egdahl and Gertman, *op. cit.*, p. 79
48. Davis, D.A., "Evidence for the effectiveness of CME: A review of 50 randomized controlled trials," *Journal of the American Medical Association*, 1992; 268(9):1111–1136.
49. "Headlines," *op. cit.*
50. *Gamble v. Board of Osteopathic Examiners*, 130 P.2d 382 (1942).
51. *Week v. State Board of Examiners in Chiropractic*, 30 N.W.2d 187 (1947).
52. *Lichtman v. Ohio State Board of Pharmacy*, Ct. App. Franklin County, Ohio, 2 August, 1974, Ohio Supreme Ct. denied cert.
53. *Harrah Independent School District v. Martin*, 440 U.S. 194 (1979).
54. *State Board of Chiropractic Examiners v. Life Fellowship of Pennsylvania*, 272 A.2d 478 (1971).
55. *Podiatry Society v. Regents*, 358 N.Y. Supplement 2d 276 (1974).
56. The following article may be of further interest: Newbern, V.B., "Mandatory continuing education in nursing: A question of constitutionality," *Journal of Continuing Education in Nursing*, 1989; 20(1):4–7.
57. Statement on Mandatory Continuing Education issued 29 April 1980, in Shimberg, B., "What is competence? How can it be measured?" in Stern, M.R. (Ed.), *Power and Conflict in Continuing Professional Education*, Belmont, CA: Wadsworth, 1983, p. 32.
58. Boissoneau, R., *Continuing Education in the Health Professions*, Rockville, MD: Aspen, 1980; p. 198.
59. *Ibid*, p. 32.
60. Cassetta, R., "House unites when faced with regulation issues," *American Nurse*, July/August 1993; p. 26.
61. Anders, G., "Nurses decry cost-cutting plan that uses aides to do more jobs," *Wall Street Journal*, 20 January 1994; pp. B1, B7.

FOUR

Ethics and Law of
Freedom (Autonomy)

TOPICS COVERED

Autonomy: For patient and for practitioner

Laws enforcing the value, Freedom

Patient

CONSENT • ADVANCE DIRECTIVES • TRANSPLANTS •
HIV/AIDS • SUICIDE

Practitioner

ADVANCED PRACTICE NURSE LAW • FUTILITY • PATIENT
DEMANDS FOR CARE • ASSISTED SUICIDE

AUTONOMY—THE VALUE AND CONSEQUENCES

▽

"The only freedom which deserves the name is that of pursuing our own good in our own way, so long as we do not attempt to deprive others of theirs, or impede their efforts to obtain it."
—**J.S. MILL,** *On Liberty*

△

The words *freedom, power*, and *choice* are often used synonymously with the value, autonomy.

The individual's autonomy (freedom to do things) is not absolute.

Laws enforce, protect, and also limit the individual's power to decide and to act.

The philosophy underlying the value of freedom is individualism (contrasted with the philosophy of collectivism).

Philosopher Kant's *categorical imperative* emphasizes individual freedom; he mandates that one should treat other people, not as means to an end, but as important for their own sake.

Philosopher Mill's explanation of freedom as a negative (freedom *from*, not freedom *to have*) would eliminate any conflict between individual autonomy and justice in illness care.

Freedom. Autonomy. Power. Choice. The value, Autonomy, is known by all these terms.

Some nurses would always rank the patient's autonomy (or the nurse's own autonomy) first—over doing good, not harming, being fair—over life itself. Others believe that, depending on the situation and the person, any of the values can be most important at any given time.

The value, Freedom, underlies all the law that expresses the individual's power to choose and act in his or her own life. The real world expressions of the abstract ethical value, Autonomy, are the laws made to enforce the value; these laws enforce and protect the individual's power to decide and to do what is wanted. In a democracy, freedom is limited only by restrictions mandated by the society (law) and restrictions that the individual nurse voluntarily assumes (ethics).

Freedom Is Relative

Autonomy is not absolute. Limits are placed on the individual's power to act. If this were not so, only the temporarily strongest would be temporarily safe—a condition of anarchy. Everyone's freedom, it may be said, is relative to their general condition; for example, children, persons declared incompetent, prisoners, people in the military, students in school, or workers on the job, have less freedom. The word *autonomy* comes from the Latin; *auto* means "self," and *nomy* means "control." Does anyone have complete control over him- or herself?

Freedom in Illness Care

Freedom is the value apparent in medical ethics cases when the patient wants one thing and the practitioner wants something different. Autonomy is not only important to the patient, it is valued by nurses for themselves, too: Must the nurse provide care considered to be useless? Must she care for patients whose diseases endanger her? Can she assert her own autonomy and refuse to assist patients to commit suicide?

In general, both practitioners and patients have obvious self-interests in protecting their own freedoms. Beyond self-interest, nurses also have an interest in protecting the patient's freedom. Nurses value control, power, choice—all synonymous with freedom—for themselves. However, such a value for individuals is possible in a civilization only if it is also granted to all others. If the nurse grants freedom only to "self," that would be anarchy. The nurse would be free, but only as long as she or he remained the most powerful individual. It is only by granting limited autonomy to others who are weaker that people can also claim it for themselves—as a right.

The philosophy underlying the value, Autonomy, is individualism—the individual's control over his or her own body (self, life, death). The philosophy that most contrasts with individualism is collectivism, in which the survival and well-being of the group as a whole is most valued.

Modern writers find autonomy (freedom) as a value in the philosophy of Immanuel Kant. Freedom to choose among various actions (free will) is implied in Kant's categorical imperative. That "imperative" (rule) incorporates the value of acting in such a way that other people are treated, not as a means, but—always—as ends in themselves. In effect, that philosopher says that one should not use other people to reach one's own goals. People should be considered more important for themselves, as equally free individuals, than for their usefulness to someone else.

Freedom Vs. Justice

Utilitarian philosopher John Stuart Mill, in his work *On Liberty*, emphasized freedom of choice. Mill's work, within the context of illness care, helps clarify what some see as a conflict between the patient's individual autonomy, and social justice in illness care. Some envision a conflict between the freedom of the patient to choose a certain expensive treatment, if that choice would then unjustly deny money to another person for another treatment. What if the patient demands a bone marrow transplant, which in turn wipes out the health department's whole budget for immunizations?

Mill would explain that "freedom" is not the freedom to have a *thing* (for example, a certain treatment), but freedom *from* having to do an action. The patient's freedom to consent to surgery, or to refuse it, is not the same as the autonomy to *demand* surgery. Autonomy is not the power to demand surgery or a bone marrow transplant: It is the power to *refuse* a treatment if it is offered.[1]

The *demand* to have a thing or a service (food, health care) is not properly called autonomy; such a demand should be termed an entitlement if it must be provided by the government or given by someone else under threat of government force.

Freedom is a negative. As Mill says, it is not a power to demand or to have, but power to be left alone. Thus, the patient's autonomy doesn't allow him to demand a certain service; rather, autonomy allows refusal of a service offered.

In discussing laws that result from valuing freedom, laws that enforce freedom for the patient will be discussed first; after which, laws that flow from valuing freedom for the practitioner.

LAW ENFORCING THE VALUE, FREEDOM, FOR THE PATIENT

CONSENT

The legal requirement of informed consent is based on the value of patient autonomy. A competent adult can consent (or not) to what is to be done to his or her body.

Consent is the defense to a *civil*, not criminal, lawsuit for battery (battery is touching the patient without her consent).

The concept of informed consent is also an expression of another value, Telling Truth (Veracity).

People who are not competent generally must have proxies or surrogates give consent for their treatment. Consent can be assumed in an emergency situation. Or consent or refusal for a procedure may be assumed from prior statements, such as a living will.

The Latin bases of the word *consent* are *con* ("with") and *sentire* ("feeling"): to feel with (to agree with) another person. Consent is a process toward a state of mind—not one moment or a signature on paper.

Consent for "usual care" given in the agency is implied by the patient's action, entering the agency with knowledge of the care usually given there (can be written as well).

Consent for a procedure is given to the person doing the procedure, but nurses are involved in the process.

The witness's signature does not attest to the validity of the consent.

The nurse is responsible and thus liable for efforts to ensure that patients truly consent to procedures they will undergo.

Values Enforced by Consent Law. Consent law has developed from the value of autonomy. Such law also reflects the idea of telling the truth to the patient, the value of veracity. The law of consent also provides a defense to the intentional torts based on yet another value, Doing No Harm. But the legal and moral requirement of informed consent is most strongly an enforcement of respect for patient autonomy.

The Rule: A Competent Adult Can Consent to or Refuse Treatment

A competent adult can consent or not consent to what is to be done to his or her body. An often-quoted case is one in which a woman consented to a pelvic exam under anesthesia—and, instead, a hysterectomy was performed.

> "Every human being of adult years and sound mind has a right to determine what shall be done with his own body."[2]

This standard reached the level of a fundamental right under the U.S. Constitution, in the *Cruzan* decision by the Supreme Court.[3] However, exceptions and modifications can be made to the rule that consent is required, when the application of the rule leads to an unjust outcome.

Consent Is a Defense to a Suit for Battery

Consent law expresses a fundamental value, the freedom of the patient even from unwanted touch. Consent is the defense to a *civil* lawsuit for battery (not a defense to a criminal charge, see below). A lawsuit for battery can be filed if the patient is so much as touched without consent, although the patient would win only a small measure of damages for mere touching if no injury resulted. A suit for battery usually arises out of injury received from a procedure or surgery done without consent.

Consent is *not* a defense to the *criminal* charge of battery, in which the batterer is usually charged with striking the victim. The criminal charge is more serious than the civil lawsuit discussed here. Criminal charges are unlikely to arise in an illness care situation. If the patient consents to the procedure that results in injury, battery cannot be charged (since the definition of battery is *un*consented touching).

A lawsuit could still be filed for lack of informed consent, in which the patient alleges that she or he did not get adequate information with which to decide on the procedure. The law of informed consent—also an enforcement of the value of telling the truth (veracity)—is based on the practitioner's underlying duty to tell the truth to the patient.

If the patient is a competent adult, she is the only one who can consent to, or refuse treatment. People deemed not competent generally must have proxies or surrogates give consent for treatment, unless such a person's consent is *implied*, as it is in an emergency—the law assumes a person wants treatment to save his life. Consent or refusal for a procedure may also be implied from prior statements; this is the basis of honoring a living will.

The word *consent* is derived from Latin *con*, meaning "with," and *sentire*, meaning "feeling." To consent, then, is to *feel with* (to agree with) another person—usually, in illness care, to agree with performing a certain procedure. Consent may be thought of as a process of the patient's gaining information, deciding, and consenting, not as one single moment, a signature on a paper. Written consent is merely evidence of the patient's mental state of agreement, of consent—that consent is in the mind of the patient, not her signature on paper.

Who Obtains the Consent?

Consent for the "usual care" given in the agency is implied by the patient's act of entering the agency with knowledge of the care given there. In addition, increasingly agencies request a "general consent" be signed for the routine care given. Consent for other than routine care should be obtained from the patient by the person who will perform the procedure. The patient usually gives consent to the doctor for what the doctor does. The nurse, as the patient's caregiver and sometimes advocate, will be interested in, and a part of, the process of informing and considering and consenting.

In many agencies, for convenience, the nurse is the caregiver who asks the patient to sign the written evidence of the consent process. It may also be the nurse who witnesses the patient's signature. The nurse who signs as witness of the patient's signature merely signifies that he or she saw the signing, not that the consent process was valid.

But the patient's total welfare, including consent to the procedure, is the nurse's responsibility, too. It's in the patient's interest, and thus the nurse's professional interest, to see that the patient knowingly consents to any procedure to be performed. To actually consent (not just sign a paper), the patient must know enough to make an informed decision.

Since consent is a process and not merely a signature, information relevant to the patient's consent needn't come from the doctor alone. The doctor should describe procedures and answer questions that the nurse cannot. Nurses take the patient's diagnosis and translate it into the patient's terms. Nurses help the patient cope with the illness; nurses tell the patient what his or her nursing care will be, before and after the procedure and after discharge. Nursing's role has always been to help patients cope with their illnesses. Teaching/informing patients about procedures and consequences so that they can make informed decisions, must be part of the consent process.

Nurse Responsibility for Consent. The law is that nurses are held responsible for patient advocacy, including advocacy in the consent process. Nurse responsibility for consent includes communication between doctor and patient, reporting to management (and perhaps even regulatory agencies, if consent is not obtained) and ultimately (if necessary) quitting the job.[4] However, following even in that scenario, the patient might still be hurt; the nurse could still be liable. More direct advocacy for the patient may be needed.

TEXAS EXAMPLE: SIGNED CONSENT ENOUGH?

Nurses may be held to a high standard of communication in consent cases:
  Lawsuit was filed for operating on a patient without informed consent (actually without *any* consent for the procedure—battery). The nurse had told the patient that an additional procedure was to be done in surgery (appropriate truth-telling and patient advocacy). The patient several times said she would not have the additional procedure—before the surgery—*but then the patient did sign the consent for the procedure.*
  The procedure was done, and the patient sued the hospital and doctor for doing the procedure without her consent. The court thought the nurses could and should have done something; that "ordinary prudence [might] require some inquiry by a nurse into the correctness of performing a surgical procedure over the direct, unambiguous, verbal objection of the patient."
  In such a case, the nurse could have prudently "inquired" about the correctness of the procedure by bringing the patient's spoken denial of consent to the doctor's attention, informing the supervisor, and documenting those actions. In addition, the nurse could make very clear to the patient that her signature on the consent form would signal to the doctor that she *was* consenting to the procedure when she went to surgery.[5]

KINDS OF CONSENT

Consents can be express (written, spoken) or implied (by patient action, and in emergency). Written consents are the standard, so that failing to have the patient sign might constitute evidence of failure to obtain any consent.
  Some states in the United States have specific consent forms for specific procedures or situations. Management of the agency will know the details, or they can be found through the index of the state's statutes or administrative codes of the states.
  Spoken consent is valid, but to prove that a spoken consent was given requires testimony (more difficult to present as evidence, than is writing). Implied consent is given by patient action (coming to the hospital, calling the ambulance). The law makes the assumption that a reasonable person, who presents or calls for such care, wants the kind of care given.
  Consent for care and procedures done in doctors' and nurse practitioners' offices has been implied by the act of coming to the office, but the trend is toward express written consent for office care.

Consent information can be waived by the patient, but the reason should be explored and the waiver put in writing.

Mentally ill patients can consent or refuse treatment to the extent that they have decisional capacity (to understand relevant information and alternatives, to make a decision and communicate it, and to realize the consequences of the decision).

Consent can be implied in true emergency situations, where treatment is immediately necessary to preserve the patient's life or to prevent irreparable harm to the patient's health.

To be valid, consent must be informed.

The old standard for informed consent: "What does the reasonable doctor tell the patient?"

The new standard for how much and what information the patient needs: "What would a reasonable person in similar circumstances need to know to make an informed decision?"

Consents are classed as express (written or spoken) and implied (by patient action, and in emergency).

Express Consent: Written

A written consent is easier to prove in court than spoken testimony. Even though a spoken consent is valid, the agency and practitioner performing the procedure should obtain a written one. The written consent has become so standard that failure to get a signed consent in writing might be looked at as evidence of failure to follow procedure. Some states' statutes have spelled out specifics that must be included in the consent, if the consent is to serve as a defense to a lawsuit alleging "failure of informed consent" or "negligent consent." (If that is the case in a particular state, the department that does surgery or other invasive procedures will have details of the statute.)

The written consent can serve as a teaching outline and a reference for the patient. The patient can be given the consent form and have it explained a day or two in advance of being asked to sign it. Ideally the patient should be given a copy of the unsigned consent early enough so there is time to read and digest it before signing.

Short stays for surgery and day surgery procedures may make it necessary that patients receive consent forms directly from the doctor's or agency's admission office prior to the procedure. Patients can be asked to sign a receipt that they have received the written consent.

Any other written materials given to the patient can be referenced in the consent form, and should be charted. Any videotape the patient sees, or other educational classes or materials the patient participates in, should be documented.[6]

Giving the patient the written consent proposal in advance gives the patient time to learn, ask questions, weigh information, and talk with the family. If the goal is real consent (also excellent protection from lawsuit), then time for the patient to consider is necessary. If the patient does not really consent, a perfectly written and signed form means nothing. The writing and signature are seen as mere symbols of the patient's state of mind. If the patient did not understand what was signed, or did not have full information to make a decision, he or she can testify to that circumstance in court, contradicting the written consent.

The policy of always getting a written consent is supported by research that shows that most patients forget even having signed a consent form.[7] Evidence of this "forgetful" tendency on the part of patients has been admissible in court on behalf of the defendant doctor and hospital, in a case in which the plaintiff said he did not give consent.[8]

Express Consent: Spoken

Spoken consent is valid. But the evidence of a spoken consent, if necessary to be presented in a lawsuit, is the testimony of a human being. The human being (nurse or doctor) may not be available when, years later, the suit comes to trial. Even if available, their testimony may be accurately remembered and convincingly communicated, or not.

Implied Consent

Implied consent is the opposite of *express* consent (expressed by writing or speaking). The law does not say that consent is "excused," but instead that certain circumstances imply the patient has consented. Consent can be implied by patient action, such as the act of entering the hospital. Consent can also be considered as implied when the patient waives the requirement of information (this is more like "waiving" the requirement of informed consent). And consent is sometimes implied in an emergency situation.

Consent Implied from Patient Action

When the patient enters the hospital or nursing home, comes to the clinic, or allows the home health nurse into the house, the patient's consent to the usual care given in such places by such people is implied by that action. It is assumed that a reasonable person would not present himself to such place or person, unless he wanted the kind of care given there. In addition, many agencies ask patients to give express consent for ordinary care by signing a written document that says, in essence, "I consent to the usual care given in this place."

Both the implied and express consent to "usual care" given by the agency include the nursing care given. Because nursing care in earlier days was more likely benign, supportive, noninvasive, comforting, and without much potential for harm, rarely was special consent needed for a nursing procedure. There was deemed to be little risk from the care that the patient would have to consider and give consent to. This has changed, however, as nurses perform invasive procedures in intensive care. As more nurse practitioners do medical diagnosis and treatment, express consent will increasingly have to be obtained for what they do. Until recently, consent for care and procedures in doctors' and nurses' offices was implied by the act of coming to the practitioner. The trend is toward written consent for office care also.

Consent Information Waived by Patient Request

The patient has the power to waive the furnishing of information. If the patient doesn't want to hear about all the risks of a procedure, the risks needn't be given. But that wish should be carefully documented. As part of the process, the nurse should investigate why the patient is unwilling to confront the possible risks of the procedure, and the patient's waiving of this right should be obtained in writing. The writing may clarify the patient's understanding of the right to information being waived, and the writing is easier evidence to prove in court if necessary.

The patient who is mentally incapable of understanding, deciding, and communicating a decision may have consent given through another person (see Consent by Another, below), through state statutes, and case law that give another person the power to consent or refuse treatment.

Mentally ill patients are not automatically incompetent for consent purposes. A mentally ill patient can consent to or refuse treatment, to the extent that the patient has decisional capacity. The patient who has the ability to understand relevant information and alternatives, who can make a decision and communicate it, and who can realize the consequences of the decision, is competent to consent to or refuse treatment.

Consent Implied in Emergency

An exception to the rule that competent people must consent to treatment before it is done occurs in emergency treatment. In an emergency the value of the patient's freedom (autonomy) is tempered by the value of doing good for and valuing the life of the patient. If autonomy were the highest value, the patient unconscious with a head injury could not be treated until waking and consenting personally—if in fact the patient ever did awake.

These exceptions are made to rules of law because the law is based on higher ethics. The ethical (and legal) requirement for consent is implied in emergency situations because the patient's life is valued more than his autonomy. At that point the society's values are projected onto the patient. It is assumed that patients would want caregivers to ignore autonomy in favor of saving their lives. In addition, the emergent nature of the situation means that action must be taken immediately if it is to be of any help. Note: Consent will only be implied in true emergent situations, where treatment is immediately necessary to preserve the life of, or prevent irreparable harm to, the patient.

Informed Consent

In one sense, the phrase "informed consent" is one word too many: To be valid, consent must be informed. If the patient does not have adequate information about the procedure, he cannot freely agree to its performance. Thus the word *consent* necessarily implies and incorporates the word *informed*. There is no true consent to a procedure if there is not adequate information about the procedure.

Standards for Informed Consent

In the past, the standard for whether consent was adequate was based on the reasonable doctor's perspective: "What information would a reasonable doctor tell a patient under similar circumstances?" In some cases "reasonable doctors" withheld information that reasonable people would use when deciding whether to have certain procedures done. Judges and juries, through case law, have since changed that standard in many jurisdictions.

The courts (juries and then judges in appellate decisions) have said that some practitioners failed to tell the patient of a possible risk that a reasonable person would consider important, or one that a reasonable patient would use to decide against a procedure. In such cases, the patient without such information was viewed as not having freely consented to the procedure. In those courts, the standard was not judged from the perspective of the reasonable practitioner, but the law looked at the adequacy of consent from the perspective of the "reasonable patient." Now more often applied is the standard: "What would a reasonable person in similar circumstances need to know to make an informed decision?" The emphasis has changed, from what the doctor would tell the patient, to what a reasonable patient would need to know to choose or refuse a procedure.

Use of consent to procedures has begun to resemble the legal concept, "assumption of the risk." Under this legal theory, the information given patients is important. People who are informed of the risks of a procedure, and proceed to have it, in some measure have voluntarily assumed the risk of having a procedure performed on themselves (relieving their caregivers of the risk). However, since there are infinite numbers of remotely possible risks, it is impossible for the patient to be informed of them all. Thus, the standard for informing patients about procedures is still based on the information a reasonable person would need to make an informed decision in a similar circumstance.

Remember that when the patient acknowledges having received information about risk (for instance, when risks are listed in the consent form), that only signifies the patient has full information to decide. It does not mean the patient consents to negligence that produces one of the risks listed. For example, listing "ureter damage" on the hysterectomy consent does not mean the patient cannot sue if the surgeon nicks the ureter—it merely means a suit alleging "failure to inform of possible ureter damage" will fail.

Minors

> People who are dependent on others have less autonomy—fewer powers to consent or refuse treatment under the law of consent.
>
> For patients under 18, the parent or guardian must consent to or refuse treatment for the child. The parent with custody usually has power to consent for the child.
>
> Mature minors (those under 18 who are in the military, or are parents, or married, or live independently of the parents) may be able to consent for themselves.
>
> In some states, minors may be able to consent for themselves to certain treatment, for such conditions as mental health, drug addiction, sexual abuse, Sexually Transmitted Disease (STD), pregnancy, contraception, or for abortion.
>
> Each state has specific consent statutes for minors, available from the emergency department or pediatric department or from the branch library.
>
> The parent or guardian has power to consent or refuse for the child as long as the decision is in the child's best interest.
>
> The nurse's patient is the child: The ethical duty and legal responsibility is to advocate for the child's best interest.

People who have some degree of dependence on others may not be considered competent adults with full power to consent or refuse treatment. Values other than the patient's autonomy/freedom are thought of more highly for these patients. Law of consent for more or less dependent people expresses that priority of other values (usually Doing Good) over the value of their freedom. Regardless of who is empowered to give legal consent, every effort should be made to secure the consent of the dependent as well.

In most U.S. states, people are considered to be adults at age 18—thus, they can consent to or refuse treatment for themselves at that age. In general, for individuals under that age (minors), a parent or guardian must consent to, or refuse treatment for the child.

Each state has specific consent statutes for minors. Minors may be able to consent at a younger age than 18 if they're in the military, or are parents, or are married, or live independently of their parents. Usually, minors can consent for themselves to certain treatment, for example, for mental health problems (especially suicide prevention), drug use or addiction, sexual abuse, and Sexually Transmitted Disease. (In some statutes still called Venereal Disease, the term was changed to reduce the stigma of the diagnoses.)

Minors whom the practitioner suspects of having been abused may be examined without their parents' permission, under some state laws. The consent statute may also allow minors to consent to treatment for pregnancy, contraception, and in some cases, abortion. In agencies that treat minors for these conditions, the management will have policies adhering to the specifics of the state statute. If needed, a particular state's statute can be obtained from the local branch library, which has a copy of the state statutes. The statute on consent for minors is usually found in the index under Consent and under specific applicable headings—Minor, Drugs, Pregnancy, for instance.

The phrases "mature minors" and "emancipated minors" refer to those children for whom consent law provides exceptions so that they can consent to treatment or refuse treatment themselves. In many cases, children over 14 or 15 can consent to treatment that is beneficial and without much risk.[9] Such exception to the rule (that only competent adults can consent) reflects the values, Doing Good and Doing No Harm, which underlie treatment and consent law.

The details of consent law are based on the underlying ethic: The child's freedom (autonomy) to consent to or refuse treatment is somewhat subordinate to what is deemed his best interest. If the child's best interest is not being advanced in a given situation, the law is not serving in the way it was intended, even if the letter of the law is followed. As always, the nurse must act according to a higher ethic (the best interest of the child) rather than a minimum law.

The issue of the parents' right to consent or refuse for their child can be difficult when the parents' beliefs conflict with what others see as the child's best interest, for example in cases where Jehovah's Witnesses' or Christian Scientists' wishes contradict medical advice. Much of the time a legal conflict can be avoided or resolved with good communication.

The rule that the parent has power to consent or refuse treatment for a child has been modified by courts in some cases. When the parents of the child are divorced, usually the parent with custody has power to consent. If there is a conflict between parents about the child's treatment, the management of the agency should be notified for assistance. Good communication and appealing to the best interest of the child may avert problems before they become wars.

The child is the nurse's patient, to whom the nurse's advocacy is owed. If parents refuse treatment, especially when the refusal could result in harm to the child, the nurse's duty to the patient requires that she take steps to protect the patient; at minimum to involve the agency's management and the patient's doctor. Nurses can help doctors and parents step back from the power struggle, to think about what is best for the child.

Consent/Refusal for Incompetent Patients

Incompetent patients generally cannot legally consent to or refuse treatment for themselves.

People formally judged to be incompetent are wards; the person responsible for the patient is the guardian.

The guardian gives or refuses consent (the patient's best interest is still the guide).

Several states' statutes give family members authority to decide for patients who are not judged formally incompetent in court.

If the patient has not had a guardian appointed and does not fit any of the specified circumstances in the statute (or if there's no state statute), then case law may determine who consents to or refuses treatment.

The agency's policy on the incompetent patient is based on statutes and case law, and if there is no law that governs, the actions of the caregivers should follow the standard of acting in the patient's best interest if possible.

The self-interested question of the agency and practitioner is: "Who can *successfully* sue us, and for what?" If the patient receives good care that a reasonable practitioner would have done for the patient's benefit, the answer is probably no one, for any reason.

Incompetent patients generally cannot legally consent to or refuse treatment for themselves. As with minors, however, it is still important—if possible—to gain the concurrence of the patient in the consent to or refusal of treatment. If the patient has been formally judged to be incompetent—and the patient has been made a *ward* (the word used in most states) of some person (the guardian) responsible for the patient—the guardian can give or refuse consent for the ward (always assuming the guardian's action is in the best interest of the patient).

State Consent Statutes

In addition to state statutes governing who can consent for a minor, several states give various family members automatic authority to make decisions for patients who are presently unable to consent. These statutes, which give consent power to relatives, might be considered a threat to patient autonomy, but ideally they are an extension of the patient's autonomy to another person.

If the patient is unconscious or deemed "incapable" of deciding for or against treatment, such laws in some states automatically give authority for consent/refusal to a list of relatives, usually in the form of a list of descending relationships, from nearest to distant relatives.

If the state statute doesn't list exactly who may consent for whom in the event the patient can't consent, or if the patient will not fit any of the specified circumstances in the statute, then case law may determine who may consent. Case law (when judges decide individual cases) is binding on lower courts in that state or federal jurisdiction.

Most illness care agencies have policies about who consents for whom. Agency attorneys will have helped with that policy, determining under their state statutes and cases who can consent for whom, and in what circumstances.

Sometimes there is no specific law on the subject, however, neither case nor statute. In such an event, attorneys do *not* advise the agency and its nurses to "do nothing." Rather, they employ that best of guides, the one nurses use in their practice: What is best for the patient. That is the standard it is assumed the courts will use; and the courts (judges) are assumed to be reasonable people with the patient's best interest in mind also.

People who are incompetent cannot consent for procedures themselves; in a life-threatening emergency, however, consent can be implied. The spouse, children, parents, or nearest relative may consent, depending on specific state statute. The department doing surgery or other procedures will know such details of the statute, or the specifics of the consent law can be found in the statutes at the local branch library, under the index headings Consent, Surrogate, or similar words. A quick rule substituting for the statute is to do what the ethical, commonsense course of action would be—the action that is best for the patient. This rule can also be followed when the terms of the statute do not seem applicable because a substituted decision maker does not seem to be acting in the patient's best interests.

Lawyers ask a stock question of themselves and the law in any situation that has no settled law on the issue, either statute or case law: "Who can *successfully* sue us, and for what?" In most cases—if the patient receives good care that a reasonable practitioner would have done for the patient's benefit—the answer is "No one, for any reason."[10]

SPECIFIC CONSENTS

The use of consent forms specified by statute creates a presumption that consent was informed; failure to use the forms might result in the opposite presumption.

Special consents must be used when providing immunizations and when obtaining the patient's consent to research.

Refusal of treatment is considered differently in law from consent to treatment, since consent is seen as life-affirming and refusal of treatment is associated with ending life.

Exceptions to the power of a competent adult to refuse treatment may be made if the interests of other people are affected, for example, the children of a father refusing a transfusion.

The presumption that the patient who refuses treatment is incompetent could lead to abuses and forced treatment.

Leaving against medical advice (AMA) negates implied consent to treatment.

Patients who are not competent may need to be forcibly protected (kept) if leaving would endanger them.

Questions to determine competency: Can the patient
(1) understand the situation and alternatives,
(2) make a decision and communicate the decision, and
(3) understand the consequences of the decision?

The state's psychiatric commitment law gives the practitioner limited ability to act without the patient's consent; the law prescribes a process to be followed.

At minimum, evidence is needed that the patient is incompetent and would be in danger, or dangerous, if allowed to leave.

If the patient is competent or is not a danger to himself, the nurse and agency can be sued for keeping an unwilling patient.

A quick assessment for competency to leave against advice: Is the patient competent to sign a surgery consent? If not, contact the doctor, management, and/or family.

If competent, make the same contacts and get a signature on release, if patient is willing. And remember: The patient leaving against advice is still a patient until "out the door" (out of the nurse's care).

In some states, statutes create panels to write consent forms for certain procedures (common types of surgeries). If used, these consents will protect the doctor and hospital somewhat in a lawsuit based on lack of consent.[11] Using such consent forms creates a presumption that consent was informed; the presumption can still be countered by evidence presented by the patient. Failure to use the forms might result in the opposite presumption, that informed consent was not obtained.

The Center for Disease Control writes federal rules specifying what information must be provided in consent forms to patients being immunized against diphtheria, pertussis, tetanus (DPT), measles, mumps and rubella (MMR), and polio.[12]

Consent to research is a special consent which is overseen by a board with power delegated by the federal government through regulations. (The Institutional Review Board and other legal and ethical research concerns are covered in Chapter Three, Doing No Harm.)

Refusal of Treatment

It is not always the case that the individual free to give *consent*, can *refuse* treatment. The value put on freedom is high. That freedom is essentially a negative—the freedom to refuse: Allowing a patient to consent to treatment is to *offer* the freedom to refuse. But if the patient exercises the right of refusal, the right is not always respected.

In law, refusal of treatment is not considered in the same way as consent to treatment. To *consent* to treatment is seen as life-affirming; whereas, to refuse treatment is often associated with denying or ending life. The U.S.

Supreme Court said in *Cruzan* that people have a constitutional right to freedom (autonomy, power) over their bodies and may decide what they want done to them—including refusal of care. That decision is the constitutional basis for the patient's right to consent to or refuse therapy. However, the case law provided this power for many years before that.

In general, people have the power to refuse treatment if they are competent. But specific exceptions to the power to refuse treatment may involve others' interests in the life of the person refusing treatment.[13] For example, a court may consider the interests of the children of a father who refuses a blood transfusion that may result in his death; or the interests of the baby in utero (its right to Life) whose mother refuses a cesarean, may have to be balanced with the mother's right to be free to refuse surgery.

A patient's refusal of treatment by itself should not be considered evidence of incompetency. Some practitioners might characterize patients who refuse treatment as irrational ("Crazy—they must be or they'd consent!"). This form of circular reasoning was employed extensively in psychiatric hospitals, in the former Soviet Union. If citizens criticized the Communist system, they were "crazy" and thus needed hospitalization. The presumption still often is that the patient who refuses treatment is incompetent, or at least marginally competent to decide to refuse therapy. If such circular reasoning were followed extensively in medical care, soon there would be no standard of any kind to refuse treatment. The doctor and nurse would be seen as more qualified to judge what's good for the patient.

Leaving Against Medical Advice (AMA)

If the patient leaves the agency against medical (and nursing) advice, the patient has essentially refused "consent" by physically removing the body. This action (or words) negates further implied consent or consent that began when the patient entered the facility in the first place.

When patients seek to or leave the agency against advice, the first consideration of the nurse must be whether they are competent to do so. Some distinguish in law between the words *competency* (seen as a legally determined state) and *capacity* (more informally determined, and possibly not permanent). However, laws in several states are equating the terms "capacity" and "competency," so nurses can equate the two. A series of questions for determining competency or capacity can be used. Can the patient (1) understand the situation and alternatives, (2) make a decision and communicate the decision, and (3) understand the consequences of the decision? If the answer to any component is no, then the nurse has reason to believe the patient is incompetent.

If the patient is not competent, and leaving the agency might result in harm, the nurse must take whatever steps are within the agency's policy to protect the patient. Generally, the value of doing good for the patient (especially the incompetent patient) takes precedence over the patient's freedom to leave—just as when minors are not allowed to consent to or refuse treatment for themselves. One law that enforces this limited ability to act *without* the patient's consent is the psychiatric commitment law in the states. Commitment law will prescribe certain steps that can be taken in such cases. At a minimum, in order to detain a patient against the patient's will, the law will say that the nurse must have evidence that the patient is incompetent and would be in danger, or dangerous, if allowed to leave. Emergency or psychiatric departments (some now called stress units) should maintain policies reflecting those statutes. The text of such statutes can be obtained from the local branch library's set of state statutes, indexed under Mental Health, Involuntary Commitment, or similar words.

The danger to the nurse in detaining the patient is that, if the patient is competent, the nurse and agency can be sued for holding the patient unwillingly. The allegation might be that the nurse violated the patient's right to refuse treatment, and the tort would be one of False Imprisonment (discussed more fully in Chapter Three). The nurse's defense is that the assessment made, and action taken, was that of a reasonable and prudent nurse and that allowing the patient to leave was reasonably believed to be dangerous to the patient or others.

A quick assessment that can be used is this: If the patient were to have surgery, would the nurse allow the patient to sign the consent form without a surrogate? If so, then the assessment likely is that the patient is competent. If not, the nurse likely believes the patient is not competent, and steps should be taken to protect the patient, steps consistent with the agency's policy in such situations.

Assuming the nurse has assessed the patient who wishes to leave against advice and believes the patient is competent, it should be ascertained whether leaving is really *against advice*. Has the patient talked to the doctor? (Perhaps the doctor is willing to discharge the patient with some other plan of treatment.)

After the nurse has contacted the supervisor and the doctor, the agency often "requires" the patient to sign a release before leaving. This in itself can be a ticklish situation—an already unhappy patient's being further aggravated by insisting on a signature. If the nurse insists on the release and the patient won't sign, she cannot keep the patient against his or her wishes; in such a matter, again, the nurse and agency are open to a suit for false imprisonment.

When leaving against advice, the patient usually is asked to sign a release that says something like, "I hold the agency and doctor and nurses harmless for any damage from my leaving." Like all releases, however, it can be contradicted by testimony; and, depending on the circumstances, the patient doesn't give up the right to sue, even if the release says so. The nurse and agency are still legally responsible to the patient until out the door. Ethics and good nursing practice establish a duty to communicate to the patient the nurse's concern for his condition and care if possible.

Incompetent Refusal

Problems encountered in patient refusal are usually in the situations of incompetent patients, since the power of competent patients to refuse is clear.

Even greater ethical and legal problems arise when someone other than the patient wants to refuse treatment for the patient.

When refusal of treatment by someone other than the patient would result in death to the patient, the standard used to measure the rightness of the action is whether the refusal is in the best interest of the patient.

The legal fiction is that the proxy or surrogate "becomes" the patient for purpose of the consent.

The legal minimum duty might seem to be to accept the decision of the proxy; but higher ethics and good nursing practice may demand the nurse continue to act as advocate, if the patient's best interest indicates.

The nurse may have a duty to see that the guardianship process is started, for the patient's safety.

The guardian's or family's power to decide whether to treat or refuse treatment for the patient is not based on any special accuracy in knowing what the patient would want.

Nurses must be careful when they intervene in the "best interest" of the patient, to recognize their own interest in the case.

Problems that issue from patients refusing care do not usually involve the competent patient. Under good ethics, good law, and good nursing practice, competent patients who are informed of the consequences of their decision have the freedom to refuse care; "refusing care" problems almost always are about the incompetent patient. It is not usually the incompetent patient refusing care that creates the ethical problem, but rather, someone other than the patient, refusing treatment *on the patient's behalf.*

In theory, whoever can *consent* to treatment for a person, can refuse treatment also. But as noted earlier, consenting to treatment usually is a consent to maintain life.

Sometimes refusing treatment means dying. When the patient refuses treatment that will result in death, caregivers are obligated to ascertain if the patient understands the consequences of refusal. When refusal of treatment by someone "on the patient's behalf" would result in death to the incompetent person, the courts also have tried to ascertain whether the decision is a good one. In most cases, legally appointed guardians have the power to refuse treatment if it is in the best interest of the ward/the patient.

Consent by One Person for Another (Proxy)

If the patient is unable to consent (for example, is incompetent), in some cases another person may consent to a procedure "for" the patient. This person is said to be the patient's surrogate (stand-in, representative, proxy). The legal fiction is that the proxy or surrogate "becomes" the patient for purpose of the consent. Society through law has enforced the ethic that something other than the patient's autonomy is of higher value: among these, the patient's life, health, and freedom from burdensome treatment.

If the patient is admitted with a paper certifying the patient has been "adjudged" incompetent (by a judge or jury), should the nurse even assess the patient for competency? In such a case, the patient already has a *proxy*, someone else to make all decisions. In legal terms, the patient has become a ward, a dependent; someone has been appointed by the court to be guardian, to guard and look after the patient's best interests. Here, as in many areas of nursing practice, what appears to be the legal minimum may not be enough for ethical and good nursing practice.

Ethical practice almost always meets the minimum of the law; but what appears to be merely legal practice may not meet the higher ethical standard. The nurse's ethical and good nursing practice may be to do more than what appears to be the minimum the law requires here. And in some cases, the law too will require more of the nurse than merely following the guardian's orders.

In the usual case, the nurse considers the patient's guardian as the person who makes decisions. But the nurse still has an obligation to practice good nursing, which not only ethically but legally may require the nurse to be an advocate for the patient. This could be the case if a proxy for the patient seems not to be acting in her best interest; for example, if the patient is merely dehydrated and needs fluids, but the guardian refuses to have fluids given.

When a guardian or other surrogate decision maker asserts him- or herself, or when the nurse believes a guardian is needed, the nurse must assess the patient's competence. In the familiar ward/guardian situation, the patient already will have been declared incompetent by a court, the guardian appointed as the surrogate decision maker. The surrogate figuratively stands in the place of the patient.

If the patient does not have a guardian but seems incompetent under the test for decisional capacity (understand, decide and communicate, know consequences), the nurse may have an ethical and even legal responsibility. The nurse has a legal duty to report the patient's situation if the patient is a danger to him- or herself. In a home situation, the nurse may have a further duty: to see that someone starts the process to have the patient declared incompetent and a guardian appointed so that the patient's safety is assured. Some states have laws that mandate that practitioners report adult abuse or self-neglect, also an action required by good nursing care and ethics, as well as the law.

Home health or public health nurses might also be responsible under licensure law standards, ethical standards, and malpractice law, to bring the patient's situation to the attention of a social services department or other agency with authority to seek a guardian for the patient. This duty is analogous to the duty to protect children from harm.[14]

The ANA Code of Ethics says that the nurse is the patient's advocate, and the ethics requires that the nurse do good for the patient. The law (licensure law and malpractice laws) enforces that value; the law mandates that the nurse *must* do good for the patient.

(Some of the advance directives statutes will let people designate in advance someone to consent for them if they're unable to—see below, under Durable Power of Attorney [DPA].)

Accuracy of Proxy Decisions

The belief that the patient's surrogate (sometimes a relative) knows what the patient wants better than other people do, is largely an illusion. Surprisingly, research shows that a stranger to the patient would be as likely to know how the patient's life was affected by disease as the patient's surrogate.[15]

The difficulty of projecting onto others what *they* would want is documented. Research shows that proxies make the care decisions their patient "would want" only about as often as random chance—in other words, as good as flipping a coin and no better. Proxies in fact usually rate patients as more impaired than the patients rate themselves.[16] There is nothing especially reliable about letting the family decide what the patient would want, whether to be treated or to refuse treatment. Families are allowed to decide because their own interest includes their relationship (kinship and love) to the patient.

Not surprisingly, practitioners sometimes follow whatever advice they personally feel most comfortable about. Practitioners tend to promote withdrawal of treatment regardless of what patient or proxy want, an attitude expected to increase in future.[17]

Imagine a patient with a malignant, inoperable brain tumor, now comatose, who has a living will and durable power of attorney (DPA, defined below). The living will gives directions about care, the DPA names a decision maker.

The staff thinks treatment should be stopped. The attorney in fact (family member) named in the DPA says "treat." Under the law, the staff should follow the proxy's orders. But the staff thinks the proxy is not following the wishes of the patient at that point. An ethics consult is held—which the family does not attend—at which the ethics team decides that the family is not acting in accord with the living will.

The practitioners seek a court order to invalidate the agent (proxy) and have a new one appointed. It is done. By that time the family has moved the patient out of the hospital. The case is dropped. Should the practitioners have pursued the case, even though their personal problem (giving care they believe the patient doesn't want) is solved?[18] Can this be interpreted as staff intervening in the "best interest" of the patient?

If staff should intervene to counter surrogates when they believe that *stopping* treatment of the patient is in the patient's best interest, then should staff intervene to counter surrogates when they believe that *continuing* treatment is in the patient's best interest?

Nurses initially protected their patient's life in the case of Nancy Cruzan; they refused to dehydrate her to death at her proxy's request. They saw *living* as being in their patient's best interest, and they were criticized by some for not following the proxy's request. Were those nurses right?

Research shows that the people who work in illness care are sometimes informal proxy decision makers for the patient. They say they treat strangers differently (more intensively) than they would want to be treated themselves.[19] The individual nurse can ascertain his or her own feelings and desires in a given situation, but the nurse cannot know what another person would want. Nurses who treat patients exactly as they would treat themselves, must be careful lest they project their subjective bias onto the patients. The nurse must instead have some clue as to what the patient would want—such as an advance directive, discussed in the next section.

ADVANCE DIRECTIVES

In legal theory, advance directives are a *presently* made refusal (or consent) to *future* treatment.

In practice, advance directives almost always refuse some treatment anticipated in the future.

Advance directives are either living wills (written or spoken) or durable powers of attorney.

Advance directives are also seen by some as advance DNRs.

Ethics and law about advance directives in some cases do enforce the value people put on dying in preference to treatment.

The unlimited care encouraged by the payment for care by a third party (government or private insurance) may result in unwanted treatment, necessitating advance directives.

The living will document has developed since 1967 as part of a campaign by the Euthanasia Society of America.

Law journals and state statutes recognized the document starting in 1969.

The durable power of attorney for health care (which lets the patient name a proxy—surrogate—for health care decisions) developed from existing laws that allow a proxy for money decisions.

Some state laws provide that parents can make advance directives for their children, which in effect order that the child be DNR in case of arrest.

An "advance directive" must be made by a competent person, and only takes effect if and when the patient becomes incompetent.

The directives have force only when made by people who have capacity to consider their own best interest.

Advance directives are, in a legal sense, a present refusal or consent to future treatment; they are, therefore, enforcers of the value of the patient's autonomy. The advance directive statutes written in the several states enforce the autonomy of patients over their own bodies—extending even to procedures contemplated in the future.[20]

Advance directives are a category of written or spoken instructions considered as advance consent to treatment. In use, advance directives almost always refuse some treatment in advance of the procedure to be done. Even if the directives do not refuse treatment, the presence of an advance directive in some circumstances may be interpreted as refusal of treatment.

An ordinary will is an advance directive, too—about what is to happen to the person's property after death. But in the context of illness care, advance directives indicate what people want to happen to their bodies if they become both incompetent and ill. Advance directives are either living wills (written or spoken) or durable powers of attorney.

Even when advance directives instruct that the patient *wants* to consent to care, the directive or the patient's proxy may be doubted. (The Helga Wanglie case, discussed near the end of this chapter, under Futility: Prolonging Poor Quality of Life, is an example of a patient whose request for care was not respected by providers.) Or the reverse may be true: that advance directives of specific *refusals* of treatment may also be doubted.

Although not necessarily *refusals* of care, some assume advance directives are, in effect, advance orders not to resuscitate (DNRs). So in addition to inclusion under the value of patient autonomy, advance directives could also be discussed under the value, Life, in Chapter Seven. Some consider the documents a means to direct a future suicide (euthanasia), under certain conditions. The documents are seen as a way to give patients a right to die.[21]

Advance directives were intended to be a way of limiting unwanted care. Most people who write them do not intend the documents to be orders to providers to end their lives.[22] But the ethics and law about advance directives in some cases do enforce the value people put on dying. Aside from that value, advance directives enforce the patient's autonomy (power, freedom) to refuse future treatment.

Advance directives are also related to economics, in several ways. One hope of the use of directives is to limit care (the limits either stated by the writer of the living will or assumed by the provider), and thus to save money on the cost of care. The systems of care payment by a third party (government or private insurance) encourage unlimited care, a system some see as of no cost to the patient or family. Such a system provided incentive to give the patient every treatment possible—leading full circle to care that is sometimes unwanted and giving rise to the desire to refuse it in advance.

History

Living will documents are part of a long campaign by the Euthanasia Society of America. Americans—with knowledge of the Holocaust, Nazi

Germany's rendering of euthanasia—initially shunned the idea of euthanasia, but an educational branch of the American Euthanasia Society (the Euthanasia Education Council) continued to work to change the public's attitude toward euthanasia. At a 1967 meeting of the Euthanasia Education Council, Luis Kutner introduced a "living will"—a document to serve as a vehicle to advance passive euthanasia, and to allay the fear of deliberately caused death. The word *euthanasia* was converted to the phrases "death with dignity" and "right to die."[23] The Euthanasia Society of America has since changed its name to the "Society for the Right to Die" (and subsequently changed again to "Choice in Dying"), and its education council is now called "Concern for Dying."

The term "living will" was used in 1969 in the *Indiana Law Journal*. In 1976 California passed the Natural Death Act, which used the term "living will" also. Like later, similar statutes, the law provided that the directive would operate only if the person was terminally ill. Somewhat later, the durable power of attorney for health care was developed to name a proxy for health care decisions; DPA laws originated in existing laws allowing the person to name a proxy for money decisions.

The success of the "living will"/euthanasia campaign is noted: The Joint Commission for Accreditation of Health Organizations (JCAHO) facilitates the making of advance directives by patients by requiring agencies to meet standards that assure patient exposure to the concept.[24] These standards help hospitals carry out the mandates of the Patient Self-Determination Act (PSDA), below.

Some state laws provide that parents can make advance directives for their children (in effect, the parent can order that the child be DNR in case of cardiac arrest). One writer advocates that children be able to write their own advance directives,[25] while others deny that parents should have power to deny resuscitation to a disabled child in an emergency. Children must be consulted on their care, but there are legal difficulties with allowing minors the power to refuse treatment in the future.

Most nursing publications have been very supportive of the concept of advance directives,[26] and advance directives are described as being for the benefit of the patient. Yet, not all patients wish to have this "benefit."

The Competent Person Has Freedom

An "advance directive," aptly named, is made while the person is competent, in *advance* of becoming incompetent, if that ever happens. The patient must be competent at the time the directive is made, and the directive is used only after the patient becomes incompetent. Competent before, incompetent now—the only time the advance directives can be made or used. If the person is competent, the advance directive is not needed; the patient can decide now, for him or herself. The patient who is already incompetent can't then make an "advance" directive.

Advance directives have force only because they are made by people who *had* decisional capacity, in considering their own best interest. Again, "best interest" is probably one word too many; one need consider only one's *interest*. The incompetent person does not have the capacity to consider his or her interest, so can't make an advance directive.

Advance Directives About Money (Wills)

> Another aspect of autonomy is the person's freedom/power to make a will determining who will inherit property after death.
> Real wills are about property; living wills are about life.
> Nurses will hear patient questions about wills, and should understand the patient's (and their own) need for one.
> Nurses should not try to answer specific questions of patients about wills; they tell them that most people do need a will, and that they should seek an attorney's help.
> In general, the patient's will should not be witnessed by a nurse (claims of undue influence could result).

A measure of the value of freedom is reflected in laws enforcing a person's power to alienate (sell, give away) property and to direct who gets property after a person dies. The person has the freedom/power to make a will—to determine before death who will receive his property at death. Nurses are more likely to encounter "living wills" than real wills in their practice, but—because patients will ask nurses questions about wills—nurses should understand their patient's (and their own) need for a real will.

For a long time in English law (the source of American law), people had no personal right to decide who would get their property after they died. Instead, rules in the law decided (usually the family, king, or church all got some of it). Some property could not even be sold during the "owner's" lifetime.

In a more communal and less individualistic time, property belonged to a continuous family extending over generations. Property was considered to belong as much to the person's spouse, children and descendants as to the individual. If the person had no spouse or children, the property was returned to the family community—the ancestors and their descendants. Over several centuries of Anglo-Saxon law the British and their occupied territories (and other countries with similar laws) have developed law giving the individual power over property, even after death.

Law about wills is complex and includes potential liability for bad advice. Nurses should not try to answer specific questions patients have about wills, nor should they help their patient make wills. Even witnessing a will for a patient is not a good idea unless there is *no* other way for the patient to get his will signed. If the nurse were actually named in the will, her signing could invalidate the gift. If she were not named, her signing could still give rise to claims by persons disinherited that the staff exerted influence over the patient. It is sufficient and safe to tell the patient, if asked, that most people do need a will. People need wills because, if a will is not made, when the person dies the law provides that certain people (spouse, children, relatives) inherit property regardless of what the individual may have wanted. The nurse's best advice to the patient is to get an attorney—not a kit or computer program. Some people have had their wishes completely thwarted using such do-it-yourself means.

A real will is a directive—an advance directive—about what should be done with property after death. An exercise in values clarification: Realize that, the instant an individual dies, all the things and all of the money accumulated no longer belong to the individual. Death comes, property leaves, no matter how much and how carefully collected and cared for.

A living will is *not* a "will" in the same sense as a property document, because a living will may become effective before death. A living will *is* a "will" in the original sense of the word, the will or wish of the person about an event in the future, if a time comes when he can't decide for or express himself personally.

LIVING WILLS

Advance directives must be signed while competent by a person who is able to consider information, to make decisions, and to know the consequence of those decisions [rough guide: whether a patient would be allowed to sign a consent for surgery].

Specifics of the different state statutes on living wills may include:

Who decides whether the patient is incompetent (usually one or two physicians);

A form to use for the will;

Who and how to witness/notarize (nurses should not sign as witnesses);

That treatment can be refused on behalf of the patient if the patient is "terminal" or, in some states, in an "irreversible condition," and who makes that determination.

Trends in the law are to make the use of living wills and withdrawal of treatment easier.

Terms used for the living will and DPA may vary from state to state.

Refusal of treatment for the incompetent person rarely requires court action.

Courts have used the "substituted judgment" and the "best interest" standards to determine what should be done for the patient.

Courts have required that it be proven, in some cases by clear and convincing evidence, that patient would wish to refuse treatment (instead of the lower "preponderance of the evidence" standard or a higher "beyond a reasonable doubt" standard necessary to convict in criminal cases).

Informal, spoken directives are valid and have been upheld in court cases; even if the living will does not meet the statute requirements, it is useful for the decision maker to know the patient's wishes.

An advance directive, whether written or spoken, formally or casually made—whether the patient is terminal or not—should be followed if following it will be in the interest of the patient (read the directive).

The specific state statute on living wills can be found at the local branch library, indexed under headings like Death or Medical Treatment.

A living will is not the same as a durable power of attorney [DPA—see discussion, Durable (Springing) Power of Attorney]. The DPA names *who* should make decisions about illness care after incompetency. A living will speaks to all potential caregivers, saying "do" or "don't" under certain conditions. A durable power of attorney speaks to one person, saying, "Decide for me when I can't." The living will says *what* to do; the DPA says *who* is to decide.

Most states now have statutes that are classed as "living will" laws, and many have laws that provide for durable power of attorney for health care. Contrasted to the long legal history of real wills, "living wills" have been written by individuals for about twenty years. As explained earlier under History, a few people who knew of the euthanasia movement had access to the concept and wrote living wills prior to that. Most of the state statutes formalizing living wills into law have been passed within the last 15 years, so the law in this area is still developing.

Nurses may be interested to know the specifics of their state's living will statute (which may change from year to year), but knowledge of the specifics is not necessary in order to practice good nursing and act ethically. If good nursing practice, a nurse's actions will largely comply with any state's law. After the Supreme Court's *Cruzan* decision, some of the restrictions on the use of living wills that are written into state living will statutes are probably unconstitutional (such as restrictions against withholding food and water, if that's what the living will calls for).

The fact that some parts of the state statute may be unconstitutional means that knowing the specific statute may be confusing. (Which *part* is unconstitutional?) Because there are 50 different living will laws, any of which could change any day, it is not helpful to summarize them as to each state's specifics. But some provisions, found in most laws, will be discussed.

Some Specific Provisions

The laws vary, but all provide that people must sign such a document while competent. Defining "competent" (like defining "obscenity") is easier when seen, harder to define in words. Generally, a competent person is one who is able to consider information, make decisions, and know the consequences of those decisions. As noted above, a rough guide to competence is whether a patient would be allowed to sign a consent for surgery. If so, the patient can probably be considered competent to decide other things.

Some statutes designate who shall decide whether the patient is incompetent; for example, two doctors, who certify on the chart or using a certain form.

Some states specify a form to use for the will. The law may specify exactly how the will may be witnessed and/or notarized, and may forbid caregivers from witnessing. And some laws state that certain categories of doctors are needed to certify that the patient is "terminal" or in "irreversible condition."

The law may have a provision that the will operates *only if* the person is terminally ill (this provision is also possibly unconstitutional, if the patient's actual living will says differently). More such provisions now allow refusal of treatment for a patient under their living will, if the patient is in an "irreversible condition." Persistent Vegetative State (PVS), Alzheimer's, diabetes, and mental retardation are all "irreversible conditions," to some extent, so care is needed in interpreting the statute.

The state statute may have qualifications for what kind of diagnosis is needed, and that the diagnosis must be agreed to by a specific number of doctors. Sometimes the law specifies what kind of treatment can be refused.

Many living will statutes say that water and food cannot be withheld (restrictions that may be unconstitutional after *Cruzan*). Most statutes do not provide for naming a surrogate in the living will. Some provide no penalty on the practitioner for not honoring the directive. (But in Missouri, the practitioner can be charged with "unprofessional conduct" for failing to honor a directive, which could result in loss of license.)

Specific Living Will Statutes and Trends

The living will statute in Ohio says that treatment of the patient can be withheld on request of certain family members and a probate court, if the patient is diagnosed as a permanently unconscious person or will die within 12 months. A new law in Illinois is similar, but it doesn't necessitate a court decision. According to the Supreme Court's words in *Cruzan, any* restriction on what the competent person can ask her living will to withhold, including food and water, may be unconstitutional.

The Maryland Health Care Decisions Act, in effect in 1993, allows a living will to be used to withdraw hydration and nutrition in persons who are not only terminally ill, but also those in PVS. The law would also would allow withdrawal of food and water from incompetent patients who are compromised in "all areas of daily living." That definition could include many patients in nursing homes. This power to dehydrate the patient to death can proceed on the directive of a living will (made by a competent person who later becomes incompetent).

In addition, dehydration can be done to the patient who has never requested such treatment. This statute (like those discussed above under Consent, which allow surrogates to give consent or refuse treatment) allows surrogate decision makers to give the order to dehydrate.

Watch for confusion in the terms; remember the function of the documents—a living will to say "what" and a durable power of attorney (DPA) to say "who." The Maryland act, described above, calls the living will an "advance directive" despite common usage elsewhere that the latter phrase includes powers of attorney as well; the attorney in fact named in the DPA (the decision maker) is called an "agent" in that law. In Texas, the living will is called a "directive to physicians" and a surrogate (proxy, agent) may be designated in the living will, whereas in most states the DPA document is used for this.

Unwritten or Informal

The living will statutes do not give another person, even a guardian, the right to refuse treatment on the person's behalf unless the patient fits the criteria in the law (as terminal, or perhaps comatose, or perhaps in "irreversible condition"). But after *Cruzan*, even if the patient's condition does not fit the statute's criteria, the living will still may be useful. The document or spoken statement can be used by the person who seeks to refuse treatment for another, to show what the person's wishes would be if the individual could decide personally.

The preference for written advance directives is an artifact of the legal process, because a written document is easier to prove than the testimony of a witness as to what was said, and when. But spoken directives are just as valid as written directives. Informal unwritten advance directives have been upheld in some court cases. Informal, spoken expressions of the person, made while competent, have been honored, as was done in the *Cruzan* case.

At the first hearing on removing Nancy Cruzan's feeding tube, her friends testified that she didn't want to live if she couldn't be "at least halfway normal." That did not meet the Missouri Supreme Court's standard of clear and convincing evidence of what she would want. At the second hearing, after the case had been to the U.S. Supreme Court, the testimony of another friend was that Nancy had either made, or heard and didn't disagree with, the statement, "I wouldn't want to live like that." The same judge who had ordered her feeding tube removed after the first hearing, now ordered the feeding tube removed, holding that this evidence did meet the clear and convincing standard. Since the Missouri attorney general didn't appeal that second ruling, the patient was dehydrated to death. (See Chapter Seven for more on *Cruzan*.)

People do not have to write an advance directive—it can be spoken. Even if the statute specifies a form and says it should be used, another form will probably be honored. There is no perfect document that will satisfy every-one. The search for one is futile.[27] And, living wills that do not meet the specific requirements of the statute are still useful in guiding the decision maker as to the patient's earlier wishes.

Court Cases

Refusal of treatment for the incompetent person rarely requires court action. Only 60-plus cases are reported for such instances, out of some 20 million deaths from limiting treatment since 1976 (limiting treatment often refers to dying without CPR). In those relatively few cases that have been litigated, the courts use guides to decide for incompetent patients, such as the patient's "best interest" or "substituted judgment." The court may say that the decision maker should stand in the patient's shoes—should use her substituted judgment; or the court may say that the decision maker should look out for the patient's "best interest."

In those cases, the courts used varying standards of evidence to assess the patient's wishes. In the *Cruzan* decision, the Supreme Court agreed that the state could require clear and convincing evidence of the patient's wishes to refuse treatment (instead of a lower "preponderance of the evidence" standard or a higher "beyond a reasonable doubt" standard used in criminal cases). The court in such cases is usually interpreting a statute, using rules of interpretation that include looking at the clear meaning of the words, and giving meaning to the intent of the legislators in writing the law.

Practice

The rule: An advance directive—whether written or spoken, formally or casually made; whether the patient is terminal or not—should be followed if following it will be in the interest of the patient. Nurses should of course read the individual patient's document. But, as always, nurses must use good nursing judgment and common sense to tell them if honoring the advance directive is good for the patient in any given situation.

If the patient has a living will on the chart, the doctor or nurse may feel more comfortable in discussing a no-code order with the patient. (But remember that having a living will on the patient's chart does not mean that DNR is automatic—the patient may *want* resuscitation.) Many people who have a living will mean them to be used in a situation similar to Nancy Cruzan's—the very unlikely event that they are in a coma, projected to live for years with tube feedings.

The living will should say generally what treatment the patient wants and doesn't want, after becoming incompetent (if that ever happens). But some forms used by patients for living wills are now quite specific, providing that people do or do not want dialysis, IVs, intubation, CPR, antibiotics, and so on. In addition, the forms may conflict with other advance directives about organ donation. What should be done if the patient's living will says *do* resuscitate but *do not* intubate or use a ventilator? What if the patient wants organs donated, but does not want CPR or life support? (The body must be maintained on life support until organs to be donated are removed.) What about new treatments not envisioned when the living will was written?

Obviously, practitioners cannot follow directives with contradictory provisions. Once again, the rule: Good nursing practice, using ethical values, will be legal. Doing what seems to be in the interest of the patient, consulting others for their assessment, is good nursing practice. No law can absolve nurses of responsibility for their practice—nor should it. And most nurses wouldn't want it to do so.

Some authorities recommend a hybrid living will/durable power of attorney, a medical directive. The medical directive is a very specific paper listing several possible scenarios, with the potential patient's estimate of his wishes in each case.[28] But others note that it is very hard to predict exactly what the setting will be, and what the options will be, when the advance directive is put to use.[29]

Specific living wills are more likely to be "used" by practitioners—meaning that therapy is more likely to be discontinued and death to be caused when the directive is more specific.

For More Information

To find out more about living wills, the nurse can read the policy of her agency; each agency employing nurses will have a policy on such documents. Agency policy is mandatory since 1 December 1991, when the Danforth amendment (Patient Self-Determination Act) became effective (details below).

Nurses can read exactly what their state's living will law says by finding the state statutes at the local branch library, looking in the index under everything related to the topic. Indexers seem unfamiliar or uncomfortable with categorizing this new kind of statute, so the statute may be indexed under any heading from Death to Medical Treatment to Wills.

DURABLE (SPRINGING) POWER OF ATTORNEY

The origin of the DPA for health care is the state statute governing the durable power of attorney for finances.

The health care DPA appoints a person who will make decisions about treatment for the writer of the document, if the writer becomes incompetent.

The decision maker, called surrogate, agent, attorney in fact, or proxy, manages the principal's *body*, not the money.

The declaration of incompetence is not done by a court (as it is in appointing a guardian for a ward) but usually by a physician or two.

> One can request in advance that a certain person be named his guardian (or that a certain person *not* be named), if guardianship appears likely in the future.
>
> A durable power of attorney for health care can be written simply.
>
> The DPA takes effect when the patient becomes incompetent but, unlike the living will, the patient does not have to be terminal (or equivalent).
>
> The Patient Self-Determination Act (PSDA—also called the Danforth amendment after its U.S. Senate sponsor) requires that agencies receiving Medicare money ask patients if they have advance directives, inform patients of their rights to refuse treatment under state law, and educate staff and the community about those rights.
>
> Failure to comply with the law could cause the agency to lose its Medicare funding.
>
> The purpose of the PSDA was at least in part concerned with the economics of care.

All states have durable power of attorney laws for financial matters. A durable power of attorney for finances allows a person (the principal) to choose another person (called the agent or attorney in fact) to manage the principal's money, as soon as it is signed. The power continues (the durable part) after the person becomes incompetent, if that should happen.

The relatively new arrangement in the law is a durable power of attorney for *health care*. This document says that a person is appointed who will make decisions about treatment for the writer of the document, in the future. Other names for the decision maker: a surrogate, an agent, an attorney in fact, a proxy—all labels that refer to a person who manages one's *body*, not one's *money*, if the person becomes incompetent.

The use of the word *durable* is inappropriate here; the analogy to the financial durable power of attorney is flawed. In the money management durable power of attorney, the power is granted to the agent immediately and continues (is durable) after the principal becomes incompetent. The illness care power of attorney is not "durable." It first comes into being after, and only if, the person becomes incompetent.

In the law, other instances of the concept of power being created by some future contingency, are termed *springing*. Property law is an example: The power springs into existence when a certain event happens. That is the case here. The power to decide about another's sick care doesn't en*dure* (stay durable) from competence through incompetence. Only at incompetence does it *spring* into being.

On the day the power of attorney is written, the person is not giving immediate power that will endure, to someone to manage the care of the body. The person is providing for a power of attorney that may spring into effect later, on the day when (and if) the person becomes incompetent.

These laws providing for durable power of attorney for health care have been enacted in many states. All the statutes in some way provide for another person to take over and make decisions for the patient, without the need for a court to make a decision of incompetence. Declaring a person incompetent and appointing a guardian is usually power over the money *and* the life.

The attorney in fact for "health" care has power over the patient's body after the patient is incompetent. The attorney in fact (or agent) does *not* have power over the patient's financial affairs or other legal matters. That power would be given by a durable power of attorney for finances, or by appointing a guardian.

The term "attorney in fact" is related to, but different from, the term "attorney at law." The word *attorney* is Old French, based on the verb "turn," to arrange, to distribute. An attorney in fact need not be a lawyer.

If the court has not adjudged the patient incompetent, someone else makes the determination that gives the attorney in fact (agent) power to make decisions. Statutes differ, but usually the physician has that power. Nurses—the practitioners who spend the most time with the patient—must furnish information to that person who determines incompetency. Being the closest to the patient and having assessed competency in order to carry out nursing practice, the nurse indeed may be the individual who initiates the process.

Under most DPA statutes the process for determining incompetency is often only one or two doctors agreeing on "incompetence," and writing that decision on the chart. This process is far less formal and has far fewer safeguards than determination of incompetency by a court. The court procedure for determining incompetency has been developed over hundreds of years of law, and has refined safeguards for the potential ward.

If one really anticipates possible incompetence at some point in one's life—as do some who carry the gene for Huntington's or familial Alzheimer's—they may wish to write a document specifying who they want appointed as their guardian. (This is different from writing a durable power of attorney for health care, since a guardian has power over the body and the property of the ward.) The request made in advance by the potential ward is binding on the court as long as the choice of guardian is reasonable. The guardian to be appointed cannot be incompetent or a minor. One can also specify who definitely should *not* be made one's guardian, if that is important, also a request that will almost always be honored by the court.

People lose virtually *all* their rights when they become incompetent—and, yet, some assert that such patients retain a "right" that amounts to a right to commit suicide (right to die) by refusing treatment that would maintain life. This is the situation when it is assumed that people in persistent vegetative state have the "right" through proxy to refuse food and water. This assumption is at odds with the standard that an intent to suicide require the *most* evidence of competency.

Mentally ill and incompetent people are prevented from committing suicide, by force if necessary. It is said that they are not competent to decide to end their lives. But incompetent people are allowed to cause their own death by dehydration, through proxies. Here, a legal fiction is maintained—that the patient is actually competent, and is expressing his or her wish to refuse treatment by proxy.

In the situation of the minor's consent powers, discussed above under Consent, the value of the minor's life and the value of doing good for the minor are put above the value of his or her autonomy (freedom). In contrast, in the case of the incompetent patient, the value of the autonomy of the incompetent patient to choose death is valued over life and doing good for the patient. In this context, some argue that causing the patient's death is in reality doing the patient good—that death is better for the patient than living.

As noted above, in the cases of minors and incompetents, providers have turned to surrogate decision makers (spouses, parents, children, and siblings) for years as part of ethical decision making, without formal documents or law. What is new is that the procedure has become formalized in recent statutes and case law.

SAMPLE DPA FOR HEALTH CARE

A durable power of attorney for health care can be written simply (state statutes may designate a form, but most states will honor the intent of the maker, regardless of the form):

I, _____, appoint _____ as my agent to make any and all health care decisions for me, except to the extent I state otherwise in this document. This durable power of attorney for health care takes effect if I become unable to make my own health care decisions, and this fact is certified in writing by my physicians.

LIMITATIONS (Write any limitations on authority in this space.)

DESIGNATION OF ALTERNATIVE AGENT (1st and 2nd)

I hereby designate _____ as my first alternative agent if for any reason my first alternative agent cannot or will not serve.

I hereby designate _____ as my second alternative agent if for any reason my first alternative agent cannot or will not serve.

Original kept at _____.

Signed copies at _____

The document should be signed and witnessed by two or three people who are not likely to benefit from the maker's death (no potential heirs, agents, nurses, spouse, or creditors). The writing should be notarized (some statutes require it). Signatures are notarized to prevent someone from later asserting that the signature on the document is a forgery and thus invalid.

Nota Bene: The patient must be incompetent before the DPA takes effect (same as for the living will). But the patient does not have to be terminal (or equivalent) for the DPA to be effective (*un*like the living will requirements).

Danforth—OBRA '90—PSDA

Living wills and other advance directives are encouraged by the U.S. government under the Patient Self-Determination Act (PSDA) and by private organizations (Euthanasia Society, JCAHO). The Patient Self-Determination Act (PSDA) was part of the 1990 amendment to Medicare law. (OBRA '90: the Omnibus Budget Reform Act, includes many other kinds of law; the budget acts of each year, OBRA '89, OBRA '91, and so on, are handy places to tack on amendments.)

The Danforth amendment (the PSDA) enforces the value of autonomy, specifically the freedom to refuse treatment. Under that amendment, agencies that care for patients and receive Medicare money must inform patients of their rights under state law to accept or refuse medical or surgical treatment—must inform patients of their right to make (or *not* make) advance directives.

The Danforth amendment requires the agency to ask the patient if he or she has an advance directive, and to indicate the answer to that question on the chart. (Surveys say that, prior to Danforth, only four percent of hospitals asked that question of patients.) The law requires the agencies to follow state law regarding advance directives. (Of course, state laws also had required that the law be followed, but now failure to follow the state law could also lose the agency its Medicare funding.) The law also requires agencies to formulate written policies about honoring patients' advance directives, and to educate their staffs and communities about them.

A good question to ask when dealing with this or any other law: What's the penalty if it's not followed? The potential penalty in this law is not jail or fine or civil liability in a malpractice case. Instead, violation could cause loss of funding from Medicare. It is unlikely, however, that by itself, violating this section would lose an agency funds, unless the violation were flagrant and continued.

But most agencies meet state-administered Medicare requirements by complying with JCAHO accreditation standards. Too many "demerits" by the JCAHO on an inspection survey will prompt a survey by the state agency that enforces Medicare standards, which could easily find additional violations of standards. So, agencies are likely to try to comply with the Patient Self-Determination Act.

Another good question to ask when dealing with law: What is the purpose of this law? What ethical value does the law minimally enforce? Freedom? Life? Doing Good, Doing No Harm to patients?

INTENT OF THE DANFORTH AMENDMENT

In a memo written by Senator Danforth, prior to passage of his amendment and quoted in an article written by a former Danforth staffer, the Senator asked about economics, quality of life, artificial extension of life, and whether a lesser degree of care to the comatose was possible. Economics was mentioned and denied as a motivator:

> More and more it is arguable that we play God by subjecting people to unwanted and sometimes unnecessary treatment, treatment that unnaturally prolongs the dying process. Our health care system has become obsessed with extending life, at times neglecting the caring component of medicine and trampling on the rights of patients.
>
> —Senator John C. Danforth (R-Mo.)[30]

Senator Danforth had cost very much in mind when he questioned Hillary Rodham Clinton on the 1993 Clinton healthcare reform plan:

> He asked her whether the system would have 'somebody at some level in a position to say no' . . . .[and] cited a baby who was kept alive for 11 months without a brain; a separation of Siamese twins of whom one was certain to die and the other had only a 1 percent chance of living; babies with low birth weight of whom only 15 percent will be functional, and expensive efforts to prolong life for three or six months at very high cost.
> Mr. Danforth has raised this issue from time to time since 1987.[31]

Another author, after discussing the costs of maintaining Permanent Unconscious Persons (PUPs), said that reducing cost of care was not the primary purpose of the law. But he then said the PSDA would have the fortuitous side effect of reducing cost. He believes there is a state and federal interest in ensuring that PUPs do not receive long-term care that they would not want.[32]

Nursing leaders have usually advocated advance directives, therefore their pleasure with PSDA promotion of advance directives is not surprising. Increasing technology, high costs, and protection of the patient as a consumer are cited as reasons for the development of the Patient Self-Determination Act. Criticisms of the PSDA are made, in particular that the law has not changed practice in the direction of withdrawing more care.[33] Regardless, the Patient Self-Determination Act directly affects the "principles" (values) of autonomy (freedom) and beneficence (doing good, caring by nurses).[34] Some nurses who believe advance directives are used to limit care inappropriately, worry that the mandate to discuss them with patients violates *nurse* autonomy.

**SAMPLE POLICY: COMPLYING WITH
THE DANFORTH AMENDMENT**

One agency's process for complying with the mandates of the PSDA and the JCAHO standards:

1. The admitting clerk gives the patient an "Advance Directive" handbook.
2. The patient is informed that a detailed booklet is available to review at admission.
3. Any patient who wants one gets a two-part form for advance directives and is informed of her option to write an advance directive.
4. If the patient writes an advance directive, medical records "puts a fluorescent sticker on the patient's record, and the advance directive document is always kept with the record."
5. Social service helps the patient write the directive.
6. The nursing department "implements" the directive—should the patient's condition warrant—and makes sure the directive is followed.
7. If the patient is transferred to another agency, social service calls and tells the new staff. The advance directive is faxed or given to the patient/family.

In this agency, the patient is told, "Completion of one of these two directives is highly recommended for everyone."

The patient is given and asked to sign a statement: "I have been given written information, I have been informed of rights to make an advance directive, I understand I'm not required make one, I understand my advance directive will be followed."

"_____ I have _____ I have not executed an advance directive."[35]

Cautions About Advance Directives

Advance directives are not seen uniformly as good for patients.

Providers don't follow the living will in about one-fourth of cases, and are more likely to deny treatment requested than to give treatment refused in the document.

Despite years of encouragement, only eight to 15 percent of Americans have written some kind of advance directive.

Documents required by statute create more paperwork, expose providers to penalties, and may be contradictory as to the patient's wishes.

The majority of people who have advance directives don't want them followed exactly.

Some assume that a living will on the chart means the patient would prefer to be DNR in an arrest, and perhaps that the patient doesn't want treatment even if the prognosis is good.

Advance consent to or refusal of treatment (in an advance directive) violates the informed consent rules, since the patient cannot have full information when consenting or refusing treatment in advance.

African-Americans are less likely than other Americans to have advance directives or to donate organs, perhaps partly because they see advance directives and organ donation as taking away their hard-won autonomy (power, control).

Living wills are seen by some as devices to allow patients to die without expensive treatment so as to save money on care.

As with the requirement for informed consent to treatment, caregivers who suggest advance directives to a patient, or who assist a patient to prepare them, must fully inform the patient of the potential consequences.

Advance directives could allow the past interest of the person (in being in control of her future) to harm her present interest (in living).

Nurses have a legal and ethical duty to protect their patient if the surrogate decision maker is not acting in the patient's best interest.

The nurse can assess that best interest using her duty to do good, to do no harm, to preserve autonomy, and to value the life of the patient.

One criticism of living wills is that in some way they seek to make the incompetent patient responsible for his own death. The provider can rationalize: "It's not my decision to terminate care; the patient wanted it this way."

EARLY CONCERNS ABOUT ADVANCE DIRECTIVES

In its beginnings, the use of advance directives was commented on as follows:

I doubt the good sense of enshrining in statutory format an individual's attempt to anticipate a disabled future and to bind family or physicians to act as if the prior directive left them choiceless. No statute should require that family or physicians automatically implement a person's earlier choice for death without regard to their own current personal misgivings and interpersonal distress.[36]

Providers sometimes do not follow what the living will says. A 1991 study showed that, in 25 percent of situations, advance directives were not followed by providers. Treatment that the living will ordered *not* be given, was administered in seven percent of cases. And patients were *denied* treatment requested in their directives 18 percent of the time. The study showed that one-fourth of treatments are different from what the patient's living will requested.

When asked to imagine themselves with a poor prognosis and desperately ill, 30 percent of people would choose life-sustaining treatment.[37] Evidence mounts that living wills are not a panacea for treating (not treating) patients whose treatment is questionable.[38]

When deciding on whether to order feeding tubes, physicians follow families' decisions instead of living wills. Patients therefore would be wise to discuss their wishes with their families and doctor *also* if they sign a living will.[39]

As noted, the Euthanasia Society introduced the concept of living wills in 1967; living will statutes in some states have been in existence for more than 15 years; and living wills written earlier than that; and although most states have had a living will statute for longer than five years, only eight to 15 percent of Americans have written some kind of advance directive. The advance refusal of future treatment is evidently not a need felt by all people (actions are evidence of values?).

As indicated above, the forms for living wills and durable (springing) powers of attorney may be as lengthy and complex as people care to make them. They must be requested from each patient, copied, and entered on the patient's chart at each admission to the agency. And some state laws provide penalties for providers if the directives are not followed.

Just as has always been done with advance directives for funerals that the family can't stand—such as advance directives to bury people in their cars or with their pets—the directives in the living will or durable power of attorney should be followed when the directives are appropriate to the patient's situation. The directives won't be justified and shouldn't be implemented when they are not in the interest of the patient.

Studies indicate that, even if they have written one, many people don't want their advance directives followed rigidly. In a study of dialysis patients, people varied greatly in their grant of authority to practitioners and surrogates, to follow or deviate from their directives: 39 percent wanted the directives followed strictly, 19 percent granted a little leeway, 11 percent a lot of flexibility, and 31 percent say the directives need not be followed at all.

Patients varied also in how much they wanted practitioners to consider pain or suffering, quality of life, new treatment possibilities, indignity, financial problems, and religion. Most wanted these things considered when carrying out their advance directives, and a few wanted the directive followed without consideration of any other factor. The nurse's problem is determining which category the patient is in.

Remarkable for people with such a serious prognosis, only 20 percent of dialysis patients had a *written* advance directive, while 43 percent said they had a spoken advance directive. After 30 minutes of interview about advance directives, at follow-up at least four weeks later, few additional patients (four of 150) had a written directive. Nine more had made spoken advance directives.

The authors' conclusion was that practitioners should talk to patients about whether to apply advance directives, and whether to modify them.[40] This advice means that having written directives is not a substitute for communication. Patients, practitioners, and families must talk about treatment wishes. Here again, it is more important to practice ethically and sensibly than to know the letter of the law. The law follows the ethics.

People who advise patients on advance directives should be aware that those instruments may be used to justify an automatic limiting of treatment by doctors, nurses, and agencies. The person advising the patient may be both legally and ethically responsible for fully informing the patient of such potential consequences of executing an advance directive, analogous to the situation of medical informed consent.

The legal foundation of refusal of future treatment is problematic under the rules pertaining to informed consent. The refusal of consent cannot be informed, since the patient cannot know in advance all future factors relative to a fully informed judgment, at the time the decision (refusal) must be made. To refuse treatment perhaps years in advance is not an informed refusal, just as consent for treatment made that far in advance cannot be informed consent. Thus, an advance consent to or refusal of treatment cannot be informed.

When used by illness care providers, often under pressure to save money by limiting care, a living will could become a living "won't"—the patient won't live long with such a document on the chart.[41]

Living wills can be used (illegally) to limit the patient's treatment without consent even when the patient is competent, not terminal, and has a good prognosis. Some nurses and doctors assume that a living will on the chart automatically means the patient would prefer to be DNR when in cardiac arrest. Further, it may mean to many that the patient doesn't want *any* treatment even if the prognosis is good.

At present, a living will is not considered the same as a DNR order. And a DNR order does not mean that the patient wants to die. But, in future, rules may be written that mandate that patients who have living wills, or who do not want resuscitation, will not be admitted to the acute care hospital. Patients with advance refusals of treatment could perhaps be kept out of ICUs, where one of the goals is to save lives with resuscitation and all available means.

There is anecdotal evidence that a patient who presents with a living will or durable power of attorney, which is then attached to the chart, is presumed to want to be DNR. This assumption is made without knowing whether DNR is appropriate or not, and whether discussed with the patient or not. Further, many have noted that a DNR order in the eyes of many caregivers is tantamount to ordering "no treatment."

ELDERLY'S FEARS ABOUT ADVANCE DIRECTIVES

"Many older patients . . . fear that a living will, combined with their age and frailty, could be used to deprive them of care that they might want before

> the trigger event stipulated as the sign to withhold care. Indeed, some of these fears are probably justified. It is still common for many house staff and attending physicians to create a penumbra of nontreatment around orders not to resuscitate. Many still think these orders are incompatible with aggressive care. Some interpret the do-not-resuscitate provisions of a living will similarly. Concerns about the negative medical consequences of exercising one's rights as a patient may not be unfounded."[42]

Agencies serving populations of African-Americans note that often their patients are wary of the medical profession. African-Americans are thus reluctant to sign a paper or otherwise authorize withdrawing or withholding medical treatment, whether a living will or DNR. Such reservations also are generally true of people who are poor and/or uneducated. Some examples reinforce their belief: The Tuskegee experiment, of black men with syphilis left untreated as a control group between 1932 and 1972 (although treatment became available in the 1940s) is now well known.

As recently as 1984, one researcher screened 13,000 black women for sickle cell anemia without their consent. There was no prescreening, no follow-up counsel, nor could the women decline participation.

African-Americans are also less likely than other Americans to donate organs. The reasons may be speculated as religious, and that they fear their organs may be taken from them prematurely. African-Americans are also more likely to want aggressive treatment in the face of terminal illness.[43] They see living wills and other advance directives as taking their autonomy (power, control) away—the reasoning, "If I agree to a DNR, it's even more likely that I won't get the treatment I need."

They may not be wrong. Evidence exists that patients with living wills are considered to be DNR. The presence of a living will means to many providers that the patient wants virtually no treatment. Competent patients with good prognoses have been allowed to die of an arrest that probably could have been reversed successfully, because a living will prompted a DNR note on the chart.[44]

Living Wills May Not Save Money

An article suggested that HMOs could better compete by offering premium discounts for Medicare beneficiaries who sign living wills.[45] Might living wills be seen by some as devices to allow patients to die without expensive treatment, with hoped-for savings in cost?

Some state laws forbid insurance companies from requiring applicants to make an advance directive (refusing treatment) in order to qualify for insurance. Those laws seek to protect people from pressure to make a living will in return for cheap insurance. But some health insurance companies mail out living will forms with their policies, to the policy holder.[46] It can be asked, is this for the benefit of the insured or the insurance company?

Some say that laws forbidding discounts for refusal of treatment themselves interfere with the patient's freedom—interfere with the ability of the person to make a contract with the insurance company for cheaper insurance. In states without statutory prohibitions, insurance companies could require a "refuse care directive" before writing *any* insurance for the individual.

Living wills were assumed to be a "more ethically feasible approach to cost control" by the authors of another study. But the study found that advance directives did not save illness care costs[47] (an implied goal of such documents).

On the other hand, anecdotal evidence suggests that patients are resuscitated who should not be, despite a DNR order to the contrary. This is done because the patient does not have a living will. The confusion of DNR with the living will is so great that in one case a patient with a DNR order was resuscitated and the doctor was told, in effect, "We had to try to resuscitate him, he didn't have a living will."[48]

Lawyers who prepare living wills or durable powers of attorney papers for their clients should be under some duty to inform their clients of how these documents may be used—that the documents might deny or limit care inappropriately. By failing to notify clients of the risks of having such documents, lawyers could be liable for failure of "informed consent" in preparation of the document for the client.

Nurses as well as patients are put at risk by the use of living wills. If nurses fail to treat a patient who might recover, just because of the presence of a living will on the chart, a lawsuit for neglect or malpractice might be brought. As indicated, the living will statute does not operate until the patient is (1) incompetent and (2) terminally ill (or in an "irreversible condition," whatever the courts may eventually interpret that phrase to mean).

Caregivers who suggest such a document to a patient, and who assist a patient with preparing such a document (just as lawyers should), must be prepared to fully inform the patient of the potential consequences, that the living will might be used to justify denial of care. The advisor could be responsible for possible liability for the effects of such assistance or advice.

Some attorneys attach a revocation form to the living will or durable (springing) power of attorney itself, because people who are competent can revoke the document, change their minds and change the document, or change the agent they appoint to be their "attorney in fact." Unfortunately, in confusion, some individuals and their witnesses have signed *all* the documents at the same sitting, including the revocation the attorney has attached —which both establishes and then immediately revokes the instrument.

Ethical Problems of Advance Directives

An ethical problem is seen by one authority: Competent persons make advance directives to feel in control of their future, but their wishes now may conflict with their needs if they become incompetent patients. The use of advance directives fails to recognize that people have different interests at different stages of their lives.[49]

People may be unable to predict their interests, as the directives assume they can. An existence unimaginable to a 20-year-old may be tolerable to a patient at 90 (at least preferable to death). The advance directive also could remove responsibility from, or give license to, the nurse who has ethical standards different from the patient's. Such a person might carry out the directive as written without considering changed circumstances. The excuse would be, "It's not my decision; the patient wanted it this way—it says so in the living will."

When a person writes an advance directive and then becomes incompetent, she or he may not be able to change the decision about care. Some would argue that because the patient has become incompetent, they are also *in*competent to change the decision. A Florida woman was denied food in a nursing home on orders of her brother (acting on a durable power of attorney) despite allegations that she requested food from staff. An Attorney Al Litem was appointed, who reported that she did "not have the current capacity to revoke her advanced [sic] medical directives." On 3 March 1995 a judge ordered all food be withheld, and she died 14 days later.[50]

Nurses have a legal and ethical duty to protect their patients. Most illness codes of ethics mandate the professional act in the interest of the patient—to be an advocate for the patient if necessary. The nurse's duty to protect the patient means that, in some situations, the nurse acts on behalf of the patient.

If the patient's surrogate decision maker—a doctor acting according to a living will, a family member, a court appointed guardian, or an agent appointed by the durable (springing) power of attorney—is not acting in the patient's best interest, what is the nurse's responsibility? The nurse may have a legal duty to act, under statute that requires report of abuse or neglect, or under case law that imposes legal liability for neglecting the duty of care. Apart from the minimum legal mandate, the nurse may have an ethical duty to assist another human being—Doing Good and Doing No Harm. The ethical obligation is reinforced by the profession's code of ethics. The nurse acts on the personal belief it is right, not only because the profession believes it is right. Codes of ethics are not law, but reminders and reinforcers.

No book on law, nor even one on the abstract of ethics, can tell a nurse when to act on a patient's behalf. Most of the time the surrogate *will* act in the patients' interest. When the surrogate doesn't, however, the nurse will recognize it by employing the values of doing good for the patient, not harming the patient, preserving the freedom of the patient, and—last but not least—valuing the life of the patient. If the surrogate does not act in the patient's interest, the nurse has an ethical and resulting legal mandate to protect the patient. In the starvation case above, it was reported to be a nurse aide who advocated for the patient.

USING THE LIVING WILL AND DURABLE POWER OF ATTORNEY: FOUR QUESTIONS TO ASK

[The following questions are for information only; for legal advice, consult your attorney.]

START

Patient needs treatment. But, for some reason, you are unsure whether to treat (or not treat) as USUALLY indicated.

1. Is the patient competent?

   NO, the patient is not competent. Next question:

   YES, the patient is competent. Treat as indicated, unless patient refuses.*

2. Does the patient have a legal guardian?

   NO, incompetent patient has no guardian. Next question:

   YES, the patient has a guardian. Treat as indicated, unless guardian refuses.*

3. Does patient have a Durable Power of Attorney (DPA) for Health Care or other agent/surrogate/proxy/authorization?

   YES, PATIENT HAS A DPA.
   A. Document your finding that patient is unable to make decisions about her care: 1) doesn't understand information, or 2) can't make decisions and communicate, or 3) doesn't understand consequences of decision. Or all three.
   B. Treat as indicated, unless the agent named in the DPA refuses. Does the patient have a living will, too? In most states, the DPA rules, with the agent using the LW for guidance.*

   NO, PATIENT HAS NO DPA. Next question:

4. Does patient have a living will?

   NO, PATIENT HAS NO LW.
   A. Document your finding that patient is unable to make decisions about her care using criteria under DPA.
   B. Treat as medically indicated, consulting persons who know patient as to wishes to refuse treatment. Statute may say who can help decide: spouse, children, parents, nearest living relative.

   YES, PATIENT HAS LW.
   A. Document finding that patient is unable to make decisions about her care using criteria outlined above under DPA.
   B. Treat as medically indicated, unless the living will says different. If an agent is named in the living will, treat as indicated unless that agent refuses. The agent should use the LW as a guide.

*NO FURTHER QUESTIONS

Nota Bene:

The LW and the DPA are both effective after and only after the patient is declared incapable of deciding, either by a court or by the physician. The LW operates after the patient is both incompetent *and* "terminal." (Some states: "irreversible condition.")

The presence of a living will does not indicate an automatic DNR order.

A living will is not a prerequisite for a DNR order. The DNR order is made when either 1) the patient refuses CPR in advance, or 2) the doctor orders DNR because the patient's condition warrants (consulting with the patient and/or family).

The LW and DPA are guides to the treatment decision, not releases from responsibility to use judgment in treating or not treating the patient.

Law is minimal ethical behavior; doing the right thing should exceed the minimum legal standard.

The LW idea was conceived by the Euthanasia Society in 1967 (now the Society for the Right to Die).

TALK WITH THE PATIENT AND FAMILY IS MORE IMPORTANT THAN WRITING ON A PAPER.

—© 1994 J.K. Hall

TRANSPLANTS

Organ transplantation usually requires a brain-dead, ICU-maintained body. But *tissues* for transplantation (corneas, skin, bone) can be taken from dead, nonmaintained bodies.

The value most important to the recipient of the organ is fairness in distribution of body parts.

The value most important to the donor of the organ is autonomy—the donor's power over her or his own body after death (or her family's power over her body).

At the point of death, the power (freedom) of the person over the body is transferred to the family.

The person's wishes about the body usually should rule over that of the relatives, but the relatives' strong feelings may prevail.

Laws that enforce the power over the body after death include consents required for autopsy and consent to donation of the whole body (or for body parts).

Federal regulations mandate that institutions receiving funding from Medicare ask families for permission to use transplantable body parts.

Proposed laws would mandate that organs automatically be donated, unless the patient expressed an objection in advance of death.

Should there be limits on what can be done with dead bodies (cadavers)?

> Transplants also involve economics: Should body parts be distributed to the highest bidder or most advanced transplant center, or should they be equally available through a waiting list?
>
> U.S. statutes make payment to the donor for body parts illegal (different from some other countries).
>
> Body parts are in short supply; proposed law would prohibit transplanting organs donated in the United States to non-U.S. residents.
>
> Growing nonrejectable body parts in pigs could provide enough body parts, but this may raise animal rights issues.

The term "transplants" is applied to body parts as an analogy to uprooting plants and planting them in another place. Transplantation can be further differentiated, between organ and tissue transplantation: *Organ* transplantation usually requires a brain-dead, ICU-maintained body; *tissues* for transplantation (corneas, skin, bone) can be taken from dead, nonmaintained bodies. To cover both situations, the term used is "body parts."

Laws allow the taking of organs from live bodies, by changing the definition of death to "brain death." Doctors and nurses—who cut into brain-dead bodies with beating hearts and breathing lungs to take out body parts—are not deemed murderers under such laws because the patient is considered to be legally dead.

New proposals hope to change the definition of death further, so that persons who have "higher brain death" (not total brain death, but severe thinking impairment) can be declared dead. If that is done, doctors and nurses who cause death in such patients will not be considered the killers of those patients either. And, presumably, organs can be taken from them as soon as they are declared dead.

Transplant issues can be discussed under two separate values: those of the *donor* of the body part and those of the *recipient* of the organ. The donor's point of view centers on the value, autonomy—the donor's power over her own body (or her family's power over her body) after death. The organ recipient's view centers on the value, fairness—for example, equal access to available organs, or in being treated without bias because of ability to pay or because of prior medical or social history.

Because the donor is presumed to have a right to keep her organs in the first place (greater than any right of the donee to receive them), the donor's value of autonomy is paramount.

The Individual's Power over the Body Extends Beyond Death. Autonomy over one's body extends to the dead body. People can decide in advance what happens to their property *and* what happens to their bodies after they die. They can donate body parts for transplants, or they can donate the whole body to be used in research or education. Autonomy is enforced by laws that spell out the patient's power over his own body. Just as the ethics and laws of consent and advance directives enforce autonomy, so autonomy is the value in laws enforcing the power over the body after death (the autonomy or dignity of even the dead body).

Consent to Donation

Laws that enforce the power over the body after death include consents required for autopsy and for donation of the whole body, or any and all body parts.

In several states, consent for this donation of the body can be made on the individual's driver's license. Donation by drivers' licenses is done by statute law. Often families can override that donation, however, either because there is actual authority in the law to do so, or because the family is alive and the potential donor is dead. (The old maxim is noted: "The dead cannot sue, but the living do.") Some describe organ donor cards as ineffective, since few transplant teams will remove organs on the basis of a card alone.

It may be argued that the donor's wishes should rule over those of his relatives. And sometimes there is a state law to that effect. But in practice, the relatives' strong feelings may prevail. An ethical rationale for that reality is that the dead will have no feelings about it, and the survivors may be distressed by a procedure to be done on their loved one's body.

State support for obtaining bodies and parts (evident in putting donor forms on drivers' licenses to encourage donation) has long precedent. Over a hundred years ago, at least 16 U.S. states had passed laws providing for the delivery of unclaimed dead bodies to medical colleges for dissection.[51] This trend to use law to help obtain body parts for transplantation continues. Several states' laws have provisions of "presumed consent" for persons who have not declared themselves to be donors or organs. For example, a Texas law provides that if the deceased is not a declared donor, and if a person authorized to consent to donation on her behalf is not contacted within four hours after death, the medical examiner may permit the removal of a visceral organ or tissue.[52] The law may be said to directly encourage medical examiners to permit organ and tissue removal without the patient's prior donation or necessity of obtaining the family's permission.

The federal government contributes to the trend also when its law mandates that institutions receiving funding from Medicare ask families for permission to use transplantable body parts.[53] Despite the law, in many hospitals, permission for transplantation is never asked; others do so only sporadically.

Under federal law, agency protocols
1. must provide that families of potential organ donors know about and have a chance to decline donation,
2. must "encourage discretion and sensitivity" to the families' beliefs, and
3. must require that the area's organ procurement organization be notified of potential donors.[54]

Agency protocols that put the law into practice require nurses or doctors to ask the relatives of anyone who is a potential donor about donation. A potential donor is anyone dying with some healthy body parts. Even though the individual is said to have the right to donate or refuse to donate her own organs, at the point of death the person's power over the body is transferred to the family.

Asking for body parts requires great sensitivity to the feelings of the relatives. Not only is it unethical to pressure people to donate organs, it could exacerbate any existing ill will toward the provider. The result might be a malpractice suit, where none would have resulted had tact been exercised.

A worst-case scenario: A father says he was billed for the cost of care required to preserve his daughter's organs for donation. (Federal law says that survivors are not liable for such expense.) In this case, the father said he was told within 35 minutes of entering the emergency room that his daughter was dead, yet $13,000 of the bill was attributed to emergency care. Emergency care given before death *would* be properly charged.[55]

If donation is made, the patient's estate or the family must not be billed for any charges incurred after the patient is declared dead. This is so even if the donor remains in ICU for organs to be taken. (For more information, consult the policy on organ donation that any agency receiving Medicare funds is required to have; that policy will follow both state and federal law.)

It is proposed that U.S. laws mandate that organs automatically be donated, unless the patient expresses a negative objection in advance of death. (This is the case in some European countries.) It is argued that society gives too much attention to individual rights, and too little to individual responsibility—such as responsibility to donate body parts.

Note: The word *cadaver* is frequently used in place of the word *body*. *Cadaver's* use may be an attempt to avoid the emotion attendant on the word *body*, or it might be merely an attempt to be more accurate, since bodies may be alive or dead. Interested individuals may want to observe whether the word *cadaver* is more often used when someone proposes what might be considered a violation or indignity, or if the word *body* is used when the speaker/writer advocates merely embalming and burial.

The legal and ethical use of bodies or cadavers is an issue that may become more intense. Heidelberg University in Germany has used cadavers in research on car crashes.[56] The conflict in such a case is protection of human dignity versus freedom in scientific research.

Some argue that there should be a limit to what can be done with cadavers. The body is held sacred, in part to maintain at least a vestige of respect for the person who lived therein while the body was alive. The use of dead bodies to practice intubation might violate such "respect for the person," just as performing CPR on some patients (those essentially dead, since it is known they cannot survive the procedure) might violate that respect.

Transplants Are Expensive

Transplants are also about economics. Most agree that body parts should be available under a fair procedure of allocation. If transplants are paid for by taxpayers (as in Medicare and Medicaid), then social justice may dictate equal outcomes for all.

The cost of transplant to the recipient is high. Liver transplant patients at one center must deposit at least $150,000, or have insurance that guarantees that payment, or be on Medicaid.[57] Should a 72-year-old man receive a liver transplant, at a cost in excess of $1,500,000 for hospital charges alone? Should he have been transplanted before younger patients? Should the governor of Pennsylvania have received a heart and liver transplant in 1993 without entering on a waiting list? Should Mickey Mantle, acknowledged former alcoholic, have received a transplanted liver?

Some argue that the social value of the transplant recipient (age, wealth, dependency) be a factor; others that the behavior that caused the need for the transplant be considered. These are the same issues as arose when dialysis was a scarce treatment, before the U.S. Congress voted to pay for all who needed dialysis. As payment for illness care moves to the private sector, such issues will become more intense and may again extend to who gets dialysis or body parts.

Payment for Donors

The ethics and the law say that the person is free (or the relatives are free) to do what the person wants with the body after death. The word *free* can be used in another way on this issue, however. Statutes make it illegal for the donor to receive payment for body parts; the donor or relatives are asked literally to *donate* body parts, not sell them. Some argue, however, that if the patient and family really are free, in the sense of having autonomy, they should be able to accept money for what is obviously so valuable. Moreover, they argue that this would help solve the problem of a shortage of body parts. Body parts are sold by the donors for payment in some countries, notably in India.

Others answer that allowing people to sell their body parts would lead to exploitation of poor people, who might endanger themselves in return for the money. And it can be argued that selling a part of oneself is a form of slavery; in the United States, people are not allowed the "freedom" to enslave themselves for money.

In some cases, body parts have been used without patient consent. Some hospitals' obstetrics units sell the placentas that their patients deliver, without consent or compensation to the mother. Placentas may be a major source of blood-generating stem cells, needed in the future for bone marrow transplants.[58]

Fair Allocation of Organs

Federal law (1984 National Organ Transplant Act) mandates fair allocation of organs.[59] A government study has concluded that the present allocation system of body parts violates that law by denying the parts to sicker patients, and makes some patients wait longer than others. The study said that the needs of transplant centers were favored over the needs of patients.

The United Network for Organ Sharing (UNOS), operated under federal contract, has a single waiting list of patients needing organs. Use of the network is not mandatory at present, but federal regulations could require it. In general, organ banks oppose such regulation, saying that local arrangements are better and that organ banks coordinate competing hospitals and surgeons.

The number of people waiting for transplants grows faster than the number of organs available. A single area-wide waiting list would mean the next *patient* on the list would get the next organ, instead of distributing organs to the next *hospital* on the list.[60]

Rationing Organs

The shortage of organs for Americans has prompted proposals for legal solutions. One proposed law would prohibit transplanting donated U.S. organs to non-U.S. residents. It would require organ transplant centers to place non-U.S. residents lower on a waiting list—lower in priority than U.S. residents, which would effectively shut out foreign citizens who come to the United States for heart and liver transplants. The law in past limited non-U.S. residents to a maximum of ten percent of a hospital transplant program's patients.[61]

Transplants are not available in many other countries—often, the United States is the only place that some people can go for transplants. Since the foreigners seeking transplants are wealthy enough to afford transplants, denying organs to foreigners might be called discrimination against a minority (wealthy aliens). The other end of the money scale is the possibility of refusal by state Medicaid programs to pay for any kind of treatment for illegal aliens. That could be called discrimination against that minority (poor aliens). Is discrimination against all aliens wrong, or only wrong if against poor aliens? Is such discrimination permissible (ethical and legal), regardless of whether the aliens are rich or poor?

Transfusions Are Transplants

Transfusion of blood is a transplant issue (although the issue is not so controversial, because it is not connected with death). Live people donate blood, and there's no serious shortage of the "transplant." But ethical controversies do exist; for example, religious groups such as Jehovah's Witnesses object to receiving blood. The law will protect their autonomy to refuse except in extreme cases, in which the life of the person needing the blood supports the life of another (a pregnant woman or father of children). Even in those extreme cases, good communication and alternative treatments may avoid a need to seek a court order to treat.

The discovery of the HIV virus in the blood supply created the need to protect the public from harm as well as to tell people the truth. These ethical values (enforced by law) were violated in scandals uncovered in Germany and France, in which HIV-infected blood was given to patients while bureaucrats knew of the infection. The cover-ups by officials were discovered and the people responsible were prosecuted, but not before many people were infected.

Transplantation Issues Involving Animals

Technological developments could solve the problem of donors for body parts. For example, proteins exist that could keep the body from rejecting organs. Genetically altered pigs could incorporate these proteins into kidneys, hearts, lungs, and livers safe for transplant into humans—at a relatively inexpensive cost—and this would relieve the shortage of human donor body parts. Xenotransplants—from one species to another—could be routine by the end of the millennium.[62] Such developments might solve the donor problem for humans, but does the *ability* to kill the pigs and take their organs give humans the right to do so? Although many objected when a baboon was killed so its liver could be transplanted into a human, the issue of killing pigs seems different because pigs are already killed for humans to eat, and pigs seem "less related" to the human species than baboons.

AUTOPSIES

The ethics and law of autopsy incorporate autonomy issues.

The law dictates that an autopsy be performed under some circumstances of death (violent, suspicious, or unknown causes). Consent cannot be withheld in those conditions.

The statute law on autopsies also specifies who can consent for an elective autopsy; that law can be obtained from the employer where autopsies are done, in the local library's statutes indexed under Autopsy, or from the county coroner or medical examiner's office.

Autopsy issues are relative to the ethics and law of autonomy. The value of freedom is reflected in law giving power over the body, respecting either the person's or family's wishes. The autopsy issue is of interest here in the sense of having the body "violated." (Some people and cultures are more sensitive to the idea of autopsy than others.) Patients can specify before death whether they will refuse an autopsy, assuming it is elective at that point. The patient's refusal may be honored (or it may not, just as his wish to donate his organs may be honored or not).

Autopsy procedures look less invasive if compared to the process of embalming. If they ask, patients and families can be assured that the body that has undergone autopsy can be restored by the embalmer for viewing. Nurses could better counsel families as to the relatively less-destructive nature of autopsy if they understood the process of embalming.[63]

In some circumstances of death—violent, suspicious, or unknown causes—the law dictates that an autopsy be done. Autopsies may also be indicated and sought by the agency and/or the family if a lawsuit is anticipated. In some states and in some facilities, a death after admission of less than 24 hours requires an autopsy. (Supervisors or risk managers can provide specific information, and state statutes governing this subject can be found in the local library. In addition, the county coroner or medical examiner's office is a good resource for the specific law in a particular state if needed.)

The statute law on autopsies will also specify who can consent for an elective autopsy. If an autopsy is desired by the medical staff, the medical staff should do the explaining and obtain the consent. The situation is similar to that of obtaining consent to treat the patient, but here there is no benefit to the patient. The nurse may still feel obligated to the family; in that case, such explanation can be justified as a nursing function.

HIV/AIDS AUTONOMY ISSUES

HIV/AIDS is discussed as an autonomy issue because:

1. The issue is one of freedom/autonomy for the person who engages in the risky behaviors that are the cause of most infections.
2. The issue is one of freedom/autonomy for the nurse who cares for the patient, since the nurse's life might be endangered by caring for this patient.

The chance of contracting AIDS is small except by IV drug use and promiscuous anal intercourse; transmission by heterosexual non-anal intercourse is very difficult.

Laws could prohibit destructive behavior that hurts society (the cost of care, to all individuals as a group); and could prohibit acts that hurt other individuals (the sexual partners of HIV/AIDS-infected people, infected if the partner does not inform them of the infection).

The future concentration of new AIDS cases in people of color will intensify ethical and legal conflicts about the control and treatment of the condition.

The ethics and law around Auto-Immune Deficiency Syndrome (AIDS) and infection with the Human Immunodeficiency Virus (HIV) give rise to many issues that cut across several values. The issues around HIV/AIDS and TB recreate controversies that have surrounded illnesses throughout history, including leprosy and bubonic plague. The conflict today is often between the autonomy of the patient to behave freely, the autonomy of the patient to have care when needed, and the autonomy of the nurse to exercise judgment in her nursing practice. The behavior of patients and whether they will be held responsible for their own health is relevant not only to people with *HIV/AIDS*, but also to smokers with lung cancer, alcoholics with cirrhosis, and other illness in which behavior freely chosen is a factor (a discussion of whether *any* behavior is freely chosen is beyond the scope of this book).

A majority of individuals infected with HIV/AIDS, or at risk of the infection, are often thought to be in that condition as a result of freely chosen behavior. U.S. HIV infections leading to AIDS have occurred overwhelmingly in two populations—homosexual males and IV drug users.[64] Only a small percent of people infected did not get the infection as a result of their own actions. Data indicate that nonpromiscuous, non-IV drug using people, of any sexual orientation and of any color, ethic background, or either sex, have little risk of HIV infection.[65]

But in future this fatal disease will likely be concentrated in groups now considered minorities; almost half of all new AIDS cases occur among blacks and hispanics. This will intensify ethical and legal conflicts about the control and treatment of HIV/AIDS.

For example, the Oregon Medicaid system (and other states with similar plans) limits care for HIV-infected people by rationalizing that their average longevity is short (but it is as long as, for example, patients with congestive heart failure). And already, a sizeable minority of African-Americans now believe that AIDS is an attempt at genocide of their people.

Nurses Fear HIV/AIDS Patients

Some nurses, reluctant to care for HIV/AIDS patients, may find that the law enforces the duty to care for all patients.

Nurses may refuse to compromise their own safety and ethical standards, but they have a professional responsibility to ensure that the nursing needs of patients are met on an emergency basis.

Whether the nurse has a duty to care for all patients combines the nurse's ability, the requirements of the patient, and the degree of risk.

Nurses may consider the risk of nursing some patients in the light of whether there is risk to themselves, their families, and their personal ethics. If the risk is minimal or low, the legal duty of the nurse is high. The more actual risk, the less the legal duty becomes.

Specific (and varied) state statutes provide for informing patients about HIV testing, obtaining consent, reporting HIV-positive patients, and informing partners. The agency's infection control department or the local library will have information on specifics. The statute will be indexed under HIV/AIDS, or the spelled-out forms of the words.

Nurses have been no better, nor worse than doctors in refusing to care for patients who were infected with deadly disease. Today, fearing infection, some nurses are reluctant to care for patients with HIV/AIDS. Law enforces a minimal ethical duty owed toward all patients, including those infected with HIV/AIDS.[66]

Some statutes, in forbidding discrimination by nurses, may impinge on the nurse's ability to decline to care for certain patients. In addition, nurses may be obligated to give care under their employment relationship, under the code of ethics, and enforcement of such ethics by state boards of nursing.

Nurses do have options *not* to care for certain patients if the nurse's own ethical standards are compromised. But nurses have a professional responsibility to ensure that the nursing needs of such patients are met, at least on an emergency basis.[67]

Whether the nurse has a duty to care for a patient is a combination of factors, including the nurse's ability, the requirements of the patient, and the degree of risk to the nurse of giving such care.

If the risk of harm to nurse from patient is minimal or low, the nurse's legal duty is high. The more actual risk, the less the duty becomes. The law would not enforce a duty on the part of the nurse to save a patient if the act meant certain death for herself. The law would not force the nurse to throw him or herself in front of the bullet aimed by a patient's assassin. Although in such instance the nurse might be a hero, there is no minimum ethic (no enforced legal duty) to do so.

The nurse has an obligation to self and perhaps to family to minimize the numbers of situations in which she is at real risk. If the patient needs a nurse and no other is available, the nurse has an obligation to care for that patient until relief is found. The nurse further has a duty not to impose his or her own values on the patient cared for through her professional actions, although of course she or he is free to express values in a personal setting.

Nurse managers especially need to understand the legal parameters of their staff's action in caring for patients with HIV/AIDS. The ethics and law they need to know is more detailed and workplace-oriented than that the practicing nurse needs.[68] The nurse as worker has another perspective on the issue.[69]

Testing patients who may have HIV/AIDS is more problematic than doing an ordinary blood count, because the possible consequences of the information the test reveals are so much more serious (stigma, death). Nurse managers should know the reliability factors (sensitivity and specificity) of the various tests for the infection (especially in low-risk populations, the test's accuracy is poor), and the specifics of their state law on counseling and confidentiality.

Some states allow or require informing the infected patient's spouse or partner. The hospital's attorney or the infection control department can furnish information; or the state statutes can be found at the local library, indexed under HIV/AIDS or the spelled words.[70]

Patients Fear Nurses

> There is only one recorded incident of HIV infection by a healthcare practitioner but patients wish to have no risk of infection.
> The risk of transmission from patient to nurse is also very small; the hepatitis virus is much more likely than HIV to be transmitted from (and to) patients.

Patients fear AIDS and, therefore, seek to avoid HIV infection from the caregiver. People want to know that they will not have *any* risk since the infection is deadly. The risk is very small; only one instance of a practitioner infecting patients has been documented (the mode of transmission is suspected to have been deliberate). No other cases of transmission of HIV/AIDS from worker to patient are known. Some workers have gotten the infection from patients, however, and some assert that nurses should have a right to know their patient's HIV/AIDS status.[71]

The nurse wants to avoid contracting the virus from infected patients. That's still small risk, but much more likely than transmission the other way, from nurse to patient. The hepatitis virus is much more likely than HIV to be transmitted from (and to) patients.

Universal precautions—gloves, masks, eye shields, and gowns, depending on the degree of danger—have been instituted for all practitioners in contact with body fluids possibly carrying the HIV virus. That's just about all body fluids usually encountered from patients, except urine without blood in it.

The risk of transmission from patient to practitioner has prompted demands that all patients be tested, so that practitioners can take appropriate precautions. But testing without consent violates the freedom and possibly the confidentiality of HIV-infected patients. So universal precautions are used on all patients to protect workers from the few who might be HIV-infected. This cost, which all pay for in their care, must be weighed against the freedom and confidentiality interests of those infected.

Nurses too have autonomy interests in not being tested without consent. The fear of HIV by the public, many of whom believe they can get HIV from practitioners, has caused proposals for laws that require testing and disclosure of the HIV status of all practitioners. Existing law has been tougher on illness care workers than on patients, despite the fact that the worker is more likely to be infected by the patient than vice versa. Instances exist of

HIV-positive practitioner confidences being violated, jobs lost, and privileges to practice denied, all because of HIV status. Inclusion of HIV-infected people under the Americans with Disabilities Act may protect them from some of these circumstances.

Americans with Disabilities and HIV/AIDS

HIV-positive practitioners are considered to have a disability under the Americans with Disabilities Act (ADA).

If practitioners are tested, then the value of fairness might require that patients be tested as well.

Lawsuits with HIV/AIDS as the issue are frequent and will continue to make law in this area.

Projections for increases in the numbers of women infected with AIDS, and for an epidemic of heterosexual AIDS in the United States as has occurred in Africa, must be examined for factual basis.

Education to prevent HIV/AIDS among young people with high-risk behavior has been unsuccessful.

HIV-positive practitioners are protected to some extent by the Americans with Disabilities Act (ADA). Under the ADA, HIV-positive practitioners are considered to have a disability. The law requires that such persons can't be discriminated against in their work, unless they present a substantial risk of transmitting the disease. The population at large is not at substantial risk from the disease, absent some high-risk behavior.

Aside: Note the words used in the title of the Americans with Disabilities Act. It is said to better refer to a person *with* a condition, such as a person with developmental disabilities, than to a developmentally disabled person. The reason given is that one should notice the person first, and that the person is disabled or challenged second. Is the use of "disabilities" and "challenges" an attempt to change attitudes with words?

Some judicial decisions have converted the phrase "substantial risk" to "*any* risk," of transmission. That limits the protection of the ADA law. Some state laws now require physicians and other providers, who are HIV-positive, to disclose that fact to their patients before performing exposure-prone procedures.[72]

If practitioners are required to be tested, then the value of fairness might require that patients be tested as well. The Center for Disease Control at one time suggested a blanket requirement, that all HIV-positive practitioners stop invasive procedures, regardless of circumstances. The CDC now recommends that a committee in the practitioner's institution address the specifics of where, how, and what procedures an HIV-infected practitioner should perform.

The agency administering another law, the Occupational Safety and Health Act (OSHA), has issued regulations extending universal precautions to all agencies where employees are covered by the act (all employers of ten or more people).

Lawsuits over HIV/AIDS

Literally thousands of lawsuits have had HIV/AIDS as an issue, in process in all areas of law; they are based on the usual ethical values enforced in law—for example, doing good, doing no harm, autonomy, telling truth, protecting confidentiality.

Statistics

Statistics should be examined closely for the effect they have on ethics, law, and public policy. For example, some evidence shows that HIV/AIDS occurs largely in only two groups, both of which engage in the risky behavior that allows transmission of the disease. Data show that it is far easier for a man to give the disease to a woman through intercourse, than vice versa. Men who have heterosexual intercourse with prostitutes are at less risk of getting infected by the prostitute than she is from a customer who is infected.

It is estimated that by the year 2000, 40 percent of all *new* HIV/AIDS infections will be in women. It is estimated that, some time later, *new infections* of women with HIV/AIDS will outnumber new infections of men with HIV/AIDS. This is an estimate based on the "large increase in numbers of women infected" (note the need to use care in interpreting statistics, below). Even if the prediction is true, the total number of women infected may not be large.

STATISTICS ARE SLIPPERY

Imagine a headline:
WOMEN FIVE TIMES AS LIKELY TO BE NEW HIV INFECTED.

Suppose the data show a 50 percent rise in women infected, and "only" a ten percent rise in the numbers of men infected last year. Think carefully about what that means. If few women are infected at present, the proportionate rise in *rate* of infections will be greater in women. For example, if two women in a population are infected this year, and next year three women are found to be infected, there has been a 50 percent rise of infections in women in that group (1 new case ÷ 2 old cases). This statistic sounds alarming, but only a small number of women are infected.

In contrast, if 50 men of a population are infected this year, and 55 men are found to be infected next year, the rate of increase is only ten percent (5 new cases ÷ 50 old cases). In that example, five times as many men (5) as women (1) are newly infected that year. The totals: 55 men are now infected, and three women. The headline is comparing a ten percent *increase* with a 50 percent *increase*, but the actual numbers sound much different. Read statistics carefully.

Projections are that 100 million people will die of AIDS in Africa (largely in the heterosexual population), but the epidemic of heterosexual AIDS in Africa cannot be generalized to predict similar outcomes in the American population. Africans use unsterilized needles to self-administer many medications for illness, not just for drugs to produce euphoria; the drugs and needles are freely available in bars and other public venues. In addition, a multiplicity of sexual partners among some of the population is of a different order of magnitude than seen in the United States.

Although the incidence of AIDS in America seems to have reached a plateau, researchers warn that continued high-risk behavior among a few young gay and bisexual men may mean a resurgence of HIV/AIDS in the United States in the future.[73] More education does not seem to help.

Education to Prevent HIV/AIDS Infection

Education to prevent the infection has been largely unsuccessful, as demonstrated in various studies of HIV/AIDS teaching.[74] The educational approach has been to teach the general public about HIV/AIDS, though public health officials know that the majority of people are not at risk for the infection. Among young people, a small minority (three percent) engage in the high-risk behavior that can possibly lead to infection.[75] In one study, 81 percent of youths did not engage in either moderate or high-risk behavior. High-risk behavior by the three percent (intravenous drug use, prostitution, and choice of risky partners) did not moderate when they had increased knowledge about AIDS or HIV infection and prevention and greater numbers of sources of information about the disease.[76]

Tuberculosis Related to AIDS

TB is the leading single infectious cause of death worldwide; untreated TB leads to death in an average of five years—the same average prognosis as HIV/AIDS.

Ninety percent of active cases of TB are *re*activation; TB is resurgent in patients with HIV/AIDS in particular.

TB control statutes still in effect are available to control patients who will not practice infection control.

The standard for laws that interfere with patient freedom (TB laws, mental illness law): Is the patient a risk to self or society; is there a less restrictive choice?

TB is more dangerous to workers and the public than is HIV/AIDS, since it can be contracted by being in the same room with an infectious person.

TB may become a new plague, with the attendant ethical and legal questions about duty to care versus duty to self.

In addition to the common ethical and legal questions about the patient's right to treatment, and the nurse's right to refuse to subject herself to danger, tuberculosis (TB) is analogous to HIV/AIDS in other respects. The two diseases are related in some infectious, ethical, and legal aspects.

Tuberculosis (TB) is analogous to HIV/AIDS in that
1. the largest reservoir of infectious TB is in HIV/AIDS patients;
2. the patient can be infected with TB but not develop active disease (as the patient can be HIV-positive and not have AIDS); and
3. a potential analogy: Laws exist to force behavior changes and treatment on patients with TB; this also has been proposed for AIDS, and actually done, in Cuba.

First, the reservoir of infectious TB is greatest in AIDS patients who have had TB, earlier made inactive by their immune systems. The immune system suppression that occurs in AIDS allows the TB to become active again.

The second analogy of TB to HIV/AIDS is that the patient can be infected with TB (be reactive on a PPD test) but may not develop active disease, just as a patient can be HIV-positive but not have AIDS immediately.

The third (potential) analogy is that there are laws to force behavior changes and treatment on patients with TB, and these were suggested by some for patients with AIDS. In the past, laws forced people into locked hospital wards if they did not follow proper procedures in caring for their infectious disease; the behavior (the patient's freedom to act) was seen as a danger to the community and was prohibited. That disease was TB—and TB is back.

TB is the leading single infectious cause of death worldwide. Untreated TB leads to death in an average of about five years (about the same average prognosis as HIV/AIDS). Hundreds of drug-resistant TB strains exist; at least three strains now are resistant to *all* TB drug therapies.

Ninety percent of active TB cases involve *re*activation. TB is resurgent in part due to the population of people with HIV/AIDS; their reduced immunity allows for a pool of infected and infectious people. Many AIDS patients are already infected with TB that has been suppressed; the HIV/AIDS-infected patients have reduced ability to keep the TB bacillus suppressed. The TB reactivates, infecting the patient and making the patient infectious to others.

No risky behavior is required to contract TB—merely proximity to a TB-infected person who isn't practicing infection control. Old TB control statutes, passed decades ago but still in effect, are available to control difficult patients; the laws differ from state to state and include enforced quarantines. Such laws make it a misdemeanor or felony to spread TB; but some workers fear the law might deter ill people from treatment.

The 1990 Americans with Disabilities Act covers AIDS patients, prohibiting discrimination on the basis of disability. Even TB patients who don't have HIV/AIDS, might also be protected under that law. If challenged, the TB quarantine laws might be considered discriminatory under the ADA. However, courts could find an exception from the ADA if the law were necessary to protect public health (the value, Doing No Harm, placed above the value, Autonomy).

The same question can also be asked of laws that seek to control TB (or AIDS) as were asked to determine whether laws for involuntary commitment of the mentally ill are just. The question: Is the patient a risk to self or society and, if so, is there no alternative that is less restrictive? The ethical value is to protect the freedom of the patient, but that value may be tempered by the value of protecting the public (preventing harm).[77]

Practice

TB is more dangerous to workers and the public than is HIV/AIDS, because TB can be contracted by far less risky behavior—such as being in class with, or in a hospital room with, an infectious person. To be protected from TB, nurses must wear disposable particulate filter masks; standard surgical masks don't prevent bacteria transmission. The patient should be on isolation for the first two weeks of treatment.

Health departments now order "Mandatory, Directly Observed Therapy" for TB patients because of the high rate of noncompliance with the medications and infection control regimen. Workers visit noncontagious TB patients to supervise them taking their medicine, or patients come to clinics to get medications and take them under observation. The practice is recommended by the Center for Disease Control and Prevention.

Some authorities see TB as a new plague, with the attendant ethical and legal questions for the public and for people who work with patients. As with HIV/AIDS, nurses must ask whether their duty is always to care for the sick person, or whether their duty is to protect self and family.[78]

The individual's autonomy may affect others. If the "freedom" of the homosexual or the freedom of the IV drug user results in infection, the nurse may be asked to care for them. And the taxpayer may be asked to pay for care for the patient, although the taxpayer did not engage in such risky behavior.

Similar considerations may be made about the freedom to smoke, drink alcohol, eat fatty foods, and stay obese. In all autonomous behaviors, either the individual must take responsibility for the consequences of behavior or someone else gets that responsibility. The root of the word *autonomy* is control of self; the emphasis has been on the right to act, but focus may change to responsibility to control one's own actions.

Suicide

The ethics and the law of suicide, euthanasia, and assisted suicide are based on the value put on *being free* (having power over one's life).

Does a person's right to die extend to the right to kill oneself under some or any circumstances? Perhaps this "ultimate" in autonomy means that the freedom to die extends to the right to be killed by doctors or nurses. It has been assumed in illness care that people who want to kill themselves are in some degree mentally ill (or, at least depressed); and such people have been rescued, restrained, and treated for depression. The practitioner's question is whether such patients need help to live, or to die.

The issue of suicide is treated fully in Chapter Seven, Life. But note that the ethics and the law of suicide, euthanasia and assisted suicide, and the intent behind living wills, are all in some manner reflections of the value put on *being free*, of having power over one's life and death. The value placed on *life* is the counterbalancing weight to the value of dying or being dead; in some cases the value of living does not outweigh the value of dying.

AUTONOMY FOR THE NURSE

Not only patients, but also nurses possess autonomy (freedom, power over self).

Nurses need independence as professionals, especially from doctor and employer control, when control conflicts with professional practice.

Nurse practitioners are classed as Advanced Practice Nurses (APNs) along with nurse midwives, nurse anesthetists, and clinical nurse specialists.

Nursing autonomy matters to the degree that it benefits the patient, whether or not the profession benefits.

The issues raised in caring for HIV/AIDS and TB patients show that not only patients, but nurses, too, have autonomy (freedom, power over self). Under democratic political systems which value individuals, every person has a measure of freedom.

Nurses seek independence as professionals—independence from doctor control and also independence from employer control—when such control presents a conflict with good practice. Nurse practitioners (NPs) are the most visible examples of the autonomous nurse, but nurses in general must make constant efforts toward independence when it benefits their patients. The discussion of independence of nurse practitioners/advanced practice nurses applies to all nurses in some degree.

Nurse practitioners are now considered in a group called Advanced Practice Nurses (APNs), which also includes nurse midwives, nurse anesthetists, and clinical nurse specialists. Nurse practitioners have been working at least since the 1970s, when a shortage of doctors prompted the American Medical Association to propose that some nurses become "physician's assistants" (able to do medical care at some level). The American Nurses Association leadership objected to the AMA proposal, saying the patients needed nurses, not junior doctors. But market demand and the interests of some nurses led to the training of nurses in that and other nontraditional roles.

It has been asserted that the APN "doctor-like" role confuses the distinction between doctors and nurses, making nurse autonomy harder to perceive. On the other hand, the "doctor-like" role of APNs might actually strengthen that perception of nurse independence. It must be remembered that nursing autonomy matters when it benefits the patient, not the profession.

Nursing Autonomy/Freedom in History

The ethics and law of nursing autonomy can be better understood and predicted by knowing its history.

Nursing philosophy and theory (and resulting nursing ethics and law) rest on the basic human activity of providing care to a person who cannot provide it for self.

Being paid to do nursing work is the base for legally mandating nurses to do good and to prevent harm; others in the society are not obligated to do so.

Nursing's roots in prehistory provide understanding of the autonomy of nursing in the modern era.

The ethics, law, and economics of nursing are inextricable from the economic condition of women in the culture, as seen in the evolution of nursing law from independent to supervised to autonomous and back to more controlled.

Under managed care almost all doctors and nurses are employees and less independent; but the return to self-paid care in the home may restore the ethic, law, and economics in which the nurse's primary relationship, contract, and responsibility is to the patient.

The ethics and law of nursing autonomy can be better understood and predicted by knowing the history of independent nursing. The distinction between professional and nonprofessional nursing is a cornerstone of modern nursing, but nursing is recognized as a continuum of activity that all human beings do for each other. Florence Nightingale wrote that every woman is at some time in her life a nurse (it should be added, so is every man). She wrote "Notes for Nurses" for lay persons who some time in their lives would inevitably nurse someone; not for people who care for sick people as their paid work.

The word *nurse* comes from, and is related to, "nourish" and "nurture." To nurse a baby is to feed it. Nursing philosophy and theory (and resulting nursing ethics and law) rest on the most basic of human activity: to provide life-giving sustenance and other care to a person who cannot provide it for self. Originally a "nurse" was a person who substituted for the mother, providing milk for the baby when the mother did not. The person who was a "nurse" in the centuries prior to this one might actually suckle her young "patient" in place of the biological mother.

Nursing very early involved taking care of helpless people, not only babies. In addition to feeding the helpless, nurses did other basic things to keep them alive. The idea evolved that a nurse is a person who cares for sick (often helpless) people. To nurse someone is not merely to feed, but to care for the person who is unable to care for him or herself.

In the long process of economic development, divisions of labor meant people began to pay specialists to do nursing work, instead of doing it themselves for their families. Nurses were "professionals" in the sense that they worked for pay, to differentiate them from people who nursed the family for no pay. Only later did the work come to include a specialized body of knowledge and other attributes, constructed to distinguish professions from other kinds of work. The payment for nursing work is the basis of imposing on nurses, through law, a duty to do good and to prevent harm; higher duty than others in the society have.

It is still true that many professionals are no different from their amateur counterparts except in that they get paid, making the activity their vocation instead of their avocation. Professional athletes and professional artists are examples.

Nursing is probably an older activity in human behavior than medicine. Caring for people who were sick doubtless preceded the attempt to cure those people with magic and its successors, science and medicine.

Economic Basis of Nurse Autonomy Law

The knowledge that nursing is such an old activity makes it easier to understand the autonomy of nursing in the modern era. All along, the nurse has been autonomous, working sometimes with and sometimes without physicians. The ethics, law, and economics of nursing are inextricable from the economic condition of women in the culture.

Women worked as private duty nurses in the homes of their patients in the early part of the twentieth century. They worked also as visiting nurses for insurance companies and public health agencies—in the patient's home. These nurses worked with doctors, but they were also usually entrepreneurs, hired by the patient and responsible to the patient (not the doctor or an employer). The nursing in hospitals was done by students learning to be nurses, and by the faculty of the schools.

The Depression of the 1930s speeded the development of hospital alliances such as Blue Cross and physician alliances such as Blue Shield, payment plans (insurance) that let people pay small amounts monthly to have large amounts available to pay doctors, nurses, and hospitals, if needed. The increased technology that developed and was accelerated by WWII in the 1940s meant that care was better done in the hospitals than the home; graduate nurse work moved to the hospital. The nurse was in closer proximity to, and more likely supervised by, physicians; she now had a legal and ethical duty to the employer as well as the patient, and more legal supervision by doctors.

The wage and price controls of the war years made employers unable to use pay increases to recruit scarce workers; the employers instead gave a new benefit, health insurance. The system of getting insurance through the workplace accelerated. The nurse now added a fourth legal relationship to her existing duties to patient, doctor, and employer: to the third-party payer.

Looking back, nurses in the 1950s are perceived as handmaidens to physicians. If true, this attitude was part of the economic need of people of that period to see women primarily as homemakers. After the World War II, returning soldiers needed the jobs that women had held during the war.

Because the economics and lower tax structure of the time allowed one worker to earn enough to support the average family, society readily accepted that few women should work outside the home. When they did work for pay, nurses and other women in society were perceived to be subordinate to men (for example, to doctors). This dependence was reflected in law, in nurse practice acts that said that nursing was done under the supervision of the physician. This economic necessity of the time was to a large degree tacitly agreed upon.

Another women's movement in the 1970s and 1980s resulted from the reacceptance of women working outside the home, as many had done in the wartime '40s. Again women were needed in the work force, and many women needed to work to maintain family standards of material consumption. The nurse licensure laws were duly amended in the 1970s and '80s to reflect the independent role of women/nurses; references to physician supervision were deleted.

After organized nursing declined to adopt the AMA's proposal for making nurses "physician assistants," the doctors began to educate them anyway— recruited from among nurses and paramedics. This had the additional effect of employing soldiers returning from the Vietnam War with paramedic skills; another war, another economic need and opportunity. Early programs for nurse practitioners developed as intensive nonacademic one-year certificate programs, for nurses who had a basic nursing education; more recently the programs have moved into academic settings and result in a master's degree.

It is axiomatic that economic needs dictate the success of women's movements and, with them, nurse autonomy. When economics dictate that women not occupy jobs, ideas are accepted that women are better off at home with the children. The current period of "family values" endorses women to again work at home; this trend may satisfy a need to focus away from material goals that have proven unsatisfying for many. Or it may be that the material goals have proven unattainable for many.

Following the women's movement of the 1970s, nursing law that recognized nurse autonomy (deleting physician supervision) has gradually changed again to provide for more medical practice (prescribing drugs). The nursing/medical practice is under increased supervision, by administrative agency or physicians, or is done by collaboration.

Studies show that alternative providers (meaning nurse practitioners and physician assistants, in this case) give primary care as competently as their doctor counterparts, for less money. NP patients are screened for complexity; the more complex, difficult, expensive cases are referred to the doctor or specialist. NPs do as well as doctors at a basic level of primary care.

Nurses themselves are not unanimous in acceptance of nurse control over nursing practice—at least not control of their own practice by other nurses. An Illinois study found that most nurses supported nurse autonomy, independent practice, and third-party reimbursement. But a large minority did not—especially not independent practice for nurses.[79]

ECONOMICS, NURSES, WOMEN

Tying together APN economics and how the present culture views nurses (97 percent of whom are women), a majority of the public will accept nurses (versus doctors) as autonomous primary care providers. A 1993 study found that, of all Americans surveyed, 66 percent would support receiving primary care from a nurse, while 31 percent opposed and three percent were unsure. While 76 percent of men would support receiving primary care from a nurse, only 58 percent of women would do so.[80]

The trend toward managed care may make the controversy over independent nurses moot for the immediate future; almost all practitioners (doctors and nurses) might be more like employees (not independent). The economic forces that reduce specialist salaries also bring doctor pay closer to that of the lesser-educated nurse. Nurses may have to compete economically with doctors earning about the same pay.

The downsizing of hospitals and likely return to more out-of-pocket payment by the patient could have two results: More care is and will be given in the patient's home, and the nurse will be paid directly by the patient. The ethic, law, and economics, in which the nurse's primary relationship (and contract/responsibility) is with the patient, may return.

Nurse Autonomy: Legal Concerns

> The fraud and abuse "anti-kickback" provisions of the Medicare law can be violated when any independent provider is recruited to an agency relationship—nurses too.
>
> Legislative changes that removed nursing from doctor supervision were seen as inadequate to cover NP practice; newer changes were generally more doctor-supervised than the basic nursing statutes.
>
> Several states require NPs to obtain what amounts to a second separate license, in addition to the basic nursing license.
>
> Changes in the substance of nursing practice must underlie any meaningful change in the form of the law.

Fraud and Abuse. APNs (and any nurses who are independent contractors of any kind) must worry about the same things doctors worry about. One legal worry: the fraud and abuse "anti-kickback" provisions of the Medicare law, which is possibly violated when any independent provider is recruited to an agency relationship.[81]

> *The fraud and abuse statute*: "Whoever knowingly or willfully offers or pays any remuneration (including any kickback, bribe, or rebate) directly or indirectly, overtly or covertly, in cash or in kind to any person to induce such person . . . to refer an individual to a person for the furnishing or arranging for of any item or service for which payment may be made in whole or in part under [Medicare] shall be guilty of a felony . . . ."[82] "Soliciting and receiving" is a felony too.

NPs who work for salary, instead of fee for service payment from the patient, must still be aware of the economics of payment for their services. References are available to help NPs through the reimbursement maze for their advanced practice.[83]

Licensure and Credentialing. Questions about the legal scope of practice in reality are often professional/ethical questions. Some NPs ask the board of nursing in their state if it is legally permissible to perform certain practices, as a result of uncertainty about their educational preparation and experiential ability to perform the act.[84]

In the 1970s licensure laws for nurses were changed to eliminate requirements of working under doctor supervision. But the power and freedom that all nurses formally obtained through those legislative changes were not considered adequate to cover this new practitioner of nursing/medicine. Subsequently many changes in nurse practice acts were passed to define the practice of NPs; in some cases these were more restrictive and doctor-supervised than the basic nursing statutes.[85]

Several states require "certification" in order to practice as an advanced practice nurse. This certification may be state administered, or it may be obtained by examination available from The American Nurses Association (master's degree required). The American Association of Nurse Practitioners (AANP) conducted its own certification exam in the fall of 1993.

Some believe a second license is needed for advance practice in nursing (the ANA opposes this).[86] The argument for a second license is that the knowledge and experience needed for that practice is so different from the "basic" nurse's practice, that the safety of the public demands different competencies and passage of a different examination. Nurse practitioners in several states already have what amounts to a separate license, in addition to the basic nursing license.

New NPs now must get a Master's degree. Several state nurses associations are moving to change the licensure law to recognize not only NPs, but to include NPs under the broader category of APN practice. Such category of practice would require a master's degree for advanced practice and for writing prescriptions. Under some proposed state statutes, clinical nurse specialists who are not primary care providers might be legally able to write prescriptions, while nurse practitioners without a Master's degree could not.

The licensure division of RNs, proposed in the past, was between "professional" nurses who have BSNs, and nurses with AD or diploma education. Instead, licensure differences in future may be made between MSNs and all other lesser-educated nurses.

Some ANPs and other nurses see changes in law as curing whatever ails their practice. But, as can be seen from the economic and legislative history of independent nursing, law follows experience. Good practice that serves the patient well is the substance that underlies the form of the law. If there is no change in substance, there will be no change in law, no matter what words are passed by the legislature.

An example of change of substance (not merely form) is this amazing about-face by a state medical association.

The Missouri Medical Association had long been leery of advanced practice by nurses. But the doctors' association president wrote the following, after some of their members working with NPs were disciplined by the medical board in that state:

Many of these nurses [NPs] are providing prenatal care, family planning, well-baby care and immunizations in areas where such services are not available and patients would not get care if [NPs] were not available through these agencies . . . . If the Board of Healing Arts continues to pursue its disciplinary actions against physicians who sign into protocols with advanced nurse practitioners, Missouri will continue to see a deterioration of basic medical services in rural and indigent inner city areas . . . . It is time for physicians in Missouri to decide whether or not we can forge a relationship with other health care professionals to move basic health care into the reach of more patients.

This change in attitude came because nurses are performing a real substantive service in Missouri, working with doctors who are members of the Missouri State Medical Association; not because of a change in the law, or a public relations campaign.[87]

Autonomous Nurse Practice Negligence Liability

In a democratic society, each individual has power over him or herself (autonomy). The law of nursing practice recognizes that autonomy, except for the restrictions that NPs themselves requested and passed. The other side of the autonomy coin (in a sense, the payment for the freedom) is responsibility. The nurse has autonomy to act, and as a result *must* act responsibly. The nurse has responsibility for acts if they harm, or do not help as intended.

Freedom that leads to responsibility is the reason for allowing malpractice lawsuits against nurses. That concept of responsibility is challenged by ideas of tort reform that would make the employing enterprise liable, not the practitioner.

The nurse undertakes to do good as an independent, autonomous practitioner. He or she then has a responsibility to do good: If not, the nurse will be penalized. In return for the freedom (power, autonomy, independence), the nurse must accept the responsibility to act as a reasonable and prudent nurse (in the case of the NP, sometimes as a reasonable prudent doctor). If not, the nurse will be liable to the patient for any damage that results.

The standard of care for nurses is: "That action which a reasonable prudent nurse in similar circumstance would do." The standard of care for nurse practitioners, who practice medicine in addition to nursing, is different: "That action which a reasonable prudent practitioner of medicine in similar circumstance would do."[88]

A general discussion of nurse responsibility is found under malpractice law in this book in Chapter Two. Further discussion, and cases that underlie that responsibility, can be found in any law library or law encyclopedia such as the American Law Reports (ALR),[89] in which several cases that created negligence case law for nurse practitioners are reported, beginning about twenty years ago.[90]

The relative independence of nurse practitioners and their authority flows in most states from the nursing board, not the medical board. This nursing board control over NPs was upheld in Arkansas.[91] In some states, NP licensure gives medical and nursing boards joint control.

As discussed above, when the NP is acting in the capacity of physician, the nurse practitioner standard of care is the same standard of care as a physician would give. Whether this is an appropriate standard may be questioned, but the public sees the primary care practitioner as they have in the past—as a doctor—even if the care is given by a nurse.

The landmark case for nursing independence is an illustration that some of the statutes written broadly, for all nurses' practice, are less restrictive and doctor-supervised than are the statutes written specifically for nurse practitioners: *Sermchief v. Gonzales*[92] is a 1983 Missouri Supreme Court case in which obstetricians objected to NP practice in a family planning clinic. The doctors' licensing board sought to charge the nurses with practicing medicine without a license. The *Sermchief* case completely upheld the broad language of the nurse practice act that had been passed seven years before over a governor's veto, the first veto override in that state for the previous 138 years.

Nurse Practitioner Prescriptions

Prescriptive authority for nurses involves, to varying degrees, the practice of nursing, of medicine, and of pharmacies and pharmacists.[93] More than half the states have granted NPs legal authority to prescribe drugs. In some, NPs have authority to prescribe without the supervision of a physician. In most states, nurses may prescribe only in collaboration with a supervising physician.

One author has proposed a two-part proposal for reform: One would be an "authorized prescriber" statute, requiring a provider who wants to prescribe drugs to pass an examination on pharmacology and prescribing. Second, a proposal to eliminate the prohibition against "unauthorized practice" in the various statutes that license providers. That is, anyone could do doctoring, but couldn't prescribe drugs without the "authorized prescriber" status.[94]

Economic efficiency is enhanced by eliminating artificial barriers to the ability of the individual to work. Others propose to enhance patient choice in drug therapy by eliminating the requirement of prescriptions for patients to obtain medications, and to enhance patient freedom by eliminating licensure of all providers, allowing patients free access to the provider of their choice.[95]

The Drug Enforcement Administration has ruled that "mid-level practitioners" (MLPs) may obtain a DEA number, which is necessary to prescribe controlled substances. This is allowed only in states where the attorneys general have determined that eligible providers actually do have prescribing authority.[96]

Increasingly, the question of whether nurses can independently write prescriptions is becoming moot. Insurers, governmental agencies, and health plans are issuing their own drug formularies that limit not only NPs but doctors as well. Only medications listed within that formulary may be prescribed.[97] As medicine becomes more regulated, so will nurses who practice it.

Nurse Autonomy/Patient Autonomy

The nurse's exercise of freedom (autonomy) may conflict with the patient's freedom. The nurse has an interest in doing what is seen as his or her best practice. The nurse is interested in using the best judgment, doing the best work, and being free personally. The nurse has a professional interest in maintaining integrity (wholeness). Nurses won't do just anything their employer asks them to do. They are free professionals.

But will nurses do whatever the *patient* asks them to do? Would they assist in removing the patient's healthy leg, because the patient who is a beggar wants more sympathy? In removing the patient's breast, because the patient believes she might get breast cancer? If she has no relatives with cancer? If every woman in her family has developed cancer?

What will nurses do for the patient who requests abortion? Sterilization? In vitro fertilization? Circumcision? Cesarean? These usually are procedures patients want, not always procedures that are medically necessary for life and health.

The prototype patient demand for medically unnecessary care is cosmetic surgery. The majority of these procedures are not medically necessary, they are patient initiated. Some doctors assert that they can decide when treatment is futile; the patient's power to decide treatment should be limited to treatment that the doctor has decided is medically necessary. But their argument is severely compromised by actions of other physicians who give away that professional freedom (power, autonomy). Doctors who perform, and nurses who assist with, cosmetic surgery, abortion, sterilization, fertilization, cesarean sections for patient convenience—any treatment done at the demand of the patient and not of medical necessity—all erode the value of professional freedom.

The patient initiates the request for the above treatments, and some nurses and doctors comply, regardless of determination of the patient's physical need. Such compliance on the part of these practitioners hinders the ability of other practitioners to assert their professional autonomy. Others can't say they won't provide treatment that is not indicated.

The Thirteenth Amendment to the U.S. Constitution prohibits slavery; it follows that practitioners must be doing these procedures willingly on the patient's demand. It is then logically difficult to assert in other cases that the treatment that patient or family wants is futile or not medically justified, especially if continuation of the treatment wanted by the patient preserves life. Other practitioners applied no such "medical necessity" standard, when their patient demanded a prettier nose.

Is the difference *which* patient demands the procedure? The patient who wants elective procedures is up walking and talking and paying taxes and paying her own bill, probably. The patient who wants treatment just to live a little longer is old and sick and not valuable to the society. And the taxpaying practioners are actually subsidizing the care they give.

Should the patient be free to choose breast implants, at slight risk, if she knows the risk and voluntarily assumes it? Lawsuits and controversy over the danger (or nondanger) of silicone breast implants is an example of the conflict between patient autonomy and patient safety. The lack of availability of implants is now a problem for reconstruction surgery in breast cancer patients. One million women in the United States, and more in foreign countries, have had the implants, over the last three decades. The disapproval of the implants by the FDA is an illustration of the value of doing no harm (patient safety) over the value of autonomy (patient choice).

Do patients have the right to mutilate themselves? The right to ask practitioners to do it for them?

Plastic surgery is not limited to facelifts, or nose reconstruction, or breast implants. In some areas of the world, and among some peoples from those areas who have immigrated to the United States, practitioners are asked to do what some call "female genital mutilation." (Notice the prejudicial use of the word *mutilation*.) The procedure involves removing the clitoris and parts of the female genitalia, "surgically." A nicer term is *female circumcision*, but that too is misleading. The process involves a partial or total cutting away of the female external genital organs with razors, ceremonial knives, or blades, often under nonhygienic conditions without anesthesia. If the patient or her family wants it done, is female circumcision different in kind, or only in degree, from much plastic surgery? Does the patient have the "freedom" to demand it? Does the practitioner have freedom to refuse?

Autonomy to Withhold Futile Treatment

The issue of the practitioner's autonomy to refuse to give "futile" treatment is a problem of definition. Treatment is rarely characterized as "futile" unless the patient is incompetent and withdrawing treatment will end a poor quality of life. The conflict is not usually the practitioner's, but the society's and family's; doing and paying for care that does not return people to full function. In practice, "futility" is asserted only in cases of patients not competent, when withholding treatment will end what is perceived as poor quality of life. Withholding or withdrawing such care may be appropriate, but use of the word *futility* may mask the reality of the reason for the action.

Futility means different things to different people; some consider treatment futile, that merely keeps the patient alive. Some consider treatment futile if it merely returns the patient to consciousness. A treatment that doesn't return the patient to a meaningful "quality of life" may be considered futile by some. Or if treatment doesn't fully return the patient to the life experienced before the illness, some might consider the care futile.

Some distinguish futile treatment from treatment that is "inadvisable." (Another synonym for futility is "medically inappropriate.") Under that definition, *futile* treatment is treatment that will not work. It won't accomplish what it is supposed to do (for example, performing CPR on a patient who is brain dead). In contrast, *inadvisable* treatment is "not worth the effort," or treatment that restores the patient to a state in which "we would not want to 'be like that' ourselves." Some believe there is an "emerging consensus among critical care physicians on the issue of medical futility." Some disagree that there is any consensus.[98]

One writer raises the question, "What does 'medically inappropriate' mean . . . ? [S]ince laetrile's clinical ineffectiveness is a technical medical fact about which doctors are supposed to have professional expertise, it is professionally appropriate for doctors to refuse to grant a patient's request to have laetrile prescribed for cancer. But [in the *Helga Wanglie* case . . .] the parties to the dispute do not disagree about whether maintaining Mrs. Wanglie on a respirator is likely to prolong her life; they disagree about whether her life is worth prolonging. This is not a medical question, but a question of values . . . . It is as presumptuous and *ethically* inappropriate for doctors to suppose that their professional expertise qualifies them to know what kind of life is worth prolonging as it would be for meteorologists to suppose their professional expertise qualifies them to know what kind of destination is worth a long drive in the rain."[99]

One can assume that there are four reasons for limiting treatment of the patient: futility of the intervention, refusal of the treatment by the patient, the quality of life of the patient, and the cost of the treatment. Note the differences in who gets to decide about the various reasons to limit treatment.

Who decides to limit treatment, depends on why treatment is to be limited:

Refusal of treatment—patient decides.
Cost of treatment—patient and society decide.
Quality of life—patient and society decide.
Futility of treatment—practitioner decides.
Practitioners should not offer treatments if they will not work (are futile).

Refusal of treatment is decided by the patient. Quality of life and cost of treatment are not factors that the practitioner may decide alone; the patient's "society" (if someone else pays) may make those decisions.[100] Of the four reasons to limit treatment, the only one that the provider can decide is to limit (not offer) treatment because the treatment is futile.

An economic or money value also underlies all these futility cases. Although not immediately and openly stated, sooner or later will be heard: "All the money it's costing," or "it's not fair to spend all this money on these old people, when it could be spent it on prenatal care for the babies," or "no wonder our health insurance premiums are going up," or "look at the bill for the hospital/taxpayer in this case."

Considering the money is always appropriate. It should be confronted openly, not hidden under other considerations of "futility," "practitioner autonomy," or "best interest of the patient"; because the money issue is not one for the practitioner to decide alone. The discussion about futility is turning from whether treatment is futile (useless), to whether the patient is worth the cost. Is the treatment futile, or is the patient's life futile?[101]

THE "FUTILE" EXAMPLE: HELGA WANGLIE

Mrs. Wanglie was an 84-year-old woman (not conscious). In the case *In re. Helga Wanglie*, Mrs. Wanglie's physicians requested the court to protect them from liability for discontinuing her ventilator.

There was conflict between the doctors, the patient's prior expressed wishes, and with her surrogate (her husband) who wanted the treatment continued.

The doctors said the treatment was not in the patient's best interest, that the treatment was futile, although it would keep her alive (it would not restore her to consciousness, but she had been unconscious before being put on the respirator).

The court ruled that her wishes to live should prevail; the ventilator continued and she died three days later.[102]

One writer has said that he has a practical, arbitrary benchmark for stopping care: "highly improbable." A "highly improbable" chance of success he defines as a chance of less than one in 100.[103] Remember that such a number or estimate of a procedures effect is an *average* determined from a population of patients which may be different from the individual patient. Can the practitioner ever consider life-saving treatment "futile" in the sense that it's chance of success is less than optimal? Less than average?

BRITISH "FUTILITY"

In England, thoracic surgeons have refused to do lung transplants on smokers.

In another case, 47-year-old Harry Elphick didn't get bypass surgery because he smoked 25 cigarettes a day. He quit smoking but died of a second heart attack before tests and surgery could be performed; he was buried on the day his catheterization was scheduled. Doctor Colin Bray, his cardiologist, said that refusal was the policy of Manchester's Wythenshawe Hospital, and that smokers benefit less from bypass than non-smokers.[104]

Whether the patient's life is valued, and whether the patient's freedom is respected by the nurse, should not depend on whether the patient agrees with the nurse. If the patient doesn't agree that treatment is futile, then the practitioner is valuing practitioner judgment (freedom) over the patient's freedom (and life). In some cases, the practitioner has asked a court to force the practitioner's professional judgment (values) on the patient.

Freedom to choose (patient autonomy) is not just freedom to *refuse* treatment offered. If the patient is not also free to choose to have or continue a treatment that is offered, it is not really a choice. Nurses should ascertain that they are not offering a "choice" that really offers only one option. Freedom to choose does not mean freedom only to refuse.

Freedom of choice in abortion does not mean merely "free to refuse abortion," nor does it mean only "free to choose abortion." If the patient is offered a true alternative of refusing treatment, be sure that the patient understands that it's a choice, and that the other alternative (treatment) actually can be chosen.

The rule: If a practitioner offers a procedure believed to be futile, and the practitioner expects only a refusal, it probably should not be offered in the first place.

Futility: Treatment Prolonging
Poor "Quality of Life" in Incompetent Patients

With a competent patient, *futile* is never used: The physician says to competent patient and family, "There's no other treatment we can do." If there were another treatment that could work, it would be tried.

The word *futile* is only used if treatment is possible but quality of life is not: If treatment is not possible, it is not suggested. If quality of life is good, any possible treatment is worth it. The physician who says "futile" means that the contemplated treatment indeed might work, but the incompetent patient's quality of life is not perceived to be worth prolonging.

If "futile" is asserted, and if the incompetent's family does not contest the assertion, the practitioner will then decide if treatment is "futile." Futility is never decided solely on medical grounds; the decision is based on the values of the practitioner and the family, both judging the quality of life for another person. In many cases this is appropriate, but using the word may cloud the reality of what is being done.

Also noted in practice: The characterization as "futile" of life-sustaining treatment for an incompetent person, is only made if withdrawing treatment results in ending the person's life. If stopping a treatment will not result in death (for example, stopping an antibiotic that's not helping), that's not characterized as "futile" treatment; just ineffective therapy.

Consider a patient receiving an antibiotic for an infection. If the antibiotic will return the patient to an active life in the community, it is not characterized as "futile" treatment. If the drug will return the patient to a vegetative state in the nursing home, however, it may be characterized as "futile," considering the patient's quality of life. If the patient will not die, the word will not be used to characterize the treatment.

Practitioners will increasingly use "quality of life" criteria to justify their decisions about futility. "Futility" is almost always shorthand for a decision not to treat, which will result in death. The decision is made appropriately, for a variety of reasons, but few reasons have to do with actual practitioner freedom not to give futile care.

Assisted Suicide

If patients have a "right" to die, then perhaps they have a right to kill themselves. More recently, movements have been mounted to give people the right to demand assistance from doctors and nurses in killing themselves; such an initiative was approved by the Oregon voters in 1994. As with suicide, perhaps this is the ultimate in autonomy for the patient. But the autonomy of the nurse could be threatened by participation in patient suicides. The individual nurse, and perhaps the whole profession of nursing, should have some "right" to refuse to act contrary to personal and professional ethics. As with the question asked about the patient's right to suicide, it might be argued that people who want to die are mentally ill (at least depressed). The nurse must ask whether such patients need help to live, or to die.

The issue of assisted suicide is discussed in Chapter Seven. But the ethics and the law of suicide, and of causing death in patients (euthanasia and assisted suicide), are all enforcement of the value of *being free*—having autonomy over one's life and death. The patient's power over life or death may be in conflict with the nurse's power over the practice of her profession.

ENDNOTES

1. Gauthier, C.C., "Philosophical foundations of respect for autonomy," *Kennedy Institute of Ethics Journal* 1993; 3(1):21–37.
2. *Schloendorff v. Society of New York Hospitals*, 211 N.Y. 125, 105 N.E. 92 (1914).
3. *Cruzan v. Director, Missouri Dept. of Health*, 110 S.Ct. 2841, 111 L.Ed.2d 224 (1990).
4. Curtin, L.L., "Informed consent: Cautious, calculated candor," *Nursing Management*, 1993; 24(4):18–21.
5. *Urban v. Spohn Hospital*, 869 S.W. 2d 450 (Tex App 1993).
6. Hirsch, B.D., and Wilcox, D.P., "Neglecting informed consent is fuel for malpractice suits," *Texas Medicine*, 1992; 88(6):50–53.
7. "Patients' recall of preoperative instruction for informed consent for an operation," *Journal of Bone and Joint Surgery*, 1991; 73-a(2):160.
8. *Young v. Horton*, 855 P. 2d 502 (1993 Mont.)
9. Cohn, S.D., "The evolving law of adolescent healthcare," Nurses Association of the American College of Obstetricians and Gynecologists, *Clinical Issues*, 1991; 2:201–207.
10. Generally, see White, B.C., "Ethical issues surrounding informed consent. Part I. A brief history and ethical foundations surrounding informed consent," *Urologic Nursing*, 1989; 9(3):11–14.
11. *E.g.*, Medical Liability and Insurance Improvement Act, Tex. Rev. Civ. Stat. Ann. Art. 4590i §§ 6.01-6.07 (Vernon Supp. 1995).
12. 42 CFR 110.

13. Harrow, A., "The blurred intersection of beneficence, competence and autonomy," *Annals of Internal Medicine*, 1993; 119:637–638.
14. See for other home health issues: Haddad, A., "Ethical problems in home healthcare," *Journal of Nursing Administration*, 1992; 22(3):46–51.
15. McCusker, J., and Stoddard, A.M., "Use of a surrogate for the SIP," *Medical Care*, 1984; 22(9):789–792.
16. Rubenstein, L.Z., *et al.*, "Systematic biases in functional status assessment of elderly adults: Effects of different data sources," *Journal of Gerontology*, 1984; 39:686.
17. Andereck, W.S., "Development of a hospital ethics committee: Lessons from five years of case consultations," *Cambridge Quarterly of Healthcare Ethics*, 1992; 1:41–50.
18. "Explore both sides when dealing with a difficult proxy," *Medical Ethics Advisor*, August 1993, pp. 92–94.
19. Darzins, Peteris, *et al.*, "Treatment for life-threatening illness," *New England Journal of Medicine*, 1993; 329(10):736.
20. See, *e.g.*, Reigle, J., "Preserving patient self-determination through advance directives," *Heart & Lung*, 1992; 21(2):196–198.
21. Reigle, J., *op. cit.*
    Strother, A., "Drawing the line between life and death," *American Journal of Nursing*, 1991; 91(4):24–25.
22. But in support of that assumption about the purpose of the directive, the fact is that the first living will documents were created and promoted by the Euthanasia Society in 1967 (subsequently renamed Society for the Right to Die and, then, Choice in Dying).
23. New York Academy of Medicine, Dilemmas of Euthanasia: Excerpts from papers and discussions at the Fourth Euthanasia Conference 42 (1972).
24. JCAHO Standard RI.2.5 in the Patient Rights chapter of the *1993 Accreditation Manual for Hospitals*.
25. Rushton, C.H., "Advance directives for critically ill adolescents," *Critical Care Nurse*, 1992; June, 31–37.
26. Strother, A., *op. cit.*
27. King, N.M.P., "Dying made legal: New challenges for advance directives," *Health Ethics Committee Forum*, 1991; 3:187–199.
28. Emanuel, L.L., and Emanuel E.J., "The medical directive: A new comprehensive advance care document, *Journal of the American Medical Association*, 1989; 261:3288–3293; and, "Advance directives for medical care—A case for greater use," *New England Journal of Medicine* 1991; 324:889–895.
29. Brett, A.S., "Limitations of listing specific medical interventions in advance directives, *Journal of the American Medical Association*, 1991; 324:882–888.
30. McClosky, E., "Between isolation and intrusion: The Patient Self Determination Act," *Law, Medicine and Health Care*, 1991; 19(1-2), 80–82.
31. Clymer, Adam, "Hillary Clinton Raises Tough Question of Life, Death and Medicine," 1 October 1993, *New York Times*.
32. Schneiderman, L.J., *et. al.*, "Effects of offering advance directives on medical treatments and costs," *Annals of Internal Medicine*, 1992; 117:599–606.
    Also see, Greco, P.J., *et al.*, "The PSDA and the future of advance directives," *Annals of Internal Medicine*, 1991; 115:639–643.
    "The Patient Self-Determination Act: Implementation issues and opportunities," *Health Lawyer*, 1992; 6(1):1–8.
33. Pinch, W.J., and Parsons, M.E., "The Patient Self-Determination Act: The ethical dimensions," *Nurse Practitioner Forum*, 1992; 3(1):16–22.
34. McLeod, D., "Bad Time to Weigh Care Options," *AARP Bulletin*, 1994; 35(1):4–5.
35. "A new focus on advance directives," *Briefings on JCAHO*, July/August 1993, pp. 10–11.
36. Burt, R., *Taking Care of Strangers: The Rule of Law in Doctor-Patient Relations*, New York: The Free Press, 1979, p. 169.
37. Danis, M., *et al.*, "A prospective study of advance directives for life-sustaining care," *New England Journal of Medicine*, 1991; 324:882–888.
38. Block, A.J., "Living wills are overrated," *Chest*, 1993; 104(6):1645–1646.
39. Ely, J.W., *et al.*, "The physician's decision to use tube feedings: The role of the family, the living will, and the *Cruzan* decision," *Journal of the American Geriatrics Society*, 1992; 40:471–475.

"Survey finds doctors favor family wishes over living will," *Missouri Bar Bulletin*, January 1993; p. 15.

40. Sehgal, A., *et al.*, "How strictly do dialysis patients want their advance directives followed?" *Journal of the American Medical Association*, 1992; 267:59–63.

41. Hall, J.K., "Living won't," *Florida Bar News*, 15 July 1993, p. 14, and 1 November 1993, p. 2.

42. Dubler, Nancy, "Commentary: Balancing life and death—proceed with caution," *American Journal of Public Health*, 1993; 83:23–25.

43. See: "Many African-American patients shy away from advance directives," *Medical Ethics Advisor*, 1993; 9(2):13–16.

Farfel, M., *et al.*, "Education, consent, and counseling in sickle cell screening programs: Report of a survey," *American Journal of Public Health*, 1984; 74:373–375.

44. Letter, *American Medical News*, 12 July 1993: 21.

45. *Managed Care Outlook*, 13 August 1993, p. 3.

46. Personal communication from Sandy Cantrell, Denver, CO.

47. Schneiderman, L.J., *op. cit.*

48. Communication from Dr. Ted Nicklas, Amarillo, TX, December 1993.

49. Robertson, J.A., "Second thoughts on living wills," *Hastings Center Report*, 1991; 21(6): 6–9.

50. "Marjorie Nighbert: Victim of a system bent on her death," *IATEF Update*, 1995; 9(4):7–8.

51. "The anatomy bill in the District of Columbia," *Journal of the American Medical Association*, 1890; 14:546–547.

52. *Texas Health and Safety Code Ann.* §§692.001 *et seq.* (1992).

53. 42 U.S.C. §1320b-8.

54. *Idem.*

55. Associated Press, *San Francisco Chronicle*, 2 December 1992, A2.

56. Bonn, A.P., "School Promises to Prove It Had Relatives' Consent," *Amarillo, Texas, Globe-News*, 25 November 1993.

57. Cox, E.E., "A recipient's perspective of the dilemma concerning visceral organ transplantation," *Panhandle Health*, 1993; 4(1):13–14.

58. Rubenstein, P., *Proceedings of the National Academy of Sciences*, 31 October 1993, in Winslow, R., "Placenta May Be Source of Cells Vital in Bone Marrow Transplants," *Wall Street Journal*, 12 November 1993, B12.

59. 42 U.S.C. §273, regulations at 42 CFR 485.305 *et. seq.*

60. Randall, T., "Too few human organs for transplantation, too many in need...and the gap widens," *Journal of the American Medical Association*, 1991, 265(10) 1223–1227.

61. McCartney, S., "Law May Allow Few Transplants for Foreigners," *Wall Street Journal*, 30 June 1993, B1,B.

62. Associated Press, "Proteins May Allow Pig-to-Human Transplants," *Amarillo Daily News*, 4 November 1993.

63. Selzer, R., *Mortal Lessons: Notes on the Art of Surgery*, New York: Simon & Schuster, 1976.

64. For data, see Johnson, A.M., "Heterosexual transmission of human immunodeficiency virus," *British Medical Journal*, 1988; 296:1017–1020.

65. Padian, N.S., *et al.*, "Female-to-male transmission of human immunodeficiency virus," *Journal of the American Medical Association*, 1991; 266:1664–1667.

Stewart, G.T., "The epidemiology and transmission of AIDS: A hypothesis linking behavior and biological determinants to time, person and place," *Genetica* 1995; 95(1-3):173–193.

66. Ziemba, T.M., "Laws affect treatment of HIV patients," *National Medical-Legal Journal*, 1993; 4(2):3.

67. Downes, J., "Acquired immunodeficiency syndrome: The nurse's legal duty to serve," *Journal of Professional Nursing*, 1991; 7(6):333–340.

68. Kearney, K.A., and Craig-Johnson, C., "What every U.S. business should know about HIV infection," *Health Lawyer*, 1992, 6(2):20–23.

69. Karassik, I.R., and Kayser, S.V., "AIDS and the health care provider," *Health Lawyer*, 1992, 6(1):15–20.

70. Flarey, D.L., "Legal and ethical issues in HIV testing, Part 1," *Journal of Nursing Administration, 1992; 22(10):14–20.*

71. For discussion, see Brent, N.J., "Confidentiality and HIV status: The nurse's right to know," *Home Healthcare Nurse*, 1990; 8(3):6–8.
72. *Texas Health and Safety Code*, §85.204(c), (Vernon 1992).
73. Chase, M., "AIDS Case Rate Is Said to Peak in San Francisco," *Wall Street Journal*, 16 February 1994, B5.
74. Ashworth, C.S., *et al.*, "An evaluation of a school-based AIDS/HIV education program for high school students," *Journal of Adolescent Health*, 1992; 12:582–588.
75. Stiffman, A.R., *et al.*, "Changes in AIDS-related risk behavior after adolescence: Relationships to knowledge and experience concerning HIV infection," *Pediatrics*, 1992; 89:950–956.
76. Stiffman, A.R., *et al.*, "The influence of mental health problems on AIDS-related risk behaviors in young adults," *Journal of Nervous and Mental Disorders*, 1992; 180:314–320.
77. See: Bayer, R., *et al.*, "The dual epidemics of tuberculosis and AIDS: Ethical and policy issues in screening and treatment, *American Journal of Public Health* 1993; 83(5):649–654.
78. See generally, for TB information: Kamitsuka, P., "Tuberculosis," *Harvard Intensive Review of Internal Medicine*, vol II, Boston: Harvard Medical School, 1993.
    Frieden, T.R., *et al.*, "The emergence of drug-resistant TB in New York City," *New England Journal of Medicine*, 1993; 328:521–6.
79. Schoen, D.C., "Nurses' attitudes toward control over nursing practice," *Nursing Forum*, 1991; 27(1):27–34.
80. "Support for nurses," *Nursing, 1993*, 23(12):8.
81. Fein, W.S., "The murky waters of physician recruitment," *Unique Opportunities*, 1993; March/April 1993, pp. 7–10.
82. 42 U.S.C. 1320a-7b(b)(2).
83. Mittelstadt, P., *The Reimbursement Manual: How to Get Paid for Your Advanced Practice Nursing Services*, Washington, DC: American Nurses Publishing, 1993.
84. See Hadaway, L.C., "State boards of nursing and issues of advanced practice," *Journal of Intravenous Nursing*, 1991; 14(4):274–279.
85. Hall, J.K., "Analysis of nurse practitioner state licensure laws," *Nurse Practitioner*, 1993; 18(8):31–34.
86. Casetta, R., "House unites when faced with regulation issues," *American Nurse*, July/August 1993, p. 26.
87. Williams, C., "Physician extenders," *Missouri Medicine*, 1992; 89(12):835.
88. See: Hirsh, H.L., "Medico-legal considerations in the use of physician extenders," *Legal Medicine*, 1991:127–205.
89. Annotation, Nurse's Liability for Her Own Negligence or Malpractice (1957 & Supp. 1987 & 1991), 51 ALR 2d 970.
90. See *e.g.*, *Flickenger v. United States*, 523 F. Supp. 1372 (W.D. Pa. 1981).
91. *Arkansas State Nurses Association v. Arkansas State Medical Board*, 677 S.W.2d 293 (1984).
92. *Sermchief v. Gonzales*, 660 S.W.2d 683 (Mo 1983).
93. Carson, W., "Gains and challenges in prescriptive authority," *American Nurse*, 1993; 25(6):19–20.
94. Hadley, E.H., "Nurses and prescriptive authority: A legal and economic analysis," *American Journal of Law & Medicine*, 1989; 15(2–3):245–299.
95. Hall, J.K., "Analysis of nurse practitioner state licensure laws," *op. cit.*
96. "Final rule published on DEA numbers for mid-level practitioners," *American Nurse*, July/August 1993, p. 22.
97. See, for examples: *National Pharmacy Program: Drug Formulary*, Detroit, MI: Blue Cross-Blue Shield of Michigan, 1994.
    Premier Rx: Drug Formulary, Scottsdale, AZ: PCS Health Systems, 1994.
98. Hansen-Flaschen, J., "When life support is futile," *Chest*, 1991; 100(5):1191–1192.
99. Ackerman, Felicia, "The significance of a wish," Hastings Center Report, 1991; 21(4):27, 28.
100. Lo, B., and Jonsen, A., "Clinical decisions to limit treatment," *Annals of Internal Medicine*, 1980; 93:764–768.
101. Ross, J.A., "Judgments of futility: What should ethics committees be thinking about," *Hospital Ethics Committee Forum*, 1991; (3)4, pp. 201–210.

102. *In re*. Helga Wanglie, Fourth Judicial District (District Court, Probate Division) PX 91-283, Minnesota, Hennepin County.
103. Schneiderman, L.J., *et al.*, "Medical futility: Its meaning and ethical implications," *Annals of Internal Medicine*, 1990; 112:949–953.
104. Schmidt, W.E., "Death of Briton Denied Operation Fires Health Care Debate," *New York Times*, 21 August 1993, p 4.

FIVE

Ethics and Law of
Fairness (Justice)

TOPICS COVERED

Ethical principles of justice

Various theories of justice: social justice

Rawls's "original position" and the nurse's "knowledgeable position"

Economics of illness care law

Effects of legal entitlement to illness care

Nursing economics

Labor law enforcing the value, Fairness

FAIRNESS (JUSTICE)

▽

"No, no!" said the Queen. "Sentence first—verdict afterwards."
—**LEWIS CARROLL,** *Alice's Adventures in Wonderland*

△

> The value, Fairness (Justice), requires treating people fairly; the law enforces that value by requiring due process (no taking of life, liberty, or property without good reason). Fairness is also enforced in law as equality of opportunity.
>
> Equating law (a minimum) exactly with justice (a higher ethical value) may result in the mistaken idea that all laws are just (that legal behavior is ethical behavior).
>
> Illness care ethics discussions may use the word *justice* to describe the concept of "social" or "distributive" justice (not based on fairness to the individual, but instead on the value of doing good for the group).
>
> Theories of fairness range from "each person should have equal outcomes" (social justice) to "each according to need" (Marx) to "each according to effort" (voluntary market) to "each according to contribution to society" (market, or social justice?) to "equal opportunity for each person."
>
> Systems of distributive or social justice promote the equality of outcomes, not necessarily equality in *the process*. Ultimately, the maxim most exemplifying social justice is "the end justifies the means."
>
> Tension exists between people who most value social justice (doing good for the group) and people who most value autonomy for the individual, since attaining equal outcomes of property (goods and services) necessitates forced distribution of property, from people who have it, to people who don't.

The value of fairness (justice) is taught to children early, by parents and teachers in their oft-repeated advice, "Play fair." (Perhaps people do know all they need to know about ethics by the time they finish kindergarten.) The value, Fairness, requires treating people fairly under the law (applying the same process to everyone, without bias). This value is assumed to underlie *all* law in the society.

The statue of Justice—prominent in many U.S. courthouses—wears a blindfold and often holds a scale that can't be unfairly weighted (symbolizing that Justice treats all people the same). The *outcome* need not be equal (one side of the scale *will* be heavier), but the process must work without bias, for or against anyone (symbolized by the blindfold).

In a democracy, being fair (being *just*) does not mean giving all people the same *things*; it does mean treating all the same, at least within the legal process.

The words *justice* and *law* are often used interchangeably, although they do not mean the same thing. *Justice* is but one of the values the law should reflect and enforce just as law reflects and enforces every other value highlighted in this book; as seen throughout, the minimum of law enforces to some degree *all* the values, not merely Fairness (Justice). Law should be fair (be just), but it should also enforce the nurse's duty to do good and not harm; law should allow Freedom and enforce Being True (Keeping Promises, Keeping Secrets, and Telling Truth). Law should also enforce protecting Life (punishing murder, for example), and should enforce the minimal ethic of the right of people to their property (the results of their work), which will be discussed in this chapter, under Labor Ethics and Law.

There is some danger in equating what is law (a minimum) exactly with Justice (a higher ethical value). That danger arises in assuming that *all* laws are *fair* (a higher ethic) merely because they are laws. Ethical behavior is almost always legal; but legal behavior does not always rise to the higher standard of being entirely just, ethical: the right thing to do.

> "If law and justice are identified [treated as identical], if only a just order is called law, a social order which is presented as law is—at the same time—presented as just; and that means it is morally justified. The tendency to identify [treat as identical] law and justice is the tendency to justify [call just] a given social order."[1]

But the words *law* and *justice* are usually indexed together, often used together, and discussed synonymously by philosophers. Under the value of fairness/justice, this book will discuss the ethics and law of justice both as equality of opportunity (the labor laws, later in this chapter) and as fairness in the legal process (due process, covered in the first chapter, Values in Ethics and Law). There is not much controversy or conflict about the value of fairness; all would agree, at least in theory, that being fair is the "right thing" to do. Exactly what behavior or action is "being fair" can be debated, however.

The laws of fairness seek mainly to "undo" wrongs; to restore conflicting parties to a status or state equal to that which existed before.

In criminal law, the "wrong" is a crime. People start out unharmed by each other, but one wrongs another (called the victim). At this point, the victim cannot be "*un*wronged"; therefore, so as to restore "balance" to the parties, a punishment is administered to the wrongdoer—in essence, to make him equally harmed.

In civil law, the wrong is called a tort. Parties start out unharmed; then one does a wrong to the other (victim). The victim (in a lawsuit, the plaintiff) may seek to be "unwronged," for example, by receiving money. To make the parties equal again, the wrongdoer (now the defendant) pays money to the plaintiff. The wrongdoer here doesn't have to be "punished" (as for crime), because—through financial restitution—the victim/plaintiff is restored to his or her prior status.

Using law to do *more* than punish wrongs (in other words, to do good) however, may result in unintended consequences.

One sense of the word *justice* means "equality or fairness under the law": fairness in *process*, not in *outcomes*; equal opportunity of action, not equal shares of a good or service.

Fairness of process under the law—guaranteed under the Constitution in the United States—need not receive lengthy discussion here, since that value is not controversial. (Laws that enforce the value of fairness are those that enforce fair treatment in the legal process, discussed under Due Process in Chapter One.) Equality of opportunity as a value is enforced in laws that forbid discriminatory treatment on the basis of some nonbehavioral status or perceived individual condition.

It is not considered fair to discriminate against people because of some characteristic they cannot change; but, to discriminate among people on the basis of their voluntary *actions* is not only fair, but even necessary. It is not considered fair to discriminate because of sex or race (an innate or inherent condition), but it is considered fair to discriminate on the bases of attitude, skill, and education.

Several statutes, at both national and state levels, forbid discrimination on the bases of specific conditions: Those conditions are not about behavior but about ascribed conditions that people cannot change by behavior (race, color, sex, ethnic origin, age, disability). Controversy arises, however, when the line between conditions and behaviors blurs—where, for example, to draw a line between an innate condition and a disability? Some conditions could be seen as behaviors *or* as conditions unable to be changed (for example, obesity).

In the United States, the law and ethic of fairness is so strong *against* discriminating on the basis of individuals' conditions, that sometimes if for some technical reason the court cannot invoke one of the laws against discrimination, they will find another law.

PUNISHING DISCRIMINATION WITH MALPRACTICE LAW

A federal appellate court held that a nurse did not illegally discriminate under the civil rights law. But it found the nurse was negligent—had committed professional malpractice—for calling the patient "[RACIAL SLUR]."

—*Hall v. Bio-Medical Applications, Inc.*, 671 F.2d 300 (8th Cir. 1982)

Note that, in the case above, there was no law that the nurse could have read and followed; the court used a tenuous connection to malpractice law. But the nurse could have practiced good nursing (calling patients names is *not* good nursing) and that would have been ethical—and prevented the legal problem.

Note that discrimination itself is not bad; people discriminate daily in choosing food, travel, and clothes. They also discriminate among people regarding whom to associate with: friends, clubs, hiring. *Discriminating* itself is not at issue, but the *basis* of discrimination is.

The value people put on fairness—and more specifically, equality of opportunity—results in laws that forbid people to discriminate, in hiring and other work situations as well as public situations, on the basis of some inherent condition or status. Most equal opportunity laws are made by statutes, and most of them enforce fairness in the workplace—to be discussed in the latter part of this chapter.

Instead of the noncontroversial concept of fairness of opportunity, a different meaning of Justice is used in many discussions of nursing ethics and law. In those discussions the word *justice* is used to describe the concept of "social" or "distributive" justice. [Much of this chapter will be concerned with what is called social justice (distributive justice) in the context of the ethics and proposed laws of illness care.] The concept of social justice seems not so much a part of the traditional value, Justice (Fairness to the individual), but a part of the value, Beneficence (Doing Good, for the group). When Beneficence is enforced in law, economic consequences result, so some basic laws of economics are described in this chapter.

Theories of Fairness

Different theories of justice are written; in addition to the definition of equal treatment under the law and of equal opportunity, some call it "just" if each person has an equal share of something. Another different theory of justice would give to each according to individual need (Marx).

Or justice may be defined as "reward according to effort expended" (as in the voluntary free market). Or justice could be described as achieved, if each received benefits according to her contribution to society. Or justice could be considered achieved when people receive benefits according to merit—a meritocracy—but, in any system, some[one?] must judge merit.[2]

Englehardt believes that philosophers of justice come in roughly three camps:

Egalitarians—people who believe that fairness in equal opportunity is the highest value. The philosophy of egalitarians desires equal access to opportunity for all.

Libertarians—people who focus on social and economic rights. (Libertarians might believe the government should not interfere with individual action, even to insure equal opportunity.)

Utilitarians—people who wish for the greatest public and private utilization of resources—may necessitate government action to assure some form of equal outcomes.[3]

The concepts of "distributive justice" or "social justice" are usually applied in terms of the philosophy of socialism; the terms, as used presently, have actually been in use about 100 years, and often used interchangeably.[4] No less a utilitarian than John Stuart Mill equated the terms. The theory of social justice underlies all proposals for tax-paid illness care. So understanding it is vital to nurses who practice in such a system.

Beyond 100 years ago, these concepts were "seen" in visions of a utopia (a perfectly equal peaceful place). Within these concepts, the equality of *outcome* (not necessarily of *process*) is the goal. For instance: In the area of race, equality of outcome (social justice) is attained when there are numbers of African-Americans in a community's school proportional to the numbers of African-Americans residing in that community. To some who desire "social justice," the fairness of process used to achieve that proportion is not as important as whether the *outcome* is equal.

Another example: Equality of outcome is achieved if the proportion of women working for a company is roughly equal to the proportion of women in the community. That outcome might be considered socially just.

A "socially just" basketball team might have 80 percent European Americans, 50 percent women, and short people in proportion to their number in the community.

Sir Friederich Hayek, economist and philosopher, dislikes the substitution of the concept of social justice for the original meaning of justice: "[Social justice] is an abuse of the word [justice] which threatens to destroy the conception of law which made it the safeguard of individual freedom."[5]

Can only conduct be just, not the rewards of conduct?

Social justice flows from the idea that all people deserve some material necessities in addition to freedoms/rights simply because they are human. The idea that all humans have basic rights (freedom from control on individual behaviors) is extended to encompass rights (entitlements) to tangible things: food, housing, transportation, service of illness care. The concept of social justice extends the idea of a right (to do an action) to an entitlement (to have some physical property or service performed).

If all people are to have a socially just share of illness care (or cars, or houses), all should have equal shares. As it is now, there is an inequality of kinds and amounts of illness care (as there is of cars and houses). All people have "access" to care, but some cannot buy as much as others.

Justice = Rights (freedom to act)
Social Justice = Goods and Services (things)

Social/distributive justice may not be compatible with full freedom. In order to attain equal outcomes of property, it is necessary to *re*-distribute property from people who own it to people who don't. To some, in order to make illness care outcomes equal, people who can buy more illness care must be prevented from buying more illness care than the poor. People who have more money or care must be made to redistribute care to people who have less—and, to that extent, the freedom (autonomy) of people with money to purchase care would have to be denied.

Justice, however, also incorporates rights of individual ownership: that their property, the products of theirs and their parents' work, shall be protected. To take someone's property without permission is theft (the time, work, and energy used to earn that property is stolen), and the law punishes that act.

The promise and guarantee of the Fifth Amendment to the U.S. Constitution limits the federal government—the Fourteenth Amendment limits the state governments: The "taking" of life, liberty, or property by government must not take place without due process of law (without fairness). Thus is government especially held to the standard of Fairness in legal proceedings.

The concept of social justice remains controversial in the context of individual values in the United States, representing no more, nor less than the rights of the individual versus those of society.

Rawls and Justice: The Original Position

John Rawls's Original Position hypothesizes that people will be fair to each other only if they are behind a "veil of ignorance" as to whether they are in a low or high position in society.

On the other hand, the Knowledgeable Position assumes that people know they are dependent on others (either now or will be in future) and that acting fairly to others increases the odds they will receive justice, too.

Proposals for illness care "system reform" imply a planned arrangement, but payment for illness care originally took place in a voluntary market (not planned—spontaneous).

The U.S. "system" of illness care is now a combination of payment through the voluntary market and mandated redistribution (the Veterans Administration, Medicare/Medicaid, Indian Health Service, and CHAMPUS).

A *monopsony* in the illness care market would occur if there were only one *buyer*, such as the U.S. government. A monopsony is relatively the opposite of a *monopoly*, in which one *producer* (or seller) controls the market.

John Rawls, a writer on the subject of justice, has written a theory of social justice. He suggests that one can imagine what the laws of society should be, by taking what he calls the Original Position. He asks people to imagine that they are making laws for their society, working behind an imaginary "veil of ignorance." The veil keeps the lawmaker from knowing his place or rank in society. Rawls believes that, from behind such a veil, the lawmaker would make laws that indeed benefit everyone. (The lawmaker assumes that he *might* be in the lower rank.) The underlying assumption is that people operate on the basis of self-interest.

Rawls suggests that laws made by a person who adheres to this Original Position would enforce the principle that no one could work to get more of anything than another had, unless the work also benefited the lowest member of society.[6]

This theory assumes that a hierarchical (Marxian) class system exists, and that a "zero-sum" game exists that makes advancing one's self-interest detrimental to others. This is in contrast to the theory that, if people cooperate, they all advance their individual self-interests at the same time.

Nurses and the Knowledgeable Position

Instead of Rawls's Original Position (ignorance of one's position in society), nurses usually take what the author has called the Knowledgeable Position. Nurses know that some day they too may be patients. They work now to benefit patients because someone, later, will work to benefit them. If they are fair (good) to patients, they increase the odds that later they will be treated fairly, too.

The individual's interest in fairness (justice) increases the odds that he or she personally will be treated fairly in return. Such an individual also believes that a fair system keeps conflict to a minimum (conflict is painful, messy, costly). People consistently treated unfairly will eventually take to the streets. Every individual instinctively seeks fair treatment; and the surest way to obtain fairness is to support and participate in a system that continues to provide justice for all—that way, the individual will receive justice whenever needed.

The Knowledgeable Position is a realistic, practical concept. In contrast, "social/distributive" justice belongs to idealism—a goal or utopian vision that everyone will have equal shares of things.

Social Justice Applied

Social justice is the most mentioned value in any discussion of the economics of illness care. The value that social justice actually reflects is the value of doing good (beneficence) for the group—doing good in a socially just illness care system. Here, one sees distributive justice in its most appealing form; that all people should get an equal share of a good (a thing). When people don't get illness care, they are seen to be treated unfairly.

The old saying: "The end justifies the means." If true, then when the outcome is correct, whatever means (process) used was justified; see the example.

An example from a first grade reader: Jane has two cookies; at the end of the day, Jane has one cookie and Dick has the other. (Ostensibly, distributive justice has been achieved.) However, Dick knocked Jane down and took the cookie. (To Dick, "The end justifies the means," thus rationalizing his assault and theft.) What if Big Mother took the cookie from Jane for Dick?

Does the *outcome* justify the *process*?

Suppose Dick and Jane both have the same opportunity to bake cookies and Jane chooses not to. (In this scenario, both have access to a *process*.) Whatever the result (outcome), the process is fair.

Dick has baked two cookies and chooses not to share them; he feels it's his right to keep cookies produced by his own labor. To interfere with Dick's possession of two cookies—in the name of equal *outcomes*—is stealing from him, and therefore unjust.

If Dick had made two cookies and given one to Jane, he'd perhaps have performed a desirable ethical act (Doing Good). The minimum of the law as it stands, however, does not mandate that he do good to Jane. If social/distributive justice *is* mandated in law, to that extent the law would force Doing Good at the expense of Freedom.

ECONOMICS OF ILLNESS CARE LAW

The current system of price controls set by government payment (for example, Medicare) results in prices that are neither set by a free voluntary market *nor* according to social justice principles.

Mandating illness care as a legal entitlement would have economic consequences that might eventually result in provision of care by the government.

Reformers call for change in the system of illness care and propose to change the system with legal mandates. The word *system* implies some kind of human-made arrangement, but illness care started out within a free market (the same that generally operates to get food from the farm to the table). Doctors and hospitals and nurses were free to contract directly with patients. Nurses cared for patients in their homes and in the hospital, independently contracting directly with their patients.

The hospitals were staffed with student nurses and a few supervisors. People who could not pay for care were given free care—charity—giving voluntarily to others, the essence of Doing Good.

As entrepreneurs, nurses have also provided voluntary charity care: In 1935, nurses reported *giving* to patients 11 days service on average each year, without compensation. That's more than two weeks of work. The figure is even more impressive when it is remembered that these nurses were independent contractors with no sick days, no paid vacations, and no paid benefits.[7]

The Depression of the 1930s was a depression for illness caregivers, too; people couldn't afford to buy care. The experience prompted doctors and hospitals to start "insurance" companies, in their own interest; people with insurance could buy doctor and nurse services and hospital care, even when they had no job and no extra cash. The "system" was still free market, but with a third-party payor—private insurance.

The U.S. government entered as another big "third-party" payor for illness care, with Medicare in 1965 and later with more Medicaid. Government bought illness care with taxpayer money—and government became the *only* buyer (the only market influence) for some categories of people: the old (Medicare) and poor (Medicaid). A *monopsony* was created in those markets.

Gradually the illness care "system" (formerly the voluntary market) became many "systems," a combination of free market and tax-paid, the latter exemplified by the Veterans Administration, Medicare/Medicaid, Indian Health Service, and CHAMPUS on the one hand, and fee-for-service practioners on the other. Any "reform" can take one of two directions; either more social control and redistribution of illness care will be enacted, or less control and more voluntary free market will be chosen (some laws repealed). Or a combination of the two will continue (most likely).

A historical note on "socialized medicine": In 1946 an ethics/economics writer saw no harm in socialized medicine. She characterized "socialized medicine" in two ways: (1) nurses and doctors employed by public health departments; and (2) doctors and nurses on salary at state university teaching hospitals, instead of being independent contractors in communities.[8] A different degree of "socialized medicine" than more lately proposed.

The current system of payment for illness care in the United States uses neither a totally free voluntary market nor a totally socialized system paid for and controlled by the government—it is a combination of the two. For example, Medicare/Medicaid is currently the only buyer (price setter) for whole populations of the poor and elderly. This creates at least a partial monopsony, since it involves all of the people in those two categories of the population. Proposals that the government become the only buyer/controller of care (as in Canada) describe a total monopsony.

▽

"Monopsony is the term used to describe a situation in which the relevant market for a factor of production is dominated by a single purchaser."[9]

△

Monopsony is the opposite of a monopoly; a monopoly occurs when a single producer controls the market, or when only one seller or type of sellers of a service is available (for example, in doctor and nurse licensure). When a monopsony exists, the price can easily be set too low to attract sufficient and qualified providers or producers.

To use monopsony as meaning a *free market* "monopoly of buyers" is error; a true monopsony can exist only when all "buyers" have become one system. That situation cannot occur without the state enforcing the situation by threat of force (law). Neither true monopoly nor monopsony can exist in a voluntary market. When the government enforces either, a voluntary market no longer exists (again, as when licensure law enforces a monopoly in the supply of doctor or nurse services).[10]

There is no true monopsony unless all those buyers are involved. As long as physicians and nurses (and other sellers of service) are free to sell their services to buyers other than the government (or Blue Shield, for example), no true monopsony exists.

The relative cornering of the market of buyers is correctly termed *oligopoly* (not one buyer, but a smaller number of buyers of care). The anti-trust laws are generally thought to protect businesses from unfair competition ("cornering of the market" of buyers). In actual practice, anti-trust law is often used by companies to gain advantages. The effect of anti-trust laws is sometimes anti-competition, not pro-competition.

Physicians and independent nurse practitioners who would bargain with buyers of their services (such as HMOs) are now in jeopardy of being prosecuted for anti-trust violations. If buyers of services are allowed to merge and cooperate in large groups, real fairness (justice) should dictate that independent doctors and nurses should be able to do so as well. That would necessitate some changes in the anti-trust law. As presently enforced, the anti-trust law would benefit the combinations of both employers and buyers of services, but would harm independent contractors who wish to cooperate and compete more effectively in a free voluntary market.

The opposite of prices set by the free voluntary market is prices set by government; but this does not produce social justice either. Paying nurse practitioners 85 percent of what physicians receive for the same work (as Medicare does); or paying licensed practical nurses less than registered nurses for the same work, is not social justice.

In a socially just comparative worth system, it would be necessary to establish *who* decides, how *much, how* to compensate, for *what* (education, skill, experience, empathy). Massive administrative costs occur under such goals—not to mention the central authority with law and force behind it. To some extent, this is done now, but not on social justice values.

Rural hospitals—rural workers including doctors and nurses—have been paid less under Medicare than their counterparts in the cities, for the same work. That lesser payment is based, in part, on an outmoded "average market price," an amount not set by local, or even regional, supply and demand, but by bureaucrats nationally.

Is a single enforced "system" of any kind truly fair—is Fairness (Justice) a *process* or an *outcome?*

The Medicare system of payment, the Relative Value Rating Base System (RVRBS), removes the system from the free market setting of price according to supply and demand. No attempt is made to ascertain what nurses should be paid (as social justice would demand). But neither is there any attempt to set prices by supply and demand (as the volutary market would).

Proposed "caps" on the budget of the whole system would be the final acknowledgement that the government doesn't follow what the market says about payment price. Nor would capping allow for social justice concerning what people should earn for their work.[11] The amount spent for care would be what is arbitrarily decided to be the "right" amount to pay.

A global budget is the ultimate price control and wage control. The people (through the force of law) create a monopsony (one buyer, enforced through government mandate). What is paid is arbitrarily set; the only freedom (autonomy, power) left to the practitioner is to leave the profession or not.

The paradox is that open-ended entitlement programs like Medicare, Medicaid, or insurance, propose to pay for whatever care qualifies under the rules (to meet all needs; in some sense, social justice). But cost controls (as done in the VA, or in a national health system with a global budget) cannot exist with open-ended entitlement programs.

The free, voluntary market could voluntarily control costs, without mandates (higher cost reduces the demand for services). The market merely reflects what individuals are willing to pay for a given product or service.

The arguments continue about what system (or nonsystem) of illness care the United States will have in the future. The debate will not be solved the first year a "reform" is passed, nor the next, no matter what programs are tried. But basic ethical issues will be involved in the debate and will determine the law.

This topic will probably have more effect on the nurse's life as a professional (and eventual patient) than any other in the book. Through elections, referenda, committees, and participation in the agency and association, nurses can have some say in what kind of system of illness care the country adopts.

The shape of the "system" matters, very much, to nurses as citizens, workers in the system, and as potential patients of the system.

Effects of Legal Entitlements on Illness Care

A continuing ethical (and increasingly legal) question is whether illness care should be considered an entitlement, like the entitlement to a basic level of food to prevent starvation. To examine the issue from an economic point of view, substitute the words *illness care* with the word *bread* in the following scenario.

If having bread were considered an entitlement, paid for by the taxpayer through taxes or enforced premiums, the economic results can be predicted to be:

1. There would be no limit to the demand for bread; bread sales would skyrocket. The price of bread would skyrocket, too—since the government pays for it for all, people don't care what it costs and there's no incentive to keep prices low to get people to buy. (Was this the condition of costs early under Medicare?)
2. To keep the national budget from being eaten (literally?), government has to pass laws to limit the amount of bread people can buy, or else limit its price. (The illness care analogy: Under Medicare, Diagnostic Related Groups [DRGs] limited the price charged to Medicare patients.)
   a) If the price of bread is limited, the quality of bread goes down since good bakers will not stay in business if their wages/profit is too low. (Illness care analogy: U.S. physicians and hospitals are increasingly reluctant to take Medicare/Medicaid patients because of the low rates of reimbursement.)
   b) If the quantity of free bread is rationed, some bakers go out of business because the price is mandated low and so is the amount of bread they can make. The supply of bread continues to decrease. (Illness care analogy: Provider jobs decrease as hospitals downsize inpatient staff due to reduced revenues.)
3. But people want free bread (they're *entitled* to the bread in this hypothetical), so some private bakers are subsidized by government to stay in business. (Illness care analogy: The providers of illness care must be subsidized by the government.)
4. Finally, the government itself must bake bread (the quality, the efficiency, the choice will be like other government enterprises). (Illness care analogy: The only provider of illness care would eventually be "the government.")

Giving all people a "right" to free bread sounds good, but it can become a nightmare. (What the government pays for, the government must eventually control.) Did government create the "bread nightmare"? Will removal of the government money (the entitlement to free bread) get the demand and the prices back down? Is the only cure to end government payment?[12] Substitute "care" for "bread" and see how it comes out.

Ethics is involved whenever the government (the people, in a democracy) mandates a "right" (really an entitlement) to care, by passing a law. An example: The U.S. ESRD (End-Stage Renal Disease) program, created in 1972, was a result of an ethics crisis about rationing dialysis. Before 1972, suitable ages for dialysis were considered to be from 20 to 55 years of age, and few people could afford the cost. Rationing was performed by default, and by committees who agonized over which patient was most "deserving" of treatment. The U.S. Congress decided to pay for dialysis for *all*, avoiding ethical choices.

Currently, the U.S. incidence of kidney disease has increased due to the fact that greater numbers of elderly live to *be* old. (People do not live to be older than in previous eras, but more people survive infancy.) More people live to develop Non-Insulin Dependent Diabetes (NIDDM) and other diseases whose complications result in kidney disease.

Payment for dialysis was added as a benefit under Medicare and numbers of patients and cost of the program have dramatically exceeded estimates. When universal access to dialysis became available, the floodgates opened. Quality is estimated to have declined as the reimbursement rate declined. The patients are older and sicker.

In Britain, a country where free care has been an entitlement since the 1940s, it is rare for people over age 55 to get dialysis. Older patients are likely to have multiple serious disorders (which are disqualifiers for dialysis there). Britain has a lower rate of dialysis patients than does the United States.[13]

Nurse Attitudes Toward Economics of Illness Care

Is there an inherent conflict between good care and good economics (saving resources)? Some researchers find this conflict among and within nurses. One believes that tending to economics is a form of caring, because it enables the agency to support the desired care. The goals of patient care and organizational survival are mutually supportive.[14]

To understand the ethical issues, nurses must understand the economic system. In a pure market system, people pay directly for goods and services, like hamburgers and lawyers. When they don't have the money, they don't buy the goods/services. The "market" is the aggregate of what all the people value at any given moment. That aggregate of millions of decisions by millions of individuals determines demand, and thus supply, and thus cost:

> The market is not good because it works; it works because it is good. It is a plain historical fact that the treatment of man by man became conspicuously more humane side by side with the rise of capitalism.[15]

Some people believe illness care is different from hamburgers and lawyers, since "health care" is equated with health (and with life itself). People value life, at least their own. If they equate health care with life, it seems wrong to allow people to go without illness care when they don't have money to pay for it.

Theoretically, everyone in the United States today can get care, and can even buy insurance for the care. People who have the money and don't spend it for illness care or private insurance, prioritize it for their wants; they choose to use the money for something else. If they are poor and have to choose food over care, they are eligible for care under Medicaid.

Few are rich enough, however, to buy all kinds of available illness care, just as few are rich enough to buy some brands of cars. The United States does not have a pure market system. The market is modified when some people are given minimal support to live; people do not starve. (Before any welfare system was made law, charity prevented starvation.)

There is no pure market system in illness care either. Through federal, state, and local governments, U.S. taxpayers already pay for at least 42 percent of the illness care in this country. Many categories of people—the poor, elderly, veterans—receive illness care paid for by taxpayers.[16]

To many, the availability of illness care is an ethical issue, not just an economics issue. They believe that other services and goods should not be classed in the same way as illness care. Illness care seems different.

Some people believe that illness care is more like police or fire protection, than it is like food or legal services. They believe it should be available to all on an equal basis. They will tolerate differences in food, housing, and other goods and services, but they believe different levels are intolerable in illness care.

Some argue that everyone should have free preventive care, not because it expresses the ethical value of doing good, but because preventive care is a good investment. It's asserted that people who get preventive care (immunizations for children, good diabetes care) need less-expensive secondary and tertiary care. Paying for care for people early, saves money in the long run, it is argued; healthy people are an asset to an economy by being more productive. Proponents say that those are pragmatic arguments for preventive care. (In Chapter One, such arguments—proposing the greatest good for the greatest number—are identified as utilitarian.)

However, if more money is spent on *prevention* and the total amount of money available stays the same, then less money will be available for critical care. This assumes a "zero-sum" game in which less money in the pot means less to spend in another way (the situation described under a global budget, with caps on total spending). People who need tertiary care (third- or high-level) lose. Utilitarianism, therefore, is not a value-free, neutral stance.

Studies that prove that prevention actually saves money are scarce; and some even say that preventive care, allowing people to live longer, actually increases the ultimate cost (as they live to be old and cost more to the society). Others say that preventive care—even if it's available and free— will not be sought by all (as has been shown in countries where care *is* free). The example of patients counseled to stop smoking (preventive care) highlights the issue of personal freedom. Would mandating preventive illness care undermine the constitutional right to Liberty?

Government (the people) does have the power to make laws to force people to stop smoking, drinking, eating potato chips, having promiscuous sex, and working late. But, thus far, the people have not decided to cut costs of care related to such behaviors. Are the freedoms worth the cost?

Nursing Economics

The three factors in the economics of illness care (and the economics of everything else) are *demand* (for care by the patient), *supply* of care (nursing time, technology, quality), and *cost* of care.

The three factors are interrelated; changing one factor affects the other two.

INCREASE DEMAND + KEEP SAME SUPPLY = INCREASED COST

INCREASE COST + KEEP SAME SUPPLY = DECREASED DEMAND

> INCREASE DEMAND OR SHARE OF CARE + GOVERNMENT CON-
> TROLS (keep same cost, payment) = DECREASED SUPPLY (fewer
> practitioners who will take Medicaid patients)
> INCREASE COST/PAYMENTS FROM TAXES AND INSURANCE +
> KEEP SAME DEMAND = INCREASED SUPPLY OF NURSING TIME
> AND *TECHNOLOGY* (as long as the money holds out)
> INCREASE DEMAND DUE TO "FREE"/PAID SERVICES + KEEP THE
> SUPPLY OF NURSING TIME AND TECHNOLOGY PER PATIENT THE
> SAME = INCREASED TOTAL COST
> DECREASE COST + KEEP SAME SUPPLY OF NURSING TIME AND
> TECHNOLOGY = DECREASED DEMAND (fewer patients can be
> cared for at the same level)
> INCREASE DEMAND + DECREASE COST = DECREASED SUPPLY
> (less nursing time per patient)

Most nurses don't take economics as a subject in nursing school, yet much of the ethics and law of illness care involves economics. The three factors in the economics of illness care (and the economics of everything else) are demand, supply, and cost.

1. DEMAND by the patient: "Access." Patient demand for care encompasses both how many patients want care and what kind of care they want. In the United States, demand is often determined by what is paid for (many people do not expect to pay out of pocket for care). And, in the United States, people generally have access to care—practitioners are located within reasonable distance of most. But some people don't have the money or don't want to spend the money to pay for care. (To have "access" to cars, in the same meaning of "access," does not necessarily mean that one will be able to or want to pay for a car.)

2. SUPPLY by the practitioner. Supply in health care also implies *quality*: the adequacy or the level of care. (Nursing time may be substituted for any of these terms.) The level of care really means how much time is spent, or how much technology is available, because adequacy or excellence of care is hard to measure (like "competence" to practice); "quality" is subjective. To define *supply*, factors are chosen that *can* be measured, like hours of nursing time, numbers of procedures, or other quantities.

3. COST—the work/money. The cost for illness care is the amount of work, money, time, and energy to be "spent" for care; it is usually measured in money.

SOME EFFECTS OF ECONOMICS ON ILLNESS CARE

The three—demand (patient want), supply (nursing time, technology), and cost—are related. The law of economics of the illness care market is: If demand for a product or service goes up, and the supply stays the same, the cost must go up. Thus:

INCREASE DEMAND + KEEP SAME SUPPLY = INCREASED COST

In a voluntary market situation, higher cost should cause demand to decrease (people buy less bread when it is expensive). Economic feedback causes the demand to go down. Thus:

INCREASE COST + KEEP SAME SUPPLY = DECREASED DEMAND

Economic feedback doesn't work as immediately in illness care, because there's more of a constant demand. (Economists say the demand is "inelastic," since people usually can't decide *when* or *if* to be sick.) More importantly, the cost does not immediately go up when more care is demanded—especially if such care is paid for by taxpayer or insurance.

If government controls the cost, providers (nurses, doctors, hospitals, and other agencies) will give fewer goods or services because the low controlled price gives them no incentive to do so. No one willingly and long-term works longer for fewer dollars.

The law of the market triumphs eventually (the attempts to control economies in eastern Europe, the Soviet Union, and Cuba are examples; so is Medicaid). If the government keeps low the price paid to the nurse practitioner and the doctor, the result will be few practitioners willing to work for such low fees. Will the supply of care (nurses and doctors) available to the patient become limited?

A formula for government cost controls—for keeping prices the same while demand goes up (as has happened in Medicaid):

INCREASE DEMAND OR SHARE OF CARE +
  GOVERNMENT CONTROLS (mandates same cost, payment
    kept same or lowered) =
DECREASED SUPPLY (fewer practitioners who will care for Medicaid
  patients)

Increasing the cost (the amount of money available) increases the nursing time and technology. Seemingly unlimited government spending on Medicare and other taxpayer-paid systems plus private insurance, at first increased the nursing time and technology available. The result: The *cost* of nursing time and technology went up, too.

When Medicare first made money-for-care seem unlimited:

INCREASE COST BY "FREE" PAYMENTS FROM
  TAXES AND INSURANCE +
  KEEP THE SAME DEMAND =
INCREASED SUPPLY OF NURSING TIME AND *TECHNOLOGY*
  (as long as the money held out)

A system of care that provides more care for more people (for example, 37 million uninsured) would increase patient demand and thus increase the total cost. Thus, if everyone is guaranteed a "basic level" of coverage:

INCREASE DEMAND BY PAYING FOR MORE PEOPLE +
  KEEP THE SUPPLY OF NURSING TIME AND
    TECHNOLOGY THE SAME =
INCREASED TOTAL COST

If the goal is to reduce the cost, caring for fewer patients at the same level of nursing time and technology might work (Medicaid has been kept under control only by removing people from eligibility). Thus, to reduce cost without compromising quality:

DECREASE COST +
  KEEP SAME SUPPLY OF NURSING TIME AND TECHNOLOGY =
THEN DECREASED DEMAND (fewer patients can be cared for at the same level *or the level of care declines*).
  This is the scenario in "managed care" (the term referring to health maintenance organizations—HMOs—or to any other insurance plan that limits amount or kind of care). If the numbers of patients stay the same and costs are decreased, the supply of care must decrease *also* (fewer nurse hours per patient, or lower level of care).

If increased demand (numbers served) and decreased cost is desired *at the same time*, there must be a decrease in supply of nursing time, *and* less technology, fewer drugs, and pacemakers for all patients. Thus, care can be given to many (all) people cheaply (decreasing the supply/quality):

INCREASE DEMAND + DECREASE COST = DECREASED SUPPLY
(less nursing time per patient)

Those are the choices that the law of economics forces. Changing the amount of one will directly change the other two. Increasing the share of care (meaning that more people can have care) increases the cost.

Myths About Illness Care Economics:

Myth: *"Health care" is the same thing as "health."* A quick analysis shows that using the term "health care" fosters the idea that health care is needed to make one "healthy," or that without "health care" a person will die. In this sense, is "illness care" better used, since *illness care* informs without using "health" (a person without illness care may *or* may not die, depending on the underlying illness)?

Myth: *The number of uninsured is 37 million.* The figure is extrapolated from much smaller numbers and, thus, arrived at arbitrarily. Does the number change according to its intended use?

Myth: *"Uninsured" means "unhealthy" or uncared for.* "Uninsured" means merely that a person's care is not paid for by insurance; the person without coverage may *or* may not be "unhealthy." It is true that many people without insurance are less healthy, but lack of insurance cannot be said to have made the person sicker. Does the presence of insurance guarantee "health" (note continuing incidence of illness in countries with socialized medicine)?

Myth: *More insurance will solve the problem of cost of care.* Third-party payment by government and private insurers has created an enormous inflation of cost in the illness care industry (due to the perception that the paid-for care was "free"). Might more insurance, of still more people, exacerbate, or solve, the problems?

Myth: *Too much money is spent on the last year/last illness.* Just which one is going to be the patient's last year? Whether the present illness will cause death cannot usually be determined *prospectively*, but only in a retrospective analysis; therefore, it is not helpful in saving money. Even if it were possible to assess an individual and determine *in advance* that this is this person's last year or final illness of life, some assert that relatively little would be saved, even if all care were denied.

Myth: *The portion of the U.S. Gross National Product (GNP) for illness care is too high.* The GNP for illness care is the "total" of what is produced/served in *all* forms of illness care (not only "dollars spent"); in the United States the illness care GNP marks a higher percentage of the nation's overall GNP than in other industrialized countries (although other countries' percentages are growing, too). The "too high" assessment is necessarily a value judgment. It is perhaps made because people have decreasing choices about paying for care (contrasted with the choice people have about paying for the percentage of overall GNP represented by the auto industry, for example).

Illness care can be bought cheaply: low-tech and little nursing care for many *or* high-tech, intensive nursing care for fewer people. Or, it can be expensive: for a lot of money, high-tech, high nursing time care for all. People do have choices. Their participation in a democratic government will determine their future.

LABOR ETHICS AND LAW

FOR WORK-RELATED "WRONGS," CONTACT:

Personal attorney.

State nurses association or specialty nurse organization.

Equal Employment Opportunity Commission, state (information directory, state capital) or federal (phone book, U.S. government).

State Occupational Safety and Health agencies.

Federal Occupational Safety and Health Administration (OSHA), U.S. Department of Labor, Washington, D.C.

OSHA Regional Offices in Atlanta, Boston, Chicago, Dallas, Denver, Kansas City, New York City, Philadelphia, San Francisco, and Seattle.

Unfair labor practices (two or more gathered about work problems): NLRB, Washington, D.C., and in 34 regional offices; in the phone book under U.S. Government, try any agency with Labor in the name.

State employees: phone number from state capital information for any agency with "labor" or "work" in the name.

Federal employees: Federal Labor Relations Authority, Washington, D.C.; in the phone book under U.S. Government, try any agency with Labor in the name.

Employees in Declining Industry Need Labor Law

Economic indicators in illness care show an industry in decline, with resultant problems in nurse employment; but the ethics of work—that nurses should be treated fairly—are enforced in labor law.

Because economic indicators in illness care show an industry in decline, nurses need to know that the ethics of work—that they *should* be treated fairly—are reflected in laws that enforce the minimum of fairness in the work situation, that they *must* be treated fairly in specific areas.

Like the defense industry in the United States, illness care was a growth industry in the 1980s. Seemingly free care inflated use and costs of care. And, like the defense industry, U.S. illness care is now considered to consume too much of the nation's resources. Medicare price controls are still in place and will get tighter, and all segments of the industry anticipate change, if not from government, then from market forces like managed care and medical savings accounts (medical "IRAs").

The labor laws outlined below will be needed even more than previously by nurses as the depression in the illness care industry deepens. The labor laws enforce a *minimum* ethical standard of fairness. Nurses and employers who deal with each other at the higher ethical standard of fairness will not need legal mandates to force each other to be fair. But either party can confidently predict that law will provide a remedy for behavior that is not even *minimally* fair.

Independent Contractor Vs. Employee

Different agencies and different laws use different factors to determine whether the nurse is an employee or an independent contractor. No one factor is determinative, but control over one's own work is one of the most important.

Rarely do staff nurses work as employees under an enforceable written contract. More likely to do so are management nurses, nurses under collective bargaining agreements (collective contracts), and independent contractor nurses (consultants, home health nurses, traveling nurses). Such contracts, along with the employment relationship that exists without contracts—employment at will—are discussed in Chapter Six, Being True. Nurse-employer relationships covered by a collective bargaining contract are discussed below.

If there is no written contract (and even if there is a writing), is the nurse an employee or an independent contractor? The answer to that question matters, because whether a nurse is an employee or independent determines whether many laws apply. Most nurses are employees, not independent contractors, but as economic conditions change, so may the employment relationship.

> **Nurses who are independent contractors and not employees have less ethical demand on the employer and less law to mandate fairness of the employer. The decreased security is exchanged for more money or more freedom than the nurse who is an employee has.**

The principle underlying the law: People who are independent contractors exchange security for other advantages such as more money or more freedom. The employer has less responsibility for them, and the independent contractor has less responsibility to the employer. Fewer legal mandates flow from that relationship.

If the nurse is an employee, the employer must pay certain federal and state taxes. The nurse employee will have rights given and responsibilities imposed from a number of laws. The nurse, too, will be subject to tax withholding, and may be less desirable to the employer since the cost to the employer may be more.

Nurses who work for temporary agencies should ask about their status as employees: specifically, who pays what taxes, including Social Security (FICA); the federal unemployment tax (FUTA); and the worker compensation premium. The nurse also needs to know who buys the malpractice insurance. More detail is needed from the employer or contractor than in the usual employer-worker situation.

If the nurse is an independent contractor, the agency (contractor) for whom she practices may not be liable for damages caused by the nurse—that is, the agency-contractor of the home health nurse might not be liable if the nurse commits malpractice. An independent contractor nurse injured on the job, might be able to sue the agency for damages, instead of being limited to a smaller workers compensation claim for money.

Independent contractors in the United States are able to take more deductions from income for expenses related to work, to save on taxes. If the worker is classed as an employee, however, then activities promoting referrals to the hospital are legal under the Safe Harbor exceptions to the federal anti-kickback law.[17]

The standard for determining independent contractor status is complex. The courts and various agencies, such as the unemployment agencies and the Internal Revenue Service (IRS), use several factors to determine whether a nurse is an employee. Different agencies use different factors and enforce different laws; usually no *one* factor settles the question.

SOME FACTORS DETERMINING EMPLOYEE STATUS

Among the factors are:

1. Control over work.
2. Worker has other business besides just this agency's.
3. Worker has and brings own tools.
4. Pattern existing in the "industry." (An important factor in illness care—for example, physical therapists have traditionally been independent contractors with nursing homes.)
5. Paid by the "job" (independent) or hour (employee).

The IRS considers at least 20 factors to determine whether one is an employee or an independent contractor. The IRS says that no one factor is determinative, that the determination depends on a totality of the situation. (Information on the issue is available from Internal Revenue Service offices.)

As in other industries where workers lose jobs, it can be predicted that more nurses will set up their own businesses or become independent contractors for service. Nurses who open a business need to know the area of law that applies—especially if the business plans to employ people; the nurse will become an employer instead of an employee. An employer will be responsible for keeping a safe workplace, for paying worker compensation insurance and unemployment compensation taxes, and ensuring that antidiscrimination laws are not violated. The nurse entrepreneur must develop good contracts, and nurses who market products should see a lawyer who specializes in patent and trademark law. Much information is available in books and periodicals for small business owners.[18]

FAIR LABOR STANDARDS ACT

The Fair Labor Standards Act (FLSA)[19] offers protection to workers, but most nurses are exempt from its protection (even an exempt worker may be covered if pay is docked or accrued leave is taken away by the employer for partial-day absences). State labor laws may cover employees exempt from the FLSA.

Many nurses are salaried professional employees, exempt from the legal requirements of the U.S. Fair Labor Standards Act (FLSA). Other nurses, who are guaranteed a salary of over $250 a week and who are either executives or administrators, are also exempt. Nurses clearly meet the exemption for professionals in the law.

Some court decisions find that even a worker exempt under one of the above categories may be considered "hourly," if the worker's pay is docked or accrued leave is taken away for partial-day absences. The employee may be eligible for back pay based on hours of overtime. This policy can result in liability for an enormous amount of money spread over an agency's entire salaried work force. Employers may avoid liability by not deducting the partial-day absences from employees' accrued leave, and not docking employees' pay for partial-day absences.[20]

State labor laws may cover employees who are exempt (for example, because they are professionals) from the overtime pay provisions of the federal law or FLSA. Some state laws require pay for *all* hours worked; specify how often workers must be paid, and in what form the pay is made; and when the worker's last pay must be made after discharge. The index of statutes at the library will list headings for Labor or Work, or information at the state capital will list a number for the agency that administers labor law.

The ethical value that people should *be fair* is enforced in labor law as antidiscrimination statutes.

In general, all labor laws prohibiting discrimination are enforced by the Equal Employment Opportunity Commission (EEOC), either federal or state. If the EEOC does not have jurisdiction over the particular act complained of, it can guide the nurse to the appropriate agency that does.

All antidiscrimination laws are discussed in this chapter within the context of the value, Fairness. The place where nondiscrimination is enforced usually is the workplace, because jobs are about survival. Discrimination that denies the person a job affects the quality of life, and in extreme circumstances could threaten the worker's very survival.

Discrimination in *employment* is discussed below under several laws prohibiting that action. Discrimination in the *provision of services like nursing care* is prohibited, too, if done on the basis of race, color, sex, religion, national origin, age, or disability.

DRUG TESTING

In drug-testing situations, adherence to ethical standards—protecting patients, intruding minimally on the employee's life and privacy, and giving advance notice that testing is a condition of the job—results in legal action too, because the law is the minimum ethic.

Employers and managers of nurses may in some instances be responsible for the acts of their employees who take drugs. This is especially true if the supervisor knew of the danger to patients and did not act to correct the situation.[21] The ethic underlying: Protect the patient from harm.

Employers generally have a strong hand when dealing with drug-impaired employees, since the law enforces the minimum ethic that taking drugs is "bad." On the other hand, the nurse employer or manager may face liability if they violate ethical and legal constraints on their acts toward employees. The ethic underlying: The freedom of the employee, and fairness to her.

More than 17 million workers are employed by private companies that test at least some of them for drugs. All federally employed persons must undergo urine drug testing. Drugs are a particularly difficult problem in illness care, both because of the need for unimpaired action by the worker and because of the access of the worker to drugs.[22]

The reliability of tests for drugs is controversial, but employees who refuse to submit to drug tests may be fired under appropriate circumstances. The Supreme Court has never held that refusal to be tested is a right, and few new rights to "privacy" are likely to be found. But the "disabled" employee, who is not currently taking illegal drugs, may be protected under the Americans with Disabilities Act (below). Egregious conduct by the employer in testing might be actionable on various grounds. Coercion, violation of privacy in the way a sample of blood or urine is obtained, or invasion of privacy in release of information gained from a sample, might produce liability if an employee sued.

Employers can test for drugs in pre-employment screens, for fitness for the job; for suspected use, if an incident has occurred; or if the employee is to be in a "safety sensitive" position. Even random testing of all employees is allowed in jobs where the public or safety is at risk; which could be argued in regard to many positions in the illness care industry.

Minimal intrusion on the employee's life and privacy, and giving advance notice that testing is a condition of the job,[23] are ethical and so are legally sound. Routine screening of all employees is probably not efficient, even if legal, because it is costly and does not distinguish among impaired employees, one-time users, or multiple users. Nor can random testing distinguish legitimate from nonlegitimate use of some drugs.[24]

As in any area of law where the underlying ethic is unsettled, the results of legal cases vary widely. Some ethical questions can serve as a guide, however: How would one want to be treated? How could one be treated? How should a person with this behavior or history be treated? Protection of the employee is important, but protecting the patient may be more important.

AMERICANS WITH DISABILITIES ACT

ADA PROVISIONS

Generally: No qualified individual with a disability shall, by reason of such disability, be excluded from participation in or be denied the benefits of the services, programs, or activities of a public entity, or be subjected to discrimination by any such entity.

No qualified individual with a disability shall, by reason of such disability, be excluded from participation in or be denied the benefits of the services, programs, or activities of a public entity, or be subjected to discrimination by any such entity.

One who is disabled is defined as anyone who has a record of or *is perceived as* having a mental or physical impairment that substantially limits at least one major life activity. (Watch that phrase "is *perceived* as having . . . impairment" [EMPHASIS ADDED].)

Passed in 1990, the Americans with Disabilities Act (ADA)[25] went into effect in 1992 and subsequent years. The law mandates that people with disabilities be integrated into the mainstream of the work force.

The ADA mandates (among other things) that people with disabilities be integrated as much as possible into the mainstream of the work force.

The law enforces the minimum ethic of what many think a higher value: that all people should have an equal chance at a job if they can do the work with a little accommodation. The ethical principle of fairness is apparent (equal opportunity, equal chance, equality in the process), but note that equal *outcomes* are not mandated.

Disabled. The word used to be "handicapped." Before that, it was "crippled." Today it is "challenged."

The stigma will remain regardless of the new word used, unless attitudes change.

The ADA applies to all areas of life, not just work, and includes the right of people to obtain illness care regardless of disability.

Specifically for the workplace, a shorthand version of the ADA follows: "If you can fix it so a disabled person can do a job, fix it unless it's a real problem or dangerous."

People qualify as disabled if they are physically or mentally impaired in doing a major life activity, or have been so disabled before, or appear to have

324 • *Ethics and Law of Fairness (Justice)*

been so disabled. Temporary disabilities, kleptomaniacs or pyromaniacs, personality traits, and sexual function are defined as *not* disabilities. Fairness under the ADA does not mean treating all alike; some "reasonable accommodation" for handicap must be made.[26]

Application of the ADA to Licensure Law

All state licensure laws establish boards that have the power to deny licensure because of drug addiction. For example, the Texas nursing law says that every agency employing ten nurses must have a nursing peer review committee. That committee is charged with the responsibility of notifying the board if a nurse "is impaired or likely is impaired by chemical dependency." That Texas statute and others help the boards identify and punish drug use; but they may conflict with the provisions of the federal law protecting persons with disability. (This problem is discussed in Chapter Three, under Licensure.) The ADA is confusing and complicated; since it is relatively new, its meaning is yet to develop in court. That is a good reason to remember the ethic underlying the law to be fair to *all* employees, the disabled too.

With the ADA, controversy can arise over who is disabled. Current abusers of illegal drugs are specified as not protected by the law. But past abusers are protected. And so are people currently addicted to *legal* drugs or alcohol.

Regarding physical status, the prospective employer can only ask if the applicant can perform the essential functions of the job, plus a question as to what, if any, accommodations are required in order to function. After the offer of employment, the employer can require a physical exam (and drug tests, see above); then the employer can question extensively. But, if hired, the employee can't be fired based on the disability. The definition of "disability" has been extended to include obesity.

Extending the ADA to illness care: To refuse treatment to a patient because of a voluntary condition (for example, one who needs bypass surgery but smokes, who needs a liver transplant but drinks) could violate the ADA. It is suggested that institutional "wellness" programs, which reward people for losing weight and stopping smoking, may be discriminatory. Eaters and smokers might be considered to have a disability that makes them unable to qualify for the award. An employer who refuses to hire a smoker might be sued under the ADA.

Insurance companies might be considered to discriminate by charging lower premiums—for nonsmokers, exercisers, people who keep normal weight. If companies are not allowed to reward "healthy" behavior, there may be less incentive to stay healthy and thus reduce cost of illness care.

CIVIL RIGHTS

Title VII of the 1964 Civil Rights Act[27] protects people from discrimination for reasons of race, color, national origin, sex, and religion.

The prohibition of discrimination on the bases of race, color, national origin, sex, and religion are obviously based on the value of fairness. The use of affirmative action programs to reverse past discrimination, however, is being challenged as *not* being "color-blind" since such programs, in effect, discriminate *in favor* of some minorities. The protection against discrimination based on sex is said to have been inserted originally as a joke, but under this portion of the law is the prohibition against sexual harassment.

Sexual harassment can be an overt demand for exchange of sex for job privileges. This is termed *quid pro quo* (in Latin, "this for that"). Or sexual harassment can be sexual activity that results in a "hostile work environment"—dirty jokes, remarks, pin-up calendars. Plaintiffs do not have to prove psychological injury. Employers can be liable for the acts of their employees, if supervisors knew of the conduct and did not address it. Cases are being decided that will give more guidance in this uncertain area, but as a guide: Being fair to employees (the ethical standard) will certainly encompass not harassing them sexually (the legal standard).

Discrimination because of religion could be charged when employees have to work on Sunday. The employer of a Seventh Day Adventist whose religion required she not work on Saturday may have a duty to offer her other days of work rather than firing her.

Some agencies of the federal government go further than the statute, their policies saying: "This program or activity will be conducted on a nondiscriminatory basis without regard to race, color, religion, national origin, age, sex, marital status, or disability."

Note that "discriminating" itself is not the evil. The evil is discrimination based on a condition people cannot change and not affecting their ability to work (like being obese, or ugly). Discriminating against a good worker with ability is not good ethics *or* business, even if it were legal.

Civil Rights Act of 1991

> The Civil Rights Act of 1991 counters a Supreme Court ruling; the statute requires the employer, whose work force is not in the same racial ratio as the community, to prove that the work force is not the result of discrimina-

The 1991 Civil Rights Act[28] clarifies the standard of proof necessary for a person to prove discrimination. Employer groups believe the law made it easier for people to sue employers; the burden of proof has shifted back to the employer. The employer, whose work force is not of the same racial proportion as the community, has the burden of proving that the work force is *not* the result of discrimination.

Pregnancy Discrimination Act

> Under the protection of the Pregnancy Discrimination Act, neither potential legal liability nor protecting the woman's fetus is sufficient reason to practice sex discrimination.

Federal law punishes discrimination against people on the basis that they *are* or *might* become pregnant. The Pregnancy Discrimination Act (PDA) of 1978[29] prohibits sex discrimination as defined in Title VII of the Civil Rights Act of 1964. The Supreme Court, by a vote of 9–0 (in what is popularly known as "The Johnson Battery Case"),[30] said that neither potential legal liability nor protecting the woman's fetus were sufficient reason to practice sex discrimination.

> Congress mandated that decisions about the welfare of future children be left to the parents who conceive, bear, support, and raise them, and concerns about the next generation were not part of the essence of the employer's business.[31]

An analysis of the decision shows that the Supreme Court said that discrimination based on a woman's pregnancy is, on its face, discrimination because of her sex. An employer's tort liability for potential fetal injuries and its potential increased cost in employing fertile women do not preclude a holding that the law is violated.

The law forbids employers from instituting sex-specific fetal-protection policies because, if the employer fully informs the woman of the risk, and the employer has not acted negligently, the basis for holding an employer liable seems remote at best. If the employer cannot comply with both state regulation and federal law, federal law preempts that of the states. The extra cost of employing members of one sex does not provide a defense for a discriminatory refusal to hire members of that sex.

That case is specifically about the potentially pregnant woman's statutory protection against discrimination in employment.

Employers said they felt trapped between possible liability to a child born damaged from work, and the requirement under the federal law to allow women to do such work. The employer's interest in avoiding liability, however, was secondary to the ethical value of justice (a woman's having an equal chance at a job of her choice). And the value of protecting potential life was considered secondary to the value of justice in that case.

Fearing that women will be discriminated against in jobs manufacturing pesticides, it is asserted that the Food and Drug Administration will not label certain chemical pesticides as "dangerous to pregnant women"—although the pesticide may be dangerous, and babies may be injured as a result.

In illness care agencies, the law may prohibit keeping women out of areas formerly considered dangerous to pregnant women, such as anesthesia and radiology. The argument can be made that the value of doing good for the child was a shield behind which paternalism hid, keeping women out of higher-paying jobs.

Age Discrimination in Employment Act

> The Age Discrimination in Employment Act[32] prohibits job discrimination solely because of age (discrimination against people aged 40 to 70).

The chief of cardiology who makes derogatory remarks about the average (advanced) age of nurses in the ICU may open the hospital to a lawsuit for discrimination, if one of those "old" nurses is reassigned or fired. This law protects people from *job* discrimination. It does not, however, apply to discrimination in provision of illness care, so 90-year-olds could be refused bypasses on the grounds they were too old, without violating this law.

Equality in Retirement Income Security Act

> The Equality in Retirement Income Security Act (ERISA) enforces the ethical values of fairness in retirement plans and other company-funded insurance. Complying with the federal law allows employers to avoid state law requirements for insurance.

The federal pension law is the Equality in Retirement Income Security Act (ERISA). The law enforces the ethical values of fairness in retirement and other company-funded insurance—including some self-provided health care insurance. Enforcement of the law is quite complex; many employers hire experts to run benefits plans in line with its complexities. Doing the right thing voluntarily would have been cheaper and easier in the first place, because the law merely enforces the minimum ethic that employees should not be arbitrarily denied promised pensions or other benefits after many years of service.

ERISA has become an important issue in health insurance reform. Because it is a federal law, ERISA pre-empts (overrules) any state laws that might conflict. Courts have ruled that self-insurance plans for health care fall under the jurisdiction of ERISA. Such self-insurance health plans escape state regulation and taxes this way. And, under ERISA, plans can limit coverage for people with big health risks. The Supreme Court let stand a lower court ruling that allowed self-insured companies to reduce coverage for workers with AIDS—based on the ERISA exemption.

Self-insured plans are also exempt (because of ERISA pre-emption) from state laws that require many expensive procedures, such as in vitro fertilization, to be covered in group health plans. The ERISA exemption for self-insured plans is a catalyst for more business to self-insure. The trend is growing in small and medium-size firms, since it allows firms to keep closer control of employee expenses.

> *Problem:* If the self-insured company goes out of business, the employee with illness bills may be stuck with them. If there's no purchase of catastrophic insurance, the total bills of the employees may exceed the company's ability to pay. The ERISA pre-emption causes problems with state health-reform plans; many states legislate that insurers pay for specific kinds of care, such as psychiatry and substance abuse. As noted above, self-insured companies are exempt from those state law requirements because they are under ERISA. Action at the federal level would be necessary to allow states to regulate (mandate) health benefits, on companies whose self-insurance plans are covered by ERISA.

Coverage Limited

Employers have been limiting illness care coverage for decades (most began providing insurance only in the World War II years as a way to circumvent wage controls and attract workers). They limited coverage for polio in the 1950s, and now limit coverages for mental health, substance abuse, infertility, and experimental surgery. If employers must pay for big expenses (for example, if Congress "vests" benefits that employers must cover), then might more employers refuse to pay for benefits in the first place? Coverage has been mandated in other cases for employees with AIDS.

NATIONAL LABOR RELATIONS ACT

> The National Labor Relations Act (NLRA) governs collective bargaining between employee groups and their managers/employers. Not-for-profit health care institutions have been covered under the law since 1974.

The National Labor Relations Act (NLRA)[33] (originally passed in the 1930s because strikers and owners were killing each other during labor disputes) governs collective bargaining between employee groups and their managers/employers. Not-for-profit health care institutions have been covered under the law since 1974.[34] Note that the institutions covered in 1974 were not called "*non*-profit"; all agencies must effectively make a profit (or at least not lose money) to operate.

People organized into unions for a long time before the 1930s, and employers opposed that strength in their employees. The process was not always peaceful, but some resolution of differences always came. The intent of the NLRA, first passed in 1935, was to promote peaceful collective bargaining. It was yet another law to enforce a minimum of a higher ethic, that people do the right thing by one another (be fair).

One provision of the law allows union and management to force employees to join the union (this provision is not in effect in "right-to-work" states). Instead of mandatory union membership, the employee may pay fees to the union—but payment is enforced by the law. The person who does not pay loses her job, and has no remedy. Is this violative of the individual's freedom; or is it only fair that the person pay for what she got, even if she didn't ask for it? The resulting union strength (the collective good) must be measured against the loss of freedom to the individual.

Whether the national labor law has succeeded depends on whether one is pro-union or pro-management. People in labor disputes seldom shoot each other nowadays. Would they, without the labor law?

Nurse Bargaining

Are these facts related? Only about 15 percent of nurses are covered by collective bargaining contracts. The nurse shortage is over. Salary increases are lower.

The composition of the "bargaining unit" was a big issue for nurses who worked in not-for-profit hospitals—and who were protected under the NLRA, first in 1974. Nurses who wish to bargain collectively must be protected from firing on that basis, then must vote on whether they want the union to represent them (and if so, which union). To determine the outcome of the vote, the workers are grouped into bargaining units—these are groups of employees who have a community of interest. A big worry during the 1974 amending of the NLRA was whether hospitals would end up with many small bargaining units and many different unions to deal with.[35]

The NLRB by rule determined that professional nurses could have their own bargaining units; and a major case upheld the rule.[36] The issue had been an enormous one for the ANA's state affiliates, which did and do the actual organizing and negotiating for nurses. The nurse associations did not want to be "unions" in the sense that they would represent any worker who wanted representation;[37] they wanted to, and largely do represent only registered nurses[38] (although not many nurses, considering the number that could be represented).

Nurse Committee "Unions?"

Electromation, Inc.[39] was an NLRB decision that found illegal a version of Japanese worker-management teams adopted by U.S. companies and used to increase production, safety, profits, worker satisfaction, and product quality—the teams were described as "sham unions." The NLRB found that the company had set up "action committees" at the same time the Teamsters Union was trying to organize the workers.

NLRA Section 8(a)(2) makes it an unfair labor practice for an employer "to dominate or interfere with the formation or administration of any labor organization or contribute financial or other support to it. . . ."[40] That section was in the original law of 1935. Its purpose (the minimum ethic) was to counter company unions established only to avoid unionization of workers. Nurse committees that handle grievances, labor disputes, wages, rates of pay, hours of employment, or conditions of work might be found to be illegal if the nurses union challenged them.

Another issue for nurses in collective bargaining is whether nurses who supervise nursing care are classified as "supervisors" under the law and thus excluded from collective bargaining. The law classes a "supervisor" as one who is able to do at least one of 12 actions, including hiring, firing, transferring, assigning, disciplining, or responsibly directing other employees. The Supreme Court held that, in one nursing home, LVNs acted as supervisors and thus were not protected from firing when they took concerted action to improve working conditions.[41] This decision may encourage employers to seek to exclude nurses from bargaining units, as "supervisors."

As sole business people (not as employees) doctors too are considering collective bargaining, in order to deal with managed-care companies. The worries of these "professionals" sound very much like some nurses' concerns about unions.

DOCTORS WORRY ABOUT COLLECTIVE BARGAINING

"I'm concerned about the specter of a labor-union image. Even though we're saying that patient care is important, this runs the risk of a strike."

—Daniel Johnson, AMA House of Delegates Speaker, Metairie, La.[42]

ANTI-TRUST LAW (THE SHERMAN ACT)

Anti-trust law was created to enforce the ethic that groups of businesses should not combine to restrain trade (to unfairly reduce competition). To some extent, these laws now operate unfairly against groups of practitioners who would otherwise be able to combine and negotiate with buyers of care.

Anti-trust law is invoked when private enterprises get too big, or too effective at competition. The law affects illness care, and nurses, and doctors. The value expressed in anti-trust law is to do good for the consumer (care at lower prices). Also enforced is the ethic of being fair, to the practitioner or competing business. Equal opportunity to compete is the goal, not equal outcome of business. There is also in the law some minimum enforcement of the value of autonomy—both for the consumer to be free to buy what he wants and for the business person to be able to compete freely.

Anti-trust law was created to enforce the ethic that groups of businesses should not combine to restrain trade (to reduce competition). "Trust" is the term used because such a combination in restraint of trade was called a "trust" in the old days. Free competition was valued (is valued) because it results in lower prices for the consumer. It is thought that a monopoly of the free market could raise prices.

Some economists believe that a private monopoly cannot exist; that no monopoly is possible unless the government forces it—as in nurse licensure.

Nurses can use anti-trust law to prevent groups of doctors, hospitals, or even other nurses from combining in some way to the detriment of the nurses' economic interest. Nurse practitioners have used these laws to challenge physicians who kept them from getting staff privileges in hospitals; physicians have used them often to challenge their peers who do the same. Recently, physicians are using the laws to challenge accrediting bodies who arbitrarily limit exams only to doctors who have qualified in a standardized program.

Antitrust actions, when used by physicians and nurse practitioners to contest denial of hospital staff privileges, must meet Sherman Act requirement Section 1: They must prove that the hospital or doctor and another person or entity, together unlawfully "conspired" to exclude the practitioner. It takes two to tango and two to conspire.

ANTI-TRUST LAW (FROM 1901)

"Every contract, combination in the form of trust or otherwise, or conspiracy, in restraint of trade or commerce among the several States, or with foreign nations, is declared to be illegal."[43]

The follow-on law, passed in 1915, is known as the Clayton Act.[44] It provides for treble damages: that's three times the loss actually suffered— say, a year's income times three. It also provides for an injunction, which in the nurse situation is an order forbidding exclusion—for example, an order to admit the doctor or nurse to the hospital staff. These remedies were declared available to private plaintiffs in civil lawsuits, not enforceable only under the criminal law by the government.

In order for the anti-trust law to apply, the offending business (hospital or other agency) must be in interstate commerce. The problem of proving that the local hospital is involved in interstate commerce was removed in 1991.[45] In 1995, however, the Supreme Court *reversed* a 60-year trend; now laws made by Congress, ostensibly based on the power to regulate commerce, are not automatically constitutional.

Doctors are using anti-trust law against the American Board of Emergency Medicine, which certifies ER doctors. They charge that the board conspired with hospitals to monopolize the market for certified ER doctors. The board cut off experience as one route to certification; it now requires three years of residency.[46]

Nurse practitioners could use the same avenue to challenge requirement by ANA that they must have a Master's degree before taking the certification exam. They could allege a conspiracy with state licensing boards to monopolize the market for NPs. Does rational basis exist for the degree qualification, since no data show that a Master's degree produces a better or automatically safe practitioner?

FAMILY AND MEDICAL LEAVE ACT OF 1993

> If the nurse must leave work for birth and/or care of a child, for adoption or placement of a child from foster care, for care of spouse, child or parent who has a serious health condition, or if unable to perform the functions of the position due to serious health condition, she may have certain benefits under the Family and Medical Leave Act.

Nurses who need to leave work for some time may take advantage of the Family and Medical and Leave Act.[47] If the nurse must leave work for birth and/or care of a child, adoption or placement of a child from foster care, care of spouse, child or parent who has a serious health condition, or if unable to perform the functions of the position due to serious health condition, the nurse may meet one of the requirements for coverage under the act. Up to 12 weeks per year of unpaid leave may be taken, or paid leave taken if it has been earned. The employer can require the employee to use earned leave, first.

As with all labor statutes, the laws do not apply to all workers. Coverage depends on the numbers of employees, and number of hours worked. But even if exempt as management under the wage and hour laws (which require pay for overtime), nurses may be covered under this law.

Employers engaged in commerce with 50 or more employees are covered, as is any "public agency" such as state and local government. The employee must be covered if she has worked for at least 13 months and has worked 1,250 hours during the 12 months; at least half-time.

Most nurses can't afford to take unpaid leave, so the law doesn't help some of the people who it was passed to help. People who can benefit are higher-income two-job professionals who can afford to miss the income, and can take advantage of the power to retain the job.

The law requires advance notice (30 days) if the need for the leave is "foreseeable." The employer can require a medical certification of need. The employer must maintain the employees' health coverage under any existing group health plan and must return the employee to her original or equivalent position without loss of benefits. Enforcement is under the Department of Labor.

OCCUPATIONAL SAFETY AND HEALTH ACT (OSHA)

> The Occupational Safety and Health Act (OSHA)[48] requires attention to employee safety, record keeping and reporting of employee injury or illness or death due to work-related causes; ethics underlying the law are that employers should not harm their employees (at least their work should not) and should treat them fairly.

This federal law covers nearly all workers, including those in illness care, and most recently those in doctors' offices. The law requires attention to employee safety, record keeping and reporting of employee injury or illness or death due to work-related causes. Ethics underlying the law are that employers should not harm their employees (at least their work should not) and should be fair to them. People who file complaints under OSHA are held to be anonymous and are protected from release of their name—demonstrating enforcement of the minimum ethic of confidentiality and veracity. In illness care agencies, the rules requiring Universal Precautions are made by OSHA.

WORKER COMPENSATION

> Worker compensation laws are made on the state level; they provide damages (compensation) to workers for injuries sustained as a result of employment. In return for a fair compensation that is certain, the worker gives up the right to sue the employer for damages.

Formerly known as "Work*men*'s Compensation," worker compensation laws provide damages (compensation) to workers for injuries sustained as a result of employment. In return for a compensation that is certain, the worker gives up the right to sue the employer for damages.

Many other laws governing working conditions are made at the state level. Sometimes those are more favorable to the employee than laws made by the federal government. A listing of those laws can be obtained by calling the agency in the state that deals with labor and employment; the phone book, under "Government, State," should have a listing.

Source for Labor Law Information

> The nurse's personnel or human resources office is usually a good source of labor law information; in addition, state and federal government offices that administer labor law can be of help.

The personnel office (lately called "human resources") of the employing institution has details of any and all these laws and how they affect nurses in their work. The people in that office administer and assure compliance with the law within the institution and they are usually expert on the details. If more information is needed, the phone book listing, "U.S. Government, Labor," will have a phone number to call for assistance or referral, and agencies listed at the beginning of this section will also have information.

The Rule

> The ethic enforced by labor law is to treat other people the way one would personally want to be treated—fairly.

Instead of learning all the separate laws governing employees and their employers, nurses and employers can stay legal by remembering the underlying ethic: to treat other people the way they would personally want to be treated. The value implicit in labor laws is fairness (justice).

Nurses and employers should expect treatment from other people toward themselves that they would expect to give to others.[49] If the value of justice is adhered to, people will do the right and legal things without knowing all the details in the statutes. It is true that the farther lawmakers stray from enforcing a *minimum* ethic, and the more law is delegated to rule makers to write details, the harder it is for nurse or employer to anticipate the statute or regulation from knowing the ethic.

For example, being fair to employees would not automatically call for a prediction that accident records must be kept (OSHA requirement). But being fair would mean making the workplace as safe as possible, and technical violations (of record keeping) are of course far less serious than substantive violations (of having dangerous conditions).

If people do the right thing, they will *likely* never be sued nor penalized; if that small possibility occurs, they will probably (but not certainly) win their case. There is *no* certainty in this life, but if nurses are fair with the people who work with/for them, they may sleep better and may be content with their actions. Good practice (with co-workers, patients and employees) is good ethics is good law.

ENDNOTES

1. Kelsen, H., *General Theory of Law and State*, translated by A. Wedberg, Cambridge: Harvard University Press, 1945; pp. 5–6.
2. See discussions of Justice in: Beauchamp, T.L., and Childress, J.F., *Principles of Medical Ethics*, 3rd ed., New York: Oxford University Press, 1989; pp. 256–301.
3. Englehardt, T.H., Jr., and Rie, M.A., "Intensive care units, scarce resources, and conflicting principles of justice," *Journal of the American Medical Association*, 1986; 255:1159–1164.
4. Hayek, F., *Law, Legislation and Liberty: The Mirage of Social Justice*, Chicago: University of Chicago Press, 1976.
5. *Ibid.*
6. Rawls, J., *A Theory of Justice*, Cambridge: Harvard University Press, 1971.
7. Densford, K., and Everett, M., *Ethics for Modern Nurses*, Philadelphia: W.B. Saunders Company, 1946; p. 168.
8. *Ibid.*, p. 238.
9. *Permian Basin Area Rate Cases*, 390 U.S. 747, 794 n.64 (1968).
10. Ile, M.L., "When health care payers have market power," *Journal of the American Medical Association*, 1990; 263(14):1981–1986.
11. Ginzberg, E., "Health care and the market economy—A conflict of interest?" *New England Journal of Medicine*, 1992; 326:72–74.
12. Inspiration for the bread entitlement postulated here: Durante, D.L., and Durante, S.J., "National health care: Prescription for a fool's paradise," *Freeman*, New York: Foundation for Economic Education Inc., 1991.
13. Levinsky, N.G., "Lessons from the medicine end stage renal disease program," *New England Journal of Medicine*, 1993; 329(19):1395–1399.
14. Nyberg, J., "The effects of care and economics on nursing practice," *Journal of Nursing Administration*, 1990; 20(5):13–18.
15. Asmus, B., "Private sector solutions to public sector problems," *Imprimis*, 1993; 22(10):1–4.
16. "Health Spending," *The Economist*, 16 November 1991, p. 127.
17. 42 U.S.C. 1320a-7b(b).
18. Brent, N.J., "Setting up your own business: Facing the future as an entrepreneur," *Association of Operating Room Nurses Journal*, 1990; 51(1):205, 208, 210–213.
19. Fair Labor Standards Act of 1938: 29 U.S.C. 201 *et seq.*, regulations at 29 C.F.R. 541.
20. Schmitt, R., "Employers' Overtime Liability Expanding," *Wall Street Journal*, 5 November 1993, B10.
21. Fiesta, J., "The impaired nurse—Who is liable?" *Nursing Management*, 1990; 21(10):20, 22.
22. Lemon, S.J., *et al.*, "Physicians' attitudes toward mandatory workplace urine drug testing," *Archives of Internal Medicine*, 1992; 152:2238–2242.
23. Fiesta, J., "Liability for drug testing," *Nursing Management*, 1993; 24(5):22, 24.
24. Morgan, J.P., "Employee drug tests are unreliable and intrusive," *Hospitals*, 1989; 63(16):64.
25. 42 U.S.C. 12101 *et seq.*, definition of disabled at 42 U.S.C. 12102(2).
26. "Business has to find a new meaning for 'fairness,'" *Business Week*, 12 April 1993; p. 72.
27. 42 U.S.C. 2000e.
28. *Idem.*
29. 42 U.S.C. 2000e(d).
30. *International Union v. Johnson Controls*, 499 U.S. 187. 13 L.Ed.2d 158 (1991).

31. *Idem.*, at 159.
32. 29 U.S.C. 621.
33. 29 U.S.C. 151, *et seq.*
34. Gideon, J., "Unions: Choice and mandate," *Association of Operating Room Nurses Journal*, 1980; 31:1201.
35. Gideon, J., "Registered nurse bargaining units: Undue proliferation?" *Missouri Law Review*, 1980; 45:348.
36. *American Hospital Association v. National Labor Relations Board*, 499 U.S. 606 (1991).
37. Gideon, J., "The American Nurses Association: A professional model for collective bargaining," *Journal of Health & Human Resource Administration*, 1979; 2:13.
38. Popp. P.W., "Separate bargaining units in the health care industry: Crisis for professional nurses in the USA," *Medicine & Law*, 1989; 8(1):83–100.
39. *Electromation, Inc.*, 309 NLRB No. 163, 16 December 1992.
40. 29 U.S.C. 158(a)(2).
41. *National Labor Relations Board v. Health Care and Retirement Corporation of America*, 114 S.Ct. 1778 (1994).
42. Anders, G., "Collective Bargaining for Doctors Sparks Contention at AMA Annual Convention," *Wall Street Journal*, 15 June 1993, B6.
43. 15 U.S.C. 1, *et seq.*
44. 15 U.S.C. 26.
45. *Summit Health, Ltd. v. Pinhas*, 111 S.Ct. 1842 (1991).
46. *Daniel v. American Board of Emergency Medicine, et al.*, U.S. District Court, Buffalo, NY, 90–1086A.
47. 29 U.S.C. 2312.
48. 29 U.S.C. 651.
49. Luke 6:31, New Testament

SIX

Ethics and Law of
Being True (Fidelity)

TOPICS COVERED

Discussion of the ethics and value, Being True

Ethics code provisions of the general value, Being True

Keeping promises (loyalty)

Employment relationships

CONTRACTS FOR EMPLOYMENT • "AT WILL" EMPLOYMENT AND EXCEPTIONS TO THE RULE

Loyalty to the patient in a managed care setting

Keeping secrets (confidentiality)

Ethics code provisions of the value

Law enforcing confidentiality

Telling truth (veracity)

Ethics of veracity

Whistle-blowing

DISCUSSION OF THE VALUE, BEING TRUE: THE ETHICS

▽

"Who shall give a lover any law? Love is a greater law than man has ever given to earthly man."

—GEOFFREY CHAUCER,
Canterbury Tales

△

The idea of Being True (Fidelity) incorporates Keeping Promises (Loyalty), Keeping Secrets (Confidentiality), and Telling Truth (Veracity).

Laws about contracts and employment, whistle-blowing, confidentiality, and informed consent, all are enforcement of the value, Fidelity (Being True), and the values incorporated in being true.

Survival once depended on doing good and keeping promises to one another. The value of fidelity extends from family, friends, and profession, to patients.

Confidentiality is related to fidelity; *con* = "with"; *fide* = "loyal."

True is a word used in several ways in ethics and law. Incorporated into the concept of Being True are Keeping Promises (Loyalty), Keeping Secrets (Confidentiality), and Telling Truth (Veracity). The word *fidelity* is based on the Latin word *fide*: "faithful."

The ethical values discussed in this section are all based on being "true" to someone, in some sense of the word. The value is expressed in many ways: Be *true* to the school. Be *true* to oneself. Be *true* to one's ideals. "Be *true* to me," says the lover. This value may be the first and most basic of all values; it is instinctively present in wolf packs, in marriages, and in relationships between parents and children.

"True" means faithful, and true also means telling the truth. To be faithful to another also means keeping promises to her and keeping secrets she has confided. To be faithful to the patient involves telling the truth. Being "unfaithful" includes lying about what one is doing and revealing secrets. The "be true" values were learned very early. Some minimum level of the value seems innate in the human condition.

Laws enforce the value of being true. Contract law and employment law are derived from the concept of keeping promises (loyalty). Laws about whistle-blowing enforce, at a minimum level, the values of keeping promises *and* telling the truth (veracity). The laws of confidentiality and of privileged communication between nurse and patient are minimum enforcement of the value of keeping secrets. The "informed" in consent law enforces the ethic of telling the truth—veracity.

Nurses are currently taught to be patient advocates, and the law enforces that teaching. Advocating for the patient rests on the value of loyalty, of nurse to the patient; putting that loyalty above some other loyalty or other value the nurse holds.

Keeping Promises: Loyalty

Being true (fidelity) is also expressed by another action: doing good for the patient (beneficence). Humans grew up in tribes, doing good for each other, keeping promises to each other. The family, in essence, is a smaller tribe.

Humans value themselves, their family, friends, agency, their own profession. By extension, nurses value their own patients. When professionals and employers are in conflict, the underlying value being tested may be loyalty: loyalty to the employer "tribe" versus loyalty to the patient, or other professionals' "tribe."

Can technicians perform some care as well as nurses? Do nurses objectively look at outcomes, or is the first reaction, "They're not NURSES. We are." The union movement and related activity are built on the value of fidelity; loyalty to the union, to the cause, to the sisterhood. This loyalty to profession, however, can conflict with loyalty to the patient, or employer, or the law. The words used in loyalty conflicts are loaded with emotion—for example, *betray, treason, tattle, rat, lie.*

Keeping Secrets: Confidentiality

Confidentiality is sometimes listed as a separate value; but confidentiality is related to fidelity. (The word origin: *Con* means "with" and *fide* means "loyal.") Loyalty to someone may mean hiding some truth, not telling a truth that could hurt the person. Truth as a secret is known because the patient believes the nurse faithful (loyal). The patient has trust (confidence) in the nurse, and in a whole system—to be true, faithful, and loyal (to be "on my side").

The individual's self-interest in being true (fidelity) to others is elemental, derived from long ago: People take care of "their own" and take care of the individual. For a long time in human history and prehistory, strangers were the *un*usual—and they were dangerous.

The world has changed from the time when humans developed some of their values. People today must deal with "strangers" daily. Nurses must care for people without fear or hate, as if patients were one of their "own." Nurses cope with a society that is open and plural. They now must work *not* to hate and distrust the strangers.

Perhaps people also must now be less loyal to their small group. If they keep strong feeling for their "own," and stay loyal to "us," can they at the same time still love the stranger? The German word for nationalism is

Nazialismus (from which came *Nazi*); perhaps people must sacrifice even some patriotism to live in a small world in peace.

ETHICS CODE FOR FIDELITY

The codes of ethics for illness care practitioners reflect the values of fidelity in several ways. The codes of ethics of the American Nurses Association, the American Medical Association, and the American Association for Respiratory Care (AARC) are compared and contrasted in Chapter One, and examples of Fidelity values are discussed here.

Code of Ethics of the American Nurses' Association

> **NURSES**
>
> **POINT 10** *The nurse participates in the profession's effort to protect the public from misinformation and misrepresentation and to maintain the integrity of nursing.*

The effort to protect the public from misinformation and misrepresentation reflects the value of fidelity (more specifically, veracity). Beneficence and non-maleficence (doing no harm) for the public is also stressed. The last clause—"maintain the integrity of nursing"—reflects the value of loyalty to the profession.

Respiratory Care Practitioners

Note that the Respiratory Care Code was changed in December 1994 (new version available from AARC, 11030 Ables Lane, Dallas, TX 75229). Changes in wording, however, do not mean that the underlying value or ethic has changed.

> **RESPIRATORY CARE PRACTITIONERS**
>
> *The respiratory care practitioner shall uphold the dignity and honor of the profession and abide by its ethical principles. He or she should be familiar with existing state and federal laws governing the practice of respiratory care and comply with those laws.*

Upholding the dignity and honor of the profession is an example of loyalty to one's colleagues and occupation.

Physicians' Code on Loyalty

III. *A physician shall respect the law and also recognize a responsibility to seek changes in those requirements which are contrary to the best interests of the patient.*

This clause exhorts the doctor to be loyal to the patient and keep the interests of the patient foremost; not the doctor's interest but the patient's.

KEEPING PROMISES: THE LAW ENFORCING THE ETHIC

Being true: Keeping promises (loyalty) underpins all employment law. In a job relationship, there exists an implicit promise to be loyal, to mind the employer's interest as well as one's own. The employer promises to pay and to be fair—a degree of loyalty—to the employee. The employee promises to work. This work for pay grew out of the medieval system of fealty (making an oath or promise to be loyal to a lord or lady), which was an outgrowth of tribal systems. The lord or lady in turn promised to be loyal to the yeoman/serf, involving the provision of opportunity to work on land, protection, and other benefits of a relationship. Employment law remains based on the value of loyalty and is an area of legal concern for most nurses.

The relationship with the employer is a second area with numerous "legal" implications for nurses—the relationship with the patient (malpractice and licensure) is the area of the nurse's life *most* regulated by law.

Employment law can be divided into (1) contract law and (2) related labor law. To some extent, all such laws enforce the ethical values of loyalty. The laws discussed in this section were written to enforce specifically the value, Being True or one of its derivatives. Other employment law enforcing the minimum ethic of fairness (the antidiscrimination law) is discussed in Chapter Five.

CONTRACTS

The value of loyalty (keeping promises) is enforced to a minimum extent by employment law. The employment relationship is an implicit promise by both parties to be loyal to the other.

One of the oldest, most basic concepts of law is the situation in which a promise two people make to each other is enforced: Contract.

Agreements that are not written might not be enforceable in court.

When there is no third-party payment (by insurance or government), there can be a direct contract between nurse and patient; the patient promises to pay, and the nurse promises to give service.

One of the oldest, most basic concepts of all law is the contract: In essence, a contract is made when two people agree (promise) that they will each do something for the other. Contracts may have marked the beginning of civilization—a first time when one could force another to keep promises. (Some libertarians, however, assert that law should not enforce promises; that the risk of unkept promises should be a risk of doing business with untrustworthy people, and that contracts [promises] should be regulated by the free market rather than enforced by public law.)

That promise made by two parties is the value, Loyalty, enforced by contract law. The basis of contract law is an agreement (a promise); two (or more) people agree to do something for each other. It sounds simple enough, but people and their lawyers have been busy for thousands of years creating and modifying contract law, through conflicts and court cases brought to resolve those conflicts.

Agreements needn't be written, but they might not be enforceable in court if they're not. Some attorneys advise, about enforcing contracts in court: It's better to make a poor contract with good people, than to make a good contract with poor (bad) people. But today, promises must be made with strangers, and the good guys are hard to predict.

In an ideal world, a nurse might contract directly with a patient for services. (This may still be done in a private duty agreement with a self-paying patient. Such contracts may be more common in future as care moves out of the hospital and as more patients have power over their spending with medical savings accounts.) But at present, indirect payment for illness care (from taxpayer or private insurance) is the norm—a situation that interferes with that practitioner-patient contract because it interferes with both the making and keeping of promises.

With a direct contract between nurse and patient, the relationship (contract) is that the patient promises to pay, and the nurse promises to give service.

PATIENT → PROMISES $$ → NURSE → ⌐
↓
NURSE → PROMISES CARE → PATIENT

In such a contractual arrangement, the patient is the direct and best judge of the nurse's skill and quality of care. The patient ensures quality of care in the same way that one eventually gets good care for one's car; the customer refuses to pay if not satisfied, and doesn't do car repair business with that person again.

One result of the lack of nursing's direct relationship/contract with the patient is that much more documentation of care becomes necessary. Such documentation is needed to prove, to a third party who pays, that the work was done. In that case, documentation is not done to provide continuity of care (nor is it done for a potential malpractice jury). Most of the documentation now required in agencies could be eliminated if its original purpose (to provide only for continuity of care) were the motivation to chart.

In the present system of payment for illness care, patients generally do not pay directly for care. Instead, patients pay a third party (in the form of premiums to insurers/HMOs or taxes to the government), which then pays the nurse or employer. The connection (the promise between nurse and patient) is interrupted. Between the two, there is no contract and no money contact.

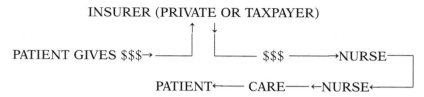

Direct promises—contracts—between nurse and patient, usual when nurses were entrepreneurs who took care of patients in their homes, are *un*usual now. But, new kinds of nurse contracts are being made. Nurse entrepreneurs do contract directly with insurers (to provide services), with other providers (as consultants), and with suppliers of services and equipment. Those promises to perform or pay are covered under contract law.

Basics of Contracts

Contracts are enforceable only if certain components are present:

1. The agreement is between two people or parties who are able to make a contract.
2. Some payment (consideration) for the promise or performance is required.

Quasi-(half-)contract and "unjust enrichment" are legal theories that courts use to prevent one party from benefiting at the expense of another who has no enforceable contract.

The Statute of Frauds is Old English law still enforced in the United States; it requires a contract to be written in order to be enforced, except in certain situations.

Spoken testimony about a contract (like testimony about patients instead of written notes) is inherently suspect because the witness's memory of what was said or done may change, whereas the writing won't.

Spoken agreements for indefinite employment are assumed to hold for longer than one year; employment agreements must be written to be enforceable.

Covenants not to compete are clauses that seek to limit the employee's power to compete after leaving employment. Such clauses must be for a reasonable duration, scope of activity (not *all* work), and area of restriction.

Dealing with people whose promises don't have to be en*forced* is better; but if legal action on a contract is needed, certain components are necessary.

REQUIREMENTS FOR AN ENFORCEABLE CONTRACT

1. The agreement must be between two people who are able to make a contract. Under law, these are people with *capacity* (for example, not minors nor incompetents). In the process of making the agreement, one party makes an offer, and the other accepts the offer. (Volumes of law are written on exactly what constitutes an offer and an acceptance. If any question about that arises, a lawyer is needed.)
2. Some "payment" for the promise or performance is required. The legal word is *consideration* and the payment can be a detriment to one party, or a benefit to the other.

Even without the requirements of a written contract, a court can find that an "implied" contract was made. In legal terms, there is a quasi-(half-) contract. If goods or services are provided for someone without making a formal agreement, the provider may still be able to be paid for the benefit (value) the other person gained.

Similarly, if one person performs a service for a second person, or relies on the promise to her detriment, the court may prevent "unjust enrichment" of the second person by making the second person keep the promise. A "legal fiction" is created that the "enriched" person *contracted* for the service or good she received. ("Legal fiction" is a way of saying the court made up a theory of law; this process is used to get to the result the court wants.)

Some unwritten contracts can be enforced. Spoken contracts—*not* about real estate—which can be performed within one year, or which are for goods valued at less than $500, may be enforced in court *as if they were written*. Spoken contracts are harder to prove than a written contract. Contracts that cannot be performed within a year, contracts for goods that cost more than $500, or contracts that deal with real estate, must be written to be enforced. Those rules derive from Old English law, originally called the Statute of Frauds. Spoken contracts are valid if they don't fall under those outlawed by the Statute of Frauds. (The specifics may vary from state to state.)

Written contracts follow the same principle that applies to written nurses' notes or surgery consents; people (juries) give more weight to written words, because spoken testimony is inherently suspect. The court assumes that the witness's memory of what was agreed may change, especially if it is in their monetary interest to do so.

Spoken agreements for indefinite employment are usually assumed to hold for longer than one year, so employment agreements must be *written* to be enforceable. Even if written, the fact that an employment contract is for an indefinite term may make the contract unenforceable.

COVENANTS NOT TO COMPETE

Some nurses who are independent contractors, some nurses who are employees, and many nurse entrepreneurs do work under the terms of a contract. The same rules apply to nurses as apply to doctors when contracting with agencies. In proposed contracts nurses should watch for overly rigid clauses labeled "covenants not to compete"; the clauses may be changed through negotiation.

HMOs and other employers of professionals often seek to write a non-competition clause into the employment contract. The details vary, but such clauses usually prohibit the professional from working at her trade within a designated area near the present employer, for a designated amount of time. If the clause doesn't specify a "reasonable" area and a "reasonable" time of noncompetition, the court may either supply such a "reasonable" clause or *not* enforce that noncompetition clause at all.

The clause might be held by a court to be "against public policy," depending on how many years and how many miles the nurse is forbidden to work in and from, competition with the agency. The "public policy" upheld is the freedom to work, a value specifically guaranteed in the Fifth and Fourteenth Amendments to the U.S. Constitution (as in life, *liberty*, and *property*).

Work is both a freedom and a property right; these values are weighed by the court against the value of loyalty to the employer by *not* competing; and against the desirability of holding someone to a freely signed agreement.

In addition to having noncompetition clause problems like their physician colleagues, NPs also may encounter problems with anti-trust law, by collaborating with colleagues in negotiations with HMOs.

Variations on the noncompete theme also include the employer who seeks to punish employees who leave an agency (the employer makes it economically punishing to leave). For example, contracts have been written that say that the resigning HMO doctor must pay $700 for each patient who follows the doctor to his new position.

A Florida court of appeals found in 1993 that such a noncompetition clause was unenforceable:

> Patients are not the property or chattel of an HMO. We believe that the public policy of this state [Florida] is violated when the business relationship an HMO has with its affiliated doctors interferes with something as fundamental as the doctor/patient relationship.[1]

Rationale: The practitioner-patient relationship is almost sacrosanct, and such contracts interfere with patients' rights to choose their own providers.

The balancing question for the court: Is the profession a business (in which any clause in a freely agreed contract is OK), or is access to care a right? Any reform or managed care system that restricts patient rights to access to particular practitioners may encounter this issue. Courts might see their role as protecting patient freedom, versus the right of business and individuals to contract freely with each other (business and providers' freedom).

Legislatures in several states have written statutes that enforce these values, by prohibiting many kinds of restrictive clauses in doctor contracts. These statutes are also generally applicable to nurses who contract. But in most states covenants not to compete are upheld, as long as they are for a reasonable duration, scope of activity (not *all* work), and area of restriction.

The courts will also weigh public-interest concerns—for example, the effect of such contract clauses on the public in an area or time of shortage. If doctors and nurses who leave the HMO cannot set up independent practices, the public in a particular locale may be left with only one HMO as a provider.[2]

Noncompetition clauses are unenforceable if the employment contract agreement is not enforceable in the first place. In one case, the independent contractor was not guaranteed any work, nor obliged to take work offered. The court found that language not to have created a contract at all. Any contract with an independent contractor may need to guarantee either that *some* work will be offered, or that some work will be *accepted*, in order to be enforceable as a contract.[3]

Nurses who are contemplating a contract, either as an employee or an independent contractor, should have legal advice from a lawyer knowledgeable about labor law in that state.[4]

Collective bargaining agreements are a special kind of contract, and only a small percentage of nurses work under such agreements. The local nurse organization and state nurse association are the best sources of advice for nurses who work under a collective bargaining contract, for nurses who would like to, or for nurses who don't want to be forced to.

The employment agreement is the promise of the nurse to work, and the promise of the employer to pay. Most nurses work without written contracts, under agreements that are unenforceable in court. That employment agreement is discussed next.

EMPLOYMENT "AT WILL"

Employment "at will" is a relationship that can be terminated at the *will* of either party; employment law upholding that freedom to act is based on the value of autonomy for both employer and employee.

Some states modify the "at will" relationship by establishing a requirement of good faith or fair dealing on the employer's part.

Personnel policy handbooks, which say that employees may only be fired for just cause, may establish a cause of action for wrongful discharge even for "at will" employees.

The promises in employee handbooks (personnel policies), *plus* verbal promises made by managers, may be held to create a contract under the theory of promissory estoppel.

Nurses who report violations of law (not merely guidelines) may be protected under the "public policy exception" to the "at will" doctrine.

The "public policy exception" to the "at will" doctrine upholds the value of doing good for the public (protecting the public from harm) over the value of autonomy of the employer.

Suits may be filed for damages caused by the employer in the course of termination (such as for slander).

Knowledge gained by the employer after a suit for wrongful firing is filed may be used in some situations to justify the firing.

Punitive damages are awarded to punish and to deter future bad conduct.

The nurse's first loyalty is to the patient, and this includes telling patients if care is needed but not available because of limits set by the managed care plan.

Managed care constraints that limit patients' care can be corrected by patients, if they are given accurate information.

Most nurses do not work under the rules of formal legal employment contracts, but under a policy known as "employment at will." This relationship can be terminated at the *will* of either party. Such freedom to act is based on the value of freedom (autonomy) for both employer and employee; courts will enforce only actual contracts that both parties have freely agreed to. The relationship between employer and employee is usually not a formal contract whose terms are enforceable in court.

This "at will" concept is applied in most states to some degree, so in most states a nurse can be fired "at will" by the employer.[5] The employer does not need a good (or "just") cause to fire the employee. A Missouri case stated the "at will" doctrine:

> . . . in the absence of a contract of employment for a definite term or a contrary statutory provision, an employer may discharge an employee at any time, without cause or reason, or for any reason and in such cases no action can be obtained for wrongful discharge.[6]

The U.S. Supreme Court declined to review the case.

States of the United States are generally free to set their own labor policies, *except* as limited by the Bill of Rights in the U.S. Constitution and federal labor laws such as those that provide for collective bargaining and forbid discrimination (described in Chapter Five).

The rightness of the ethics underlying the employment "at will" doctrine has been argued in legal articles, and different states have different law. For example, in Illinois an employee can charge that she relied (to her detriment) on the employer's promises—even though the promises were not in a contract. Employer promises can be enforced under the legal theory of *promissory estoppel* (example below). In such cases, the court may "imply" a contract. In other states (Wisconsin and California), some fired employees have won cases by establishing a requirement of good faith or fair dealing on the employer's part. Those cases enforce the value of justice (fairness) over the value of the freedom *not* to contract.

A nurse who *does* have a written contract might believe she can only be terminated for just cause—that the employer can't fire her without a good reason. But a written agreement may not be an enforceable contract unless it meets all criteria for a contract. In one case a nurse with a written agreement sued the former employer, alleging that termination was without cause. (The written agreement with the employer had said the nurse could be terminated only "with just cause.") The court of appeals found that the contract had no ending date; therefore it was a contract "in perpetuity" and wasn't really a contract at all. So the nurse was really an employee "at will" and the hospital had the right to discharge her without any "just" (good) cause.[7]

The "at will" doctrine is usually upheld by conservative state courts unless and until the legislature changes the statute. Conservative court decisions say it is the courts' job to interpret law in cases, not to make wholly new law. If a change is desired in this policy, the people through the legislature can make new statutes. More liberal courts may make the law they think is "just."

If the personnel policy handbook says that employees may only be fired for just cause, even an "at will" employee might sue for wrongful discharge on that basis. That is so even though the employee handbook states that it is not a contract and even if the handbook states that supervisors can fire and change policies without notice. (It depends on the wording, the location, and even the size of type the statement is set in.)

Exceptions to the "At Will" Rule: Public Policy

Some nurses might believe that they are protected from termination if they act to uphold nursing standards. For example, many would think that they can't be fired for reporting agency violations of standards to JCAHO inspectors. This is not necessarily so.

When upheld, this kind of job protection is called a "public policy exception" to the "at will" doctrine.[8] The theory is that the policy value of doing good for the public (in the nurse cases, protecting the public from harm) is more important than the value of autonomy of the employer. The policy usually applies only to reports of violations of law; guidelines (such as JCAHO's) are not law.

Distinguishing law from non-law: Law is *written* and made by people with *authority* to make law. Law is always in the form of a statute, a regulation, or a court case. A writing from other than those sources is a guide, not a law, and the public policy protection may not apply.

A variation of the public policy exception to employment "at will" may protect nurses who are public employees, who speak out about matters of public concern. A nurse fired from a public hospital in Illinois asserted that the First Amendment right of free speech meant that her employer had a duty not to fire her when she spoke about the danger she saw to patients in cross-training nurses without adequate supervision. Her case went to the U.S. Supreme Court, which said the public employer can fire for insubordination (which is what the employer alleged her speech was). The employer must make "reasonable" investigation of what was said before firing; and the employer can fire if it has a good faith belief that the speech is not protected.[9]

Advice

A contract with an employer must be a real contract for a specified time. Nurses seeking an employee contract should have a labor lawyer review the proposal. A contract can cut both ways; a nurse who breaches the contract by quitting before the date of termination can be made to pay damages. The employer might (but not likely) sue for damages for the cost of the breach to the employer; for example, the cost of recruiting a new employee. Sample contracts for individuals are available in the self-help section of the library and bookstore, as well as from nurse associations, but they do not replace advice of the labor lawyer.

The promises in employee handbooks (personnel policies), *plus* spoken promises made by managers, may be enough to create a contract. (The theory is promissory estoppel.) A lawyer can analyze the remedies the nurse may have. Managers must be careful about the promises they make; they may be forced to keep them.

Absent some other certainty, like a personal or collective bargaining contract, nurses and their managers can assume that employees work "at will." The nurse employee must be prepared to deal with the possibility of losing the job, preparing for that with savings, education, and skill that can be transferred to a new job.

Or the employee may sue.

Various issues of ethics and law arise in cases brought by employees against their former employers for "wrongful discharge" (defamation of the employee in the process of firing is often alleged). In such a suit, knowledge gained by the employer *after* the suit was filed may be used in some situations to justify the firing. For example, if the employee sues for wrongful discharge, and on reviewing the employee's application and work record, some misconduct (resumé fraud or work-related misconduct) is discovered, that reason might be used as an affirmative defense to the lawsuit if misconduct is severe enough.

In such a case, the employee is fired and sues. The employer then learns the employee lied on the application for work. The employee loses. Or such after-acquired evidence may merely limit damages the employee can get; the fraud or misconduct reduces the amount of recovery from the wrongful employer.[10]

When punitive damages are awarded, the intent is to punish and to deter future conduct. The average award in suits for wrongful discharge is substantial; but remember, "average" means a lot of little awards are averaged with a few gigantic ones. Experts say such cases are hard to win.

The presumption that the employee is "at will" can be avoided by several legal theories, among them public policy, promissory estoppel, and suits alleging damages by the employer in the process of the termination. In addition, several state and federal laws (statutes) specify reasons that *can't* be used to fire or otherwise discriminate among employees or applicants for a job. Neither age, sex, race, ethnicity, disability, pregnancy, nor veteran status can be used to make employment decisions. All these laws have as their ethical base the value of fairness (justice), discussed in Chapter Five.

LOYALTY TO THE MANAGED CARE PATIENT

New ways of paying for care, and efforts to limit the cost of care, place obvious restraints on providers who give care. "Managed care" is terminology encompassing the various ways to accomplish third-party payment, all with one thing in common: they limit care. All that is new in the managed care/HMO environment is the *obvious* limiting of care by insurers. Care has always been limited by what is available, what will be paid for, and what will be beneficial to the patient. But a conflict between the nurse's loyalty to the patient and loyalty to the employer may arise, as insurers and employers of providers issue rulings that patients *not* get certain kinds of care (or get less of it) from providers.

The limits on care are more obvious compared to past decades when the payment for care was *seemingly* unlimited, from premiums paid by the insured and from taxes paid by citizens. That attitude resulted in inflation in the cost of care, which resulted in the inability to continue to pay for care at that level. The limits now envisioned and encountered in managed care fall largely on the caregiver who works at the point of entry into the system: the primary ambulatory care nurse or doctor.

This "new" environment is not new for nurses. Nurses have always faced a potential conflict between their loyalty to patients and loyalty to the employer who paid them. And nurses have in the past usually not had the freedom (autonomy) to decide who gets care. Nurses who act as gatekeepers in the system may have such power/responsibility.

As professionals with a higher duty than to the present job, the nurse's first loyalty is to the patient. Nurses do have a duty to advocate for their patients within and outside of the system, if that is needed.

As further advocate, nurses have a duty to uphold the value of truth telling (veracity) with the patient. The patient must be told if and when care is needed, or indicated, but is not available because of limits set by the managed care plan (usually the HMO). In some cases, in tax-based managed care systems (as in Britain and Canada), patients are either *not* told about optional (unpaid) treatment or *are* told they don't need such treatment. Only with accurate and full information can the patient make choices based on reality.

But nurses cannot give care that is not paid for, unless they are willing to donate their time (and money, for supplies and equipment) to the patient. If managed care constraints cause patients too much pain (figuratively or literally), then in a free society with total information, patients will seek another system. They may choose to pay for care privately; but even in a free market fee-for-service system, the nurse can give only that care the patient can and will pay for—not *unlimited* care.

Providers who worry most about the limits of managed care are doctors, who (unlike nurses) have believed they alone had the power to decide what the patient needed, without reference to economics. This attitude operated in illness care only in the years since passage of Medicare and the increase in insured care in the 1960s; and it has resulted in such inflation in the industry that many people are unable to buy basic care out-of-pocket. Economic deflation/depression and more realistic attention to the cost of care may result in better care for the money—and, in the end, a "healthier" industry.

Keeping Secrets (Confidentiality)

The practical reason for nurses to value keeping patient secrets (confidentiality) is that patients are then more likely to freely give the nurse all necessary information.

Codes of ethics and laws reinforce what is learned first from the marketplace: Telling secrets learned in the nurse-patient relationship is costly to the nurse who does it.

Nurses have always held to the ethical value of confidentiality. They keep secret (confidential) the information they learn in the course of the care of their patient.

▽

"All that may come to my knowledge in the exercise of my profession or in daily commerce with men, which ought not to be spread abroad, I will keep secret and never reveal."

—Oath of Hippocrates

△

This is part of the Hippocratic Oath for doctors, written well over 2000 years ago—there is no doubt the duty was recognized before the Oath was even written.

The value of confidentiality (part of the more encompassing value of fidelity, being true) arises from the great power to harm that information about the patient gives to the nurse. The patient may not have given such information to any other "stranger." Disclosure of the information could embarrass or even harm the patient.

The practical reason for confidentiality is to increase the likelihood that the patient will freely give the nurse all necessary information. If the patient thinks the nurse will not keep secrets, the patient will be less likely to confide information needed for care.

The practitioner has a practical self-interest in keeping confidences, even without laws to enforce this value. If nurses reveal secrets, people will know the nurse is untrustworthy (unfaithful). If nurses don't keep patients' secrets, they get less information, and give poorer care, harm or don't help patients, and obtain fewer patients. People stop hiring nurses who tell patients' secrets, and legal consequences may be lawsuit or license loss.

Codes of ethics and laws reinforce what is learned first from the marketplace: It is detrimental to tell things about patients that are learned in the course of the nurse-patient relationship.

Ethics Code Provisions (Confidentiality)

NURSES

POINT 2. *The nurse safeguards the client's right to privacy by judiciously protecting information of a confidential nature.*

This code provision refers to the requirement of confidentiality (another expression of the value, Fidelity, to the patient). Implicit in confidentiality are also the values of beneficence and non-maleficence.

Note that the nurses' code assumes a "right" to privacy, which may no longer be upheld in federal constitutional law; the principle of privacy is still being upheld, but only under the Fourteenth Amendment's constitutional right to liberty (and life and property). Also note the qualifier word *judiciously* in that code section: This means the nurse must use judgment in deciding to protect patient confidence if the patient's welfare indicates otherwise.

RESPIRATORY CARE PRACTITIONERS

The respiratory care practitioner shall hold in strict confidence all privileged information concerning the patient and refer all inquiries to the physician in charge of the patient's medical care.

—from code in effect
prior to December 1994

The reference to " the physician" makes clear the dependent relationship of this occupation to physicians.

PHYSICIANS

IV. *A physician shall respect the rights of patient, of colleagues, and of other health professionals, and shall safeguard patient confidences within the constraints of the law.*

Some respect is shown above for the "rights" (freedom-autonomy) of the patient, and of nurses too under the phrase "other health professionals." Note that the physician code says the doctor's responsibility is to keep patient secrets only to the limit of the law; under this clause (contrasted to the "judgment" call of the nurses' code) doctors do not have the duty to make a decision if the law mandates otherwise.

No ethical standard is recognized here that might exceed or be counter to the law. For example, a German doctor under the National Socialist government might have been "legally" mandated to select mentally retarded patients to be killed.[11] This ethical code provision might not require the doctor to keep the patient's condition secret if the law mandated its disclosure.

Confidentiality Requirements

The patient or surrogate does not own the chart, but in most circumstances can have access to the information in the chart.

New technology makes compilation of data access easier, causing potential ethical and legal problems in patient confidentiality as well as in comparison of performance of individual practitioners and agencies.

Medical Records. The patient's chart does not "belong" to the patient; the agency has ownership of its records, and the doctor of hers. But, despite ownership, the patient or surrogate can have *access* to the information in the chart, unless there is some medical reason not to see it (an unusual situation). Nurses must remember to chart so they wouldn't be embarrassed if the patient read the notes (nor the patient's attorney).

In addition to the patient, others have access to the record: other agencies; other workers with reason to see it; the courts always; and possibly the guardian or surrogate. Another record, not in the chart, is the incident report: If the patient should sue, he likely can discover (obtain) that report. Often incident reports are self-serving, exculpating the providers from any wrong; for that reason, they may not be admissible *by the defense*, which may seek to introduce them into evidence.

Minutes of meetings, or spoken discussions at the meetings, can usually also be discovered in a lawsuit. Peer review meetings, however—where discipline of practitioners is discussed—may qualify under state or national law as protected from discovery. Complying with such law may protect the committee members from liability.

New technology in record making and record keeping allows information about patients to be easily obtained, but causes new concerns about confidentiality. The need to safeguard the patient's secrets becomes even more important.[12]

With easy computer access, broad and detailed research can now be done on patient outcomes. The potential for violation of the patient's confidence is always a danger. Proposals are being made that such research be reviewed, like other research on patients, by the Institutional Review Board of the agency.

Further, the compilation of data and easy access allows comparison of performance of individual practitioners (not only hospitals). A potential concern for *nurse* confidentiality is that the nurse's "score"—for example, 200 patients cared for during a year, 20 patients died—may in future be discoverable (and usable in a malpractice case?). Nurses' concern for patient confidentiality also extends to faxes of patient records, which could be misdirected. The ethical principle and law that enforces being true, protecting patient confidence, are the same as ever. The new specifics of technology are merely new challenges to upholding the value of loyalty.

Another area of concern for confidentiality of nursing actions and status is the National Practitioner Data Bank (NPDB). The intent of the NPDB law is to protect patients (doing no harm) by identifying bad practitioners who, before the passage of the NPDB, could move undetected to another state. Nurses are now included under the law, under which a report is compiled and kept on all practitioners reported as having been disciplined by their state's board of nursing. A malpractice suit settlement or a late renewal of license might bring discipline. If the practitioner pays out money in a malpractice case (even a small amount, a "nuisance" claim), that must be reported and recorded by the data bank.

Those data are available to any board of nursing in the state in which the nurse applies for licensure, and any agency to which the nurse applies for a job. Here again is a law whose intended consequence is good—to protect patients from bad practitioners (value: non-maleficence); but the law itself has some unintended consequences—perhaps harm to good nurses in conflict with the value of confidentiality.

The 1993 Clinton health reform plan would have made NPDB data available to the general public, so patients or neighbors would have been able to check on the nurse. Proposals also continue to be made that all complaints to licensure boards be public, even if the complaints were made anonymously.

LAW ENFORCING CONFIDENTIALITY

Cases brought under the quasi-intentional torts of "invasion of privacy" (public disclosure of private fact) are examples of the law punishing someone for telling something they knew but shouldn't have told.

Legal exceptions to the mandate of keeping patient secrets enforce the conflicting value of telling the truth. The truth telling "wins" only when it is done for someone's good (patient or public).

Statutes mandate that certain information learned in the course of practice must be reported somewhere; they enforce the ethical value of non-maleficence.

Reporting may conflict with the mandate to keep confidentiality; the rule is that the nurse cannot legally keep confidences if that causes harm to the patient or to other people.

If mandatory reporting is required, the report must be made only to the proper authority specified in the statute.

If obeying the law is counter to the ethics of the nurse, she must decide whether to obey the law or her conscience. The nurse must recognize her personal ethical values, the laws that apply, and the consequences of not following the law.

The legal duty of the nurse enforces the ethical duty to be true to the patient. Cases, statutes, and regulations enforce the minimum of ethical behavior of keeping the patient's secrets.

All the cases brought under the quasi-intentional tort of invasion of privacy—public disclosure of private fact—are examples of the law punishing someone for telling something they knew but shouldn't have told. This tort is discussed also under the value non-maleficence (Chapter Three), since it is considered to be harming someone with some intent to do so (not negligently).

There are numerous exceptions to the legal duty that enforces the ethical mandate to keep secrets. The legal exceptions to keep secrets all enforce the value of telling the truth. Truth telling "wins" only when it is done for the good of someone—the patient or the public. This is a classic prioritizing of values in which the question is: "Which value is most important in this case?"

The reason to *tell* patient secrets: The patient or other people would be harmed by *keeping* the secret. A famous case in California held a psychiatrist's employer responsible for *not* telling secrets. The patient said he was going to kill his girl friend; the girl friend wasn't warned; the patient killed her.[13]

When the patient is HIV-positive and tells a nurse he hasn't told his sexual partner, the nurse faces a conflict. The patient's interest in confidentiality is pitted against a lover's interest in the truth—and, possibly in life. The nurse has a duty of loyalty to the patient; the other duty is to prevent harm to the third person. The conflict is between the interest of keeping the patient's secrets (loyalty to him), versus not harming another.

Does the nurse have any duty to a person who is not her patient? In the above case the nurse might be in the same position as a member of the "public," having no direct duty to the third person. The minimum duty of a citizen is not to harm another person. Does the nurse "harm" the third person by not divulging information that might prevent the harm? The *Tarasoff* case, described above, would say yes. The law might view the third person as being in some minimal sense also a patient of the nurse, at least to the extent that the nurse must prevent harm that can be foreseen.

Most states have statute law that governs the HIV-positive diagnosis, including warning sex partners of HIV-positive patients. The duty to warn a third person is probably less than in the psychiatric case.

Nurses needn't learn every law in their state that might affect patient confidentiality. The rule is still that practicing good nursing and using good sense will be ethical and legal. Treating the patient as the nurse personally would want to be treated is usually ethical, legal, and good practice. The conflict arises when persons other than the patient and nurse are at risk, as in the HIV situation described above.

In such a conflict, the nurse should seek counsel: first the supervisor, the agency management and attorney if necessary, and the specific law for her state on the subject (find the statute law in the library).

Nurses in occupational health, who counsel workers with drug or other personal problems, must be vigilant in safeguarding the workers' confidentiality—just as nurses safeguard patient confidences. Occupational health nurses often serve as Employee Assistance Professionals in their work setting. Laws at the federal and state level, policies of the company, and the nurse's professional code of ethics, all can be used as guides to safe, ethical, and legal behavior in such relationships with workers.[14] Good practice will incorporate protecting worker confidentiality *when that benefits the worker* and when protecting that confidence *does not harm others*.

All states mandate that certain information learned in the course of practice must be reported somewhere. Such mandatory reporting laws enforce the ethical value of non-maleficence; they seek to prevent harm (or further harm) before it happens, not only to punish after harm is done, as most law does. But the mandatory reporting statute may conflict with another ethical value (and legal mandate) of nurses, keeping patients' information confidential.

To find which value is most important in a situation, remember: The nurse cannot ethically (nor legally) keep confidences if that causes harm to the patient or to other people.

Examples of Statutes Mandating Reports: Statutes mandate reporting certain infectious diseases (AIDS, TB), evidence of violence (as in gunshot wounds), neglect or abuse of the young, the old, or the disabled or otherwise vulnerable patient.

Nurses may be required by law to report alcoholism or drug use by colleagues. Substance abuse is the most frequent reason for discipline by state boards of nursing. Statutes that require reporting generally also give the nurse immunity from any potential lawsuit resulting from the report.

If the nurse tells a patient or a colleague's secret when the law requires, the nurse would have immunity from a lawsuit for such violation of privacy. But if mandatory reporting is required, the report must be made only to the proper authority specified in the statute. For example, the fact that suspected child abuse must be reported to the state's department of social welfare may not automatically give the nurse license to report her suspicion to any other agency such as the police, the child's teacher, or the newspaper. Violating patient or coworker confidences in other than the required manner may expose the nurse to a suit for defamation (slander or libel) or invasion of privacy.

Laws that mandate reporting of a colleague's substance abuse or a patient's actions may interfere with the value of loyalty to the colleague, and the value of confidentiality. In some situations, obeying the law may be considered unethical by the individual nurse since the law is an *arbitrary minimum ethic*—the minimum ethic of the majority as interpreted by lawmakers. The nurse may value Loyalty to patient or colleage more than Doing No Harm (the minimum ethic enforced by mandatory reporting). In that case the nurse will have to decide whether to obey the law or her conscience. To make an informed decision, the nurse needs to recognize her personal ethical values, to know the laws that apply, and be ready to endure the consequences of not following the law.

Privileged Communication

Privileged communication means that the patient can prevent the nurse from testifying in legal proceedings about private conversations between the two; but many exceptions to the privilege mean that nurses should assume that conversations with the patient can be ordered divulged in court.

Lawsuits alleging invasion of privacy enforce the value of non-maleficence and also of confidentiality; keeping the patient's physical and psychological person private is good practice (and good ethics and good law).

Further related to confidentiality is the law of privilege, theory developed from centuries of cases. In essence, the theory of privilege means that the patient has the power to prevent the provider from testifying in legal proceedings about private conversations between the two. Here the law again en*force*s the minimum of the ethical value of confidentiality. Privileged communication is the patient's privilege to invoke. The provider cannot on her own refuse to testify if the patient wants the testimony; the patient invokes the privilege (unless the patient is unable to do so; the nurse might then involve the privilege on behalf of the patient). In a malpractice or other suit in which the patient's illness is an issue, the privilege is considered to be waived by the patient; so the practitioner can testify.

Ethical and legal issues are raised by statutes that establish privileged communication. This "privilege" is an exemption from the court's ability to compel testimony about the practitioner's conversation or relationship with the practitioner.[15] It is often extended to psychiatrists and psychologists, and as a result has implications for psychiatric/mental health nursing. Psychiatric nurses in many states do not have such a privilege of *not* testifying to patient communication; some would like to have it.

Each state's law differs regarding which providers are subject to the privilege. Rarely is there specific nurse-patient privilege. The state's laws usually differ between civil suits (for damages) or criminal prosecutions (for violation of law). Physician-patient and therapist-patient communication is often privileged in civil suits, but not in criminal prosecutions. There are so many variations and exceptions to the privilege that nurses and doctors should assume that conversations with the patient *can* be ordered divulged in court, and behave accordingly.

Other Privacy Issues

The law of invasion of privacy is discussed under the value of non-maleficence (Chapter Three), since that theory of law is classed as a quasi-(half)-intentional tort. But the underlying ethic is also keeping the patients' secrets (confidentiality). It is not merely good practice, but also good ethics and law, to be sensitive to the patient's situation. One example: What seems the usual state of dress (or undress) in clinic or hospital may be very embarrassing to the patient.

Not only physical but mental or emotional privacy is important to the patient. Revealing the patient's condition or diagnosis may be extremely invasive of the patient's privacy (even to the family). Nurses who work in psychiatric settings have particular responsibility for meeting that patient need for privacy.

A related issue is whether the patient's desire for privacy (such as a woman patient who wants a nurse who is a woman) outweighs the nurse's desire for fairness (the ability of a nurse who is a man to work in labor and delivery). The argument that doctors who are men take care of women, begs the question that the woman freely chose the doctor—she may not have freely chosen the nurse. Almost always, some compromise can be reached; extremes of behavior should be avoided by both sides. Lawsuits usually are based on extreme behavior by someone.

TELLING TRUTH (VERACITY)

> The value of truth telling (veracity) is less-often mentioned, since there is no controversy that patients should be told the truth.

Telling the truth is enforced in law (the First Amendment freedom of speech, and civil and criminal actions for lying) because truth gives more information about reality, needed for good decisions.

Nurses ask patients to tell them the truth; and vice versa, nurses have a duty to be truthful to patients (truthfulness is implied in consent).

Risk is a part of veracity, both in regard to what is told the nurse, and what the nurse tells.

Criminal law enforces the value of veracity by punishing lying done deliberately to take property from another person (as in fraud on the Medicare system).

The Basis of the Law: Ethics

Another word for telling truth is *veracity* (*vera* means "truth" in Latin). This value is less mentioned than others because there is no longer controversy over whether patients should be told the truth (in the old days, nurses and doctors sometimes protected patients from the truth—lied to them). Even U.S. constitutional law (the First Amendment) protects the value of truth telling, as freedom of speech.

The guarantee of free speech in the First Amendment is not just a vague ideal without meaning in reality. And telling the truth is not just "nice." Telling the truth is *enforced* in law.

Telling truth results in more information about reality, about the world. People need truth (reliable information) to decide upon actions to take. Not telling the truth (lying) can result in great cost.

Everyone in the system benefits from truth. If the laboratory lied when asked for blood chemistries, imagine the consequences. Imagine if the RT doesn't do the blood gases, just draws and makes them up. Imagine if the nurse on the preceding shift doesn't communicate that the patient got 30 mg of morphine intramuscularly. The system would break down if people couldn't rely on others to give them true information. If nurses or doctors had to get all information for themselves, they would accomplish much less.

Nurses ask the patient to tell them the truth. To get needed information about the patient, nurses implicitly promise not to betray the patient's *confide*nce; the patient has *confide*nce in the nurse and will *confide* in them.

Informed Consent

On the other hand of veracity, nurses must also tell truth to the patient. Nurses have a corresponding obligation to be truthful to the patient, as the patient was asked to be to the nurse. That truthfulness is implied in consent (that is why it is unnecessary to add *informed* to *consent*). The topic of informed consent is elaborated in the law of the value of autonomy (Chapter Four), but the law of informed consent also enforces the minimum of value of veracity.

Risk of Veracity

More truth equals better information equals a better outcome (at least, the outcome is more likely based on reality). But more truth carries some risk. Nurses must be prepared to deal with the information they give or seek. For example, unless they know what to do with the information sought, they should not culture all the obstetrics department personnel for staphylococcus. Before the patient is given the truth about her positive HIV test, the nurse must be ready to deal with the consequences to the patient. Before patients are routinely screened for abuse (or for any other condition), the practitioner must be ready to follow up on the truth the patient tells.

The freedom of speech (truth telling) is a relative value, like all others. The classic example of its relativity is that the freedom to speak is not the freedom to speak *irresponsibly*, as in shouting "Fire!" in a crowded theater. Nurses have power over patients, gained from superior knowledge of the patient's condition. Nurses must be careful about using that power in coercive and threatening ways, legal or not. Good practice demands that the nurse *persuade* the diabetic to comply with her regimen—not that the nurse threaten to initiate competency and guardianship proceedings to coerce the patient.

Nurses must be concerned with free speech, especially nurses who provide information that might violate regulations that might be in force at any given time, depending on the philosophy of the lawmakers. In recent years, nurses in federally funded family planning were under a mandate not to inform patients of abortion options (see the *Rust* case, discussed below and in Chapter Seven under A Time to Be Born). Other nurses have had their licenses to practice endangered for exercising their free speech rights—by telling patients of therapy their physicians don't want them to hear, for example (the *Tuma* case, discussed in Chapter Three, under Licensure).

The criminal law enforces the value of veracity by punishing lying, if lying is done deliberately to take property from another person. That crime is called fraud (lying for gain). The crime of fraud, for instance, is committed if the practitioner signs a Medicare form that a service was provided when it wasn't. Through a civil lawsuit the law may also provide money damages if lying is proved in cases of defamation (libel and slander) or civil fraud.

Those penalties alone give nurses a self-interest in telling the truth. In addition, nurses who tell truth benefit in other ways: People see them as reliable sources of information; they turn to nurses, value them, and nurses are directly better off for that. Nurses then also participate in that larger system of veracity, which benefits them and everyone else.

WHISTLE-BLOWING

The ethical duty and legal mandate to report ("blow the whistle") in the patient's best interest, is required in ethical codes of several professions.

> Blowing the whistle may put the nurse at risk with the employer, but it also can be financially rewarding in a few cases.
>
> The whistle-blower should not hide behind the qualified privilege of protecting another in order to mount a character attack.
>
> Nurses may see a conflict with telling truth, in order to help the patient by false representations to the payor.
>
> Nurses must weigh the harm to patients if they don't tell the truth, against the harm that might come to themselves, their institution or patient if they do. Nurses should factor in the harm to *their own view of themselves* if they don't tell the truth.

Whistle-blowing is a new term for an old action—telling the truth; the value is veracity. Telling truth, however, may conflict with the people who put higher the value of loyalty to the employer. Or the value of veracity might be lower than one's monetary interest; or the value of confidentiality; or loyalty to a friend (such as when a nurse refuses to report drug use or other bad behavior of a friend). Another value implicit in blowing the whistle is beneficence: To tell the truth may do good for the patient or the "group" of patients, the public.

The ethical duty and legal mandate to report a colleague who uses drugs on duty is blowing the whistle. In addition, the ethical codes of several professions require that practitioners act in their patients' interest, or even advocate for patients. Some code provisions strongly encourage such advocacy, to the point of telling truth for the patient's benefit that might even cost the nurse her job.

$$\triangledown$$

"The best security for the fidelity of men is to make their interest coincide with their duty."

—ALEXANDER HAMILTON

$$\triangle$$

When self-interest and ethical behavior are made identical, ethical behavior will result. The law that awards money for telling the truth accomplishes that.

People who "tell" may suffer retaliation (firing) for their actions. In one case, a federal court judge ordered that, if a company wants to learn the identity of the whistle-blower's sources of information, the company had to guarantee lifetime employment to those whose names were revealed (the employees). That judge also ruled that reporters did not have to divulge whistle-blowers' names (the company had engaged in a large "espionage" operation against the whistle-blower). The case was settled with an undivulged award, reported to be in the millions.[16]

Loyalty does not merely mean being quiet.[17] Nurses have an obligation, as part of their loyalty, to speak up (tell truth) when something wrong occurs.[18]

Some law requires reporting adverse drug reactions.[19] And the Safe Medical Devices Act of 1990[20] requests providers voluntarily report information if a medical device caused or contributed to a patient's death, serious injury, or serious illness. Reports are to be made to the Food and Drug Administration (FDA). (The FDA has established a program walled "Medwatch," which accepts reports of adverse events and product problems—including drug reactions.)

Professional Employee: Duty to Inform

The legal duty to inform (or not) enforces the value of veracity. In some cases the law has mandated actions on the part of practitioners that also affect the value of practitioner autonomy. The U.S. Supreme Court upheld a regulation that prohibited practitioners who work in federally funded family planning clinics from advising patients about abortion.[21] This regulation can be seen as actually mandating the nurse *not* to tell the patient some truth (information).

To some, this regulation was an invasion of the nurse-patient relationship. To others, it was a reasonable exercise of employer authority to require certain policy attitudes on the part of employees. Some argue that the government does not have to pay for family planning at all, so when the government pays, it may choose to subsidize and encourage birth control through contraception in preference to abortion (which is not preventing conception, but preventing a live birth).

But in some instances, failing to inform a patient, even if the nurse was required *not* to do so by law, could theoretically result in a malpractice suit (and a failure of the standard of nursing care).

The interplay of the values of patient autonomy, practitioner autonomy, doing good for the patient, loyalty and veracity to the patient and/or to the employer, can *all* be seen in this one example of regulatory law.

The "gag" rule was changed early in 1992 for doctors, so that physicians could advise patients about abortions. Other practitioners still could not. What are the ethical implications of that differentiation between professionals? The Clinton administration rescinded the rule altogether in 1993. But with this U.S. Supreme Court case as precedent, a new rule that *required* nurses to counsel patients about abortion at family planning clinics might be upheld. Same issues?[22]

Other laws require practitioners to tell patients some "truth." Statutes require practitioners to inform patients about such treatments as electroconvulsive shock therapy, sterilization, breast cancer therapies, and about the consequences of abortion to the fetus.

Regulations that provide for informed consent for HIV testing may be seen as intervening in the practitioner-patient relationship. Some laws in some cases require counseling that promotes (or at least does not discourage) homosexual activity or intravenous drug use.

Nurses sometimes want to lie in order to help the patient. For example, home healthcare nurses may be faced with a dilemma that they believe is unique in nursing, though instances in other nurse practice situations can be cited as parallel. The conflict is between (1) documenting the patient's actual needs and care in such a way as to get payment for the work done, or (2) telling the truth and losing the patient's status as paid, thus losing him the nursing care too.[23] This conflict will increase as managed care of illness may "force" the nurse either to limit care or lie. Does the end (care) justify the means (lying)? Never? Always? Ever?

Negatives of Whistle-Blowing

On the negative side of the duty to tell the truth is the ability of the whistle-blower to be anonymous and hide behind the qualified privilege of protecting another. The "truth" teller from this position can mount a character attack.

The Sixth Amendment to the U.S. Constitution gives the accused a right to confront witnesses in a trial. That protection is there precisely because of the danger of anonymous assassination. In earlier times, other places, people could whisper an anonymous attack. And without the deterrence of knowing they'd be challenged by the accused, accusers were free to attack at will.

Anita Hill could not attack Supreme Court nominee Clarence Thomas on grounds of sexual harassment, and stay anonymous. Fairness dictated that she come forward and be examined in public on her statements.

To enforce (or at least encourage) the value telling truth/whistle-blowing, statutes in some states protect people who tell (and, as noted, judges in many cases provide protection). State laws may, through statutes and cases, encourage people to tell the truth when the public interest is at stake.

Firing an employee for following a *law*—not just an ethical code—when the law requires reporting, is prohibited. (This is a policy exception to the "employment at will" doctrine, discussed under contract law above.) Other examples of job protection for whistle-blowing are in federal laws, such as the Toxic Substances Control Act. Some states have whistle-blowing laws, too.

There always has been, and probably always will be, some danger in telling truth that other people, especially employers, don't want to hear—or truth that they don't want heard by others. Even the small taunt that one

364 • *Ethics and Law of Being True (Fidelity)*

suffered in kindergarten, "Tattle-tale, Tattle-tale," deters irresponsible informing.

It may be a good thing that "telling" or accusing is not completely free of retribution, however small. In the bad example of Germany under National Socialism, children were encouraged to report on their parents. Similar examples were uncovered more recently in Eastern Europe: A high percentage of the population of East Germany was reporting to the secret police, on their neighbors, family, and friends under the former government.

Nurses must weigh the harm to patients if they *don't* report, against the harm that might come to themselves and the institution if they *do*. In some cases, they have to remember the harm to *their own view of themselves* if they don't tell the truth.

The best ethics lesson on veracity the author ever heard was in law school. Not in the long semester of rules-learning of the "professional responsibility" course, but in the response of the professor of civil procedure to a student. The student asked, "If I do this (bad thing), who'll know?"

"*You'll* know," Professor Ross answered.

He didn't add it, but it was obvious who would be hurt most by unethical behavior. In the nursing context it is not always the patient, and not always the institution that is hurt the most—it is the nurse's opinion of *herself*.

ENDNOTES

1. *Humana Medical Plan Inc. v. Ira S. Jacobson*, 636 So.2d 120 (Fl. App. 1994).
2. Felsenthal, E., "Courts debate patients' rights, doctors' pacts," *Wall Street Journal*, 22 April 1993; B1, B7.
3. *Burgess v. Permian Court Reporters, Inc.*, 864 S.W.2d 725 (Tex. App. 1993).
4. Advice to employers: Zucker, T., "The litigation perspective: Drafting the enforceable covenant not to compete," *Texas Bar Journal*, 1993; 56(10):1000–1008.
5. See for the effect on nurse freedom: Murphy, E.K., "Professional autonomy v. 'at will' employee status," *Nursing Outlook*, 1990; 38(5):248.
6. *Amaan v. City of Eureka*, 615 S.W.2d 414 (Mo. Banc 1981), *cert. denied* 454 U.S. 1084 (1981).
7. *Main v. Skaggs Community Hospital*, 812 S.W.2d 185 (Mo. App. 1991).
8. See, for example: Cushing, M., "The right to fire v. the public interest," *American Journal of Nursing*, 1992; 92(12):18,20.
9. *Waters et al. v. Churchill et al.*, 114 S.Ct. 1878 (1994).
10. Johnson, E.P., "After-acquired evidence of employee misconduct: Affirmative defense or limitation on remedies?" *Florida Bar Journal*, June 1993; pp. 76–79.
11. For examples see: Lifton, Jay, *The Nazi Doctors*, New York: Basic Books, Inc., 1986.
12. Curran, M., and Curran, K., "The ethics of information," *Journal of Nursing Administration*, 1991; 21(1):47–49.
13. *Tarasoff v. Regents of the University of California*, 131 Cal. Rptr. 14, 551 P.2d 334 (1976). Also upholding the duty to warn: *Bradley v. Ray*, 904 S.W.2d 302 (Mo. App. 1995).
14. Mistretta, E.F., and Inlow, L.B., "Confidentiality and the employee assistance program professional," *American Association of Occupational Health Nursing Journal*, 1991; 39(2):84–86.
15. See generally: Stern, S.B., "Privileged communication: An ethical and legal right of psychiatric clients," *Perspectives in Psychiatric Care*, 1990; 26(4):22–25.
16. McCoy, C., and Schmitt, R.B., "Alyeska settles suit by a whistle-blower," *Wall Street Journal*, 21 December 1993, B8.
17. Curtin, L., "When virtue becomes vice," *Nursing Management*, 1993; 24(9):20–26.

18. Pinch, W.J., "Nursing ethics: Is 'covering-up' ever 'harmless'?" *Nursing Management*, 1990; 21(9):60–62.

19. See, for example, O'Donnell, J., "Understanding adverse drug reactions," *Nursing*, 1992; 22(8):34–39.

20. 21 U.S.C. 321.

21. *Rust v. Sullivan*, 500 U.S. 173 (1991).

22. See generally: Sugarman, J., and Powers, M., "How the doctor got gagged: The disintegrating right of privacy in the physician-patient relationship," *Journal of the American Medical Association*, 1991; 266:3323–3327.
    Physician's Financial News, 15 January 1992; pp. 15–16.

23. Anderson, K.L., "Deceptive documentation in home healthcare nursing," *Home Healthcare Nurse*, 1992; 10(6):31–35.

SEVEN

Ethics and Law
of Life

TOPICS COVERED

General discussion of the value, Life

A time to be born

Artificial insemination

In vitro fertilization

Surrogate motherhood—adoption

Contraception, fertility control, and technology

Abortion

GENERALLY • HISTORY AND LAW • WHO ABORTS AND WHY • HOW TO ABORT AND WHEN • INTERESTS

Neonates

A time to die

Who dies? The old, the sick

AGE AND DEATH BIAS • LIFE EXPECTANCY, AVERAGES, RISK PROBABILITY

Why do people die? Why should they die?

COST OF CARE • QUALITY OF LIFE • COMPETENCY/CAPACITY

How do people die?

CPR/DNR • WITHDRAWING VS. WITHHOLDING, TREAT OR LIMIT TREATMENT • DEHYDRATION • CASES/THE "RIGHT" TO DIE

What is death? What is dying?

PVS • BRAIN DEATH AND HIGHER BRAIN DEATH

When do people die—and who chooses?

NAZA EUTHANASIA • KILLING: ASSISTED SUICIDE • OTHER-KILLING: EUTHANASIA • INTENTIONAL DISTINCTION • SELF-KILLING • POSITIONS OF DOCTORS AND NURSES • THE HOLLAND EXPERIENCE • PAIN CONTROL

GENERAL DISCUSSION OF THE VALUE, LIFE

$\triangledown$

"For every thing, there is a season . . . a time to be born and a time to die. . . ."

—Ecclesiastes 3:1–2

$\triangle$

All of the work, ethics, and law of nursing is founded on the value of life. Some ethics writing emphasizes other values (autonomy, doing good, not doing harm) in preference to the valuing of the patient's life.

The value, Life, underlies the ethics and law of the two topics next discussed: being born and dying. All of the work of nursing is founded on Life and the value of life. If people didn't value life, they wouldn't be nurses. Everything that nurses do is for the life of the patient—even when giving what might be the last dose of morphine, nurses are valuing the life and comfort of the patient.

If one assumes that valuing life is something everyone does, this value needn't be separately discussed. Most of the issues identified under this value might be (and sometimes are) discussed under other values such as Freedom, Doing Good, and Doing No Harm.

The assumption that the value of life is either understood without discussion, or else not among the highest of values, seems to be the case in other texts and papers on ethics. In some, the shift has occurred *against* identifying life specifically as a condition to be valued. Life is not even mentioned as a separate value in some writing about ethics and law.

The authors of those writings might explain that the value of life underlies all the other values, as indeed it does (like self-interest). But among them, there is also a trend to emphasize other values—the patient's choice, or the choice of the surrogate, doing good and not doing harm—in preference to the valuing the individual patient's life.

For purposes of discussion here, Life is divided into two broad areas of time: a Time to Be Born and a Time to Die. It may sound strange to think of "die" as a valued act, but the state of being dead is emphasized as a positive good and preferable to being alive in some conditions, in much of the literature of ethics in illness care. The state of being dead is described as good, contrasted to the process of decline and dying, which is often seen as a period to be avoided if possible.

The specifics of the two topics are different, but nurses will recognize that the philosophical and ethical questions are much the same for issues surrounding both birth and death:

What is a person? When does a person begin to, or cease to exist? What is the value of life compared to other values, especially compared to the value of money? Whose interests prevail when the interests of people conflict (as in whose baby, whose fertilized ova, whose insurance money, whose life, whose death, whose choice prevails)?

Life as a value may also be referred to as "sanctity of life," as some religions teach that life is sanctified or blessed by God. This section of course deals with *human* life, not animal or plant life (those topics discussed briefly in Chapter Three, Doing No Harm).

Some people are characterized as adhering to an absolute value of life—of *all* life, whatever the condition or quality. Others have labeled valuing life a philosophy: vitalism. Still others believe that life should *not* be valued or preserved at all costs, which makes the value of life not absolute, but relative to other values.

The term "quality of life" is heard frequently. The implication of "quality of life" is that lives have different qualities, or different values. Is life more valued to one person, than to another? Are the last, dying days of a patient less valuable to that person, than the first few days of an infant's life? Can a number be put on the value (quality) of life? For one's self or someone else's life? What is a human life worth? (Quality of Life, as a concept, is discussed in the second part of this chapter, A Time to Die.)

The value, Life, could be divided in other ways than by time: by issues, or by whose interests are affected, for example. Because humans have a limited, finite, life span, demarked by two physical changes (birth and death), this chapter divides the issues surrounding the value into A Time to Be Born and A Time to Die. The earlier chapters of this book relate to the span of life between those two markers.

A TIME TO BE BORN

Artificial insemination

In vitro fertilization

Surrogate motherhood—adoption

Contraception, fertility control, and technology

Abortion
GENERALLY • HISTORY AND LAW • WHO ABORTS AND WHY • HOW TO ABORT AND WHEN • INTERESTS

Neonates

The work of helping mothers and babies avoid illness may be more nearly "health care" than is any other nursing work.

Artificial insemination, in vitro fertilization, and surrogate parenting, raise ethical and legal questions:

Use of technology to manipulate life.

Cost of the technology and who pays.

Parentage of the child (who "owns" the child and who is responsible for it).

Whether the result of a "perfect" child justifies whatever means are necessary to produce it.

What nurses do is give illness care, but care at the time of life around birth appears better to deserve the title "health care" than any other kind of care. Even here, however, nurses and doctors work to prevent illness (complications) and to deal with them if they occur. The only reason a midwife, nurse midwife, or doctor is needed at the birth of a healthy baby to a healthy woman is to deal with what might go wrong. Midwives and doctors and nurses who work with mothers and babies do not make things go right (don't make people healthy), but they may help people who are healthy to keep from getting sick: Giving immunizations to a "well baby" is a perfect example.

Ethical and legal issues around the beginning of human life include artificial insemination, in vitro fertilization (and use of fertilized ova), surrogate motherhood, abortion and use of aborted babies, infant mortality rates, addicted babies, women's reproductive interests, and disabled babies' treatment (or not). Note that none of these issues is about the healthy, "normal" sequence of events.

Of the values that will be discussed in this section, the first is the value, Life (the life of the fetus/child or woman). The value of freedom (autonomy) is also important within this value, for the woman or parents or surrogate—and sometimes for the nurse. And, the value of doing good (beneficence) for the ill, poor, or handicapped is present. The value of being true (loyalty), perhaps to one's sex or to one's image as a person, may also be raised within discussion of this value.

The topics discussed under Life: A Time to Be Born may not be practice issues for all nurses, only for those nurses who work specifically with those patients. But the topics in this section about the beginning of Life are concerns of all citizens, including nurses, and are part of the ethics of illness care. It is appropriate that nurses be leaders among the citizens who shape the ethics and law in these areas.

Artificial Insemination

As generally understood, "artificial" is something that humans cause—it does not come without human action. Using the *artificial* versus *natural* distinction here, as in most other areas where "artificial/natural" terms are used, is unhelpful, however.

Under *Artificial Insemination* (AI), sperm in semen is delivered to the cervix by "artificial" means (means other than sexual intercourse). Artificial insemination (AI) uses either the husband's sperm, a donor's sperm, or donor *and* husband's sperm; about 30,000 babies a year are born as a result of AI. Clinics run by ethical people use one donor for only ten women, to reduce the odds of half-brothers and -sisters unknowingly meeting, marrying, and reproducing. Such practice recognizes the human fear of breaking the incest taboo.

Incest (sex between members of the same family) violates all known ethical codes. (In the royal families of ancient Egypt, brothers and sisters married; they were considered immortal and had to marry other gods—the only other gods were their family.) In-family marriage (or incest) tends to emphasize genetic defects because mothers and fathers who are related have similar genes. The odds are greater that recessive genes inherited from both parents will be present, combine, and produce the defect carried by both parents.

The ethical and resulting legal responsibility of the agency providing semen is to check the semen donor to be sure he is free of HIV, hepatitis B, and other infections. He should be rechecked after several months to verify that he was not latently infected at the time of the first check (the sperm was frozen at collection).

Clinics have not only a higher ethical but a minimum legal duty to screen donors for disease: 44 percent of clinics test for HIV, 28 percent for syphilis, 26 percent for hepatitis, 12 percent for cytomegalovirus (CMV), and six percent for herpes. One legal case has held that CMV transmission from donor sperm could produce liability.[1] And, as in adoptive proceedings, clinics must obtain personal information about a donor's family, health history, and possible genetic diseases.

Once semen is donated, it is frozen and stored in a sperm bank. As would be expected, sperm conceivably carrying desirable, specific genetic traits is also stored. There exists a sperm bank of Nobel Prize winners, seen by some as an attempt to do "eugenics" (see Eugenics, below). One goal of the Germans of the 1930s National Socialist government was to produce a superhuman (a super race) through eugenics. Even if semen and records are kept securely by such banks, can society tolerate the use of a "superman's" sperm for multiple inseminations? What if a supply of John Kennedy's sperm were available, and many people wanted to have him as their child's father? Martin Luther King? Ronald Reagan?

Fertility clinics' potential for fraud exists. It is here where ethical ideals such as using sperm for a limited number of pregnancies, are enforced as the minimum ethic of law.

> A formerly respected physician was charged with using his own sperm to impregnate many women at his clinic.

Further potential for ethical violations, leading to legal (civil and criminal) punishment, occurs as hormones are injected to make women test positive for pregnancy (increasing a clinic's rate of success and the patient's satisfaction). Later, when the "pregnancy" fails to develop and menstruation commences, the women is told that a spontaneous abortion occurred.

Artificial insemination requires services and goods (it's expensive), and usually it must be repeated many times to produce a pregnancy. It is an elective procedure, not necessary to the health of the potential mother or father, except perhaps mentally. Some health insurance policies pay for AI; and, due to lobbying by some affected people, state laws have been passed that mandate insurance companies include AI whenever group coverage is offered.

If a particular health insurance pays for AI, other members of the insurance pool see their premiums increase for what some would consider "unnecessary" care. A couple with six children might object to paying for AI for others trying to conceive. (At least, such a couple will be insured for a service they are not likely to need.) Is the single woman, past menopause, to be mandated to share the cost of couples' baby attempts? In states where such insurance coverage is mandated (and all pay premiums for it), the conception of children by their "natural" parents is obviously considered an important social good. However, if a basic level of care were mandated through a national health insurance or system, such a question would be urgent. In the future, if all are mandated to buy insurance, an issue may be whether AI should be covered in a reproductive health care basic benefits package.

Such a mandate is not a new idea. Payment of taxes in effect mandates that all pay for (buy insurance for) illness care of the poor, the elderly, and certain other groups.

On the other hand, if AI is not in a package of basic benefits—and if a global cap on "health care" spending limits the amount that can be spent totally for such care in the United States—then even individuals who can pay for AI out of pocket might be prohibited from buying the service (limiting their freedom). This is because, under a global expenditure cap, people allowed to buy AI reduce the amount of money that can be spent elsewhere, on other people and other sicknesses.

An issue arises as to whether it is "fair" to spend money on something like AI that is not necessary to life or physical health, to satisfy some couple's (or woman's) desire to propagate their own genes (there are children of other parents to adopt). If insurance pays for AI, the entire group of premium payers will bear the increased cost.

The Roman Catholic Church opposes artificial insemination on the grounds that AI removes the sex act from procreation. The Church sees procreation as the reason for sexual intercourse in marriage.

The technology of artificial insemination would appear to give women (married or single) equality in having a child. With AI, single women can have babies without having heterosexual sex (without having to deal with a man who would then have rights in or to the child). Associated is the issue that has arisen as to whether lesbian couples should have the right to conceive a baby (one of the couple, at least) and raise a child.

The issue of fairness to the child is often raised: Is it fair to the child to grow up in a single-parent household without the benefit of a father? Would the child be better off *not* to have been born at all?

If artificial insemination is available for a price, and not paid for by mandatory insurance schemes, then the poor will be denied reproductive opportunity; and at least two levels of opportunity may result. On the other hand, prohibiting artificial insemination involves government in private affairs again.

The ethical questions are: Do people have a right to seek to have their own genetic child or a "perfect" child? Do they have a right to spend their money on that attempt? And/or, do they have a right to force other people to help pay for it?

In Vitro Fertilization

In the early 1980s, the press hailed in vitro fertilization (IVF): the ability of medical science to provide means for a baby to be conceived outside its mother's body. *In vitro* means "in glass" (*vitro* is the Latin word for "glass"); *in vivo* is the opposite (meaning, "in life"). In vitro fertilization occurs literally in a glass container: The ova are flushed from the woman's ovaries with doses of fertility drugs that cause several ova to mature at the same time; the ova are retrieved, placed in containers, and then sperm are introduced, resulting in hoped-for fertilization.

The same fertility drugs are used in infertile women to stimulate ovulation, a process that often results in multiple births. Over two million women have taken such fertility drugs since their development. Until recently, the only side effects known were temporary bloating and mood swings. However, a Stanford University report[2] has raised the possibility that women who took the drugs, even decades ago, show a three times greater risk of ovarian cancer than women who did not. The risk was greater if the drugs were taken and conception did not occur. (The risk of ovarian cancer is not high in any case.)

About 15 percent of attempted IVFs result in pregnancies (about the same rate of success as *not* using IVF). Gamete intrafallopian transfer, in which the egg and the sperm are introduced through laparoscopy into the fallopian tube for fertilization, is said to be successful about 26 times out of 100 efforts.

IVF is an even more expensive procedure than AI because of the drugs, the procedure to retrieve several eggs, the fertilization, and the implanting.[3] The same arguments arise about the ethics of insurance—forcing others to pay for the process, or preventing individuals from spending their own money for it.

The Catholic Church, among other entities, opposes in vitro fertilization techniques. In order to get at least one viable zygote (fertilized ovum), usually four are fertilized; opponents say that, at that point, several potential humans exist in the dish.[4] To increase the odds that fertilization will take place, all of the zygotes may be implanted in the uterus. If all survive implantation (now they are embryos), either there will be a multiple birth or a selective abortion of all but one (the procedure can cause loss of all embryos). Destroying the others, whether implanted or in the dish, raises the same issues as abortion.

Comment: Although it can be argued that not even *one* baby would have been born had the procedure not been done, the argument may rest on whether one believes it to be "God's will" that people have children—and whether the creation and birth of one child justifies the destruction of others.

Fertilized ova can be frozen and thawed with no apparent damage and used later. If a couple freezes zygotes and later separates or divorces, however, an issue arises as to who gets custody of such fertilized ova. Are the ova considered children, with the attendant legal rules and procedures, or are they classed as property, to be divided according to those laws?

In a Tennessee case, zygotes fertilized in 1988 were sought by their "father" in a divorce proceeding; he didn't want his ex-wife to have them implanted. The Tennessee Supreme Court gave the zygotes to the ex-husband. According to news reports, he then had the zygotes destroyed.[5]

Regardless of which one of the "parents" had gotten "custody" (or owner-ship), the other theoretically could be made to be a parent against her or his will years after donating the cells. Legal cases on the issue have differed. Because the technology hasn't been available for long, the law is still devel-oping—true of many issues where ethics (thus law) and technology interface in illness care.

After having "consented" to contribute half of a person, may one with-draw consent? Perhaps some sort of "advance directive" can be made, incorporated in a prenuptial or pre-pregnancy agreement: "If we divorce, then the following should happen to my zygotes." The same conditions could be imposed on adoption, precluding a biological parent from later reversing consent and wanting the child back. The unwed father has rights attendant to his child when the mother of the child gives the child up for adoption (see the discussion below, The Father's Interest).

The same conditions could also be imposed relative to an abortion deci-sion: Once the conditions for pregnancy are set up, a person could be deemed to have "consented" to be pregnant and prohibited from reversing the consent. Women who did not consent to sexual intercourse would still have an abortion option (not having consented to creating a pregnancy). Pregnancy is in some sense a legal "servitude" of the woman's body; whether involuntary or not is arguable, depending on the circumstances of the intercourse that risked the pregnancy.

In the frozen zygote situation, the parent with custody or ownership doesn't require anyone to be pregnant (a surrogate mother can be used). But the noncustodial person could still be made a "mother" or a "father" invol-untarily.

Other ethical and legal issues are possible if a woman can't produce her own ova. Donation of oocytes from another woman produces a situation similar to AI; but the donation process is more difficult than sperm dona-tion.[6] Allegations that clinics "stole" fertilized ova from couples in their care, and implanted them in other women, add to the legal and ethical tangles the procedures have produced.

Eugenics

Cystic fibrosis is the most common genetic illness, occurring in about one in 20,000 births among Caucasians. Zygotes fertilized in vitro from couples at high risk for cystic fibrosis were tested; researchers were able to isolate the noncarrier (desirable) zygotes from a larger sample. Other genetic de-fects—such as Duchenne's muscular dystrophy, sickle cell disease, hemo-philia A, and Tay-Sachs disease—could also be detected.

The procedure is expensive: The prenatal (pre-pregnancy) exam costs about $12,000, on embryos of eight cells or less.[7] This is arguably better tim-ing than testing after pregnancy commences, when the fetus is 11 to 16 weeks old. At that point, a positive test for CF could produce a difficult decision about abortion. Women and men with inheritable defects will be more willing to risk parenthood if testing can be done before the pregnancy begins.

If the technology improves, prospective parents who want to be sure their baby has no defects could routinely do IVF and have DNA testing, even if they could conceive without it. Then the defective zygotes could be weeded out before implantation.

In future, will only the poor have "defective" children? If so, future generations will be able to tell who was born to poor or careless parents: anyone with a disease that could have been detected in the embryo stage. Rich people's embryos with handicaps will be aborted; poor people's will be born—changing the meaning of "advantaged" and "disadvantaged."

Human zygotes have now been cloned, although the zygotes are not long-lived. Such cloned zygotes could be used to help infertile couples who have difficulty in obtaining many ova to fertilize, or whose sperm infrequently fertilizes an ovum. One ovum could be fertilized, and then many copies cloned to implant. But unless the rest are aborted, many identical babies will result.[8]

If some very great people are identified, and the technology exists to clone them from a cell—should it be done? Is this a form of immortality?

Surrogate Motherhood—Adoption

A woman who deliberately delivers a baby whom she knows she will not keep is called a surrogate mother. The term *surrogate* mother is applied only to the woman who deliberately conceives and/or carries it to term in behalf of a designated person or couple. For whatever reason, the term "surrogate mother" is *not* applied to women who have babies to give up for adoption to an agency, or to some other unknown person; such a woman is called the *birth* mother, *biological* mother, or "natural" mother (in contrast with *adoptive* mother).

Aside. The phrase *surrogate mother* is sometimes first encountered in psychology courses, in terms of wire forms used to simulate monkey mothers in Maslow's experiments on the effects of non-nurturing.

In surrogate motherhood various arrangements are possible—the mother can be artificially inseminated with the sperm of the man who will eventually obtain the child (it's *his* genetic child). Or a zygote from a couple can be implanted (it's *their* genetic child). The couple could be characterized as "renting" the surrogate's uterus; the couple could be seen as buying the baby, or buying the woman's time and risk.

Note that, in discussing this issue, instead of using *uterus, womb* is the emotion-loaded "motherhood" word preferred by opponents of the procedure. *Womb* suggests a time (only about 100 years ago) when it was thought the sperm contained the whole of the genetic material—that the woman was merely the bearer of the man's "seed," containing all of the material of the baby (as in "she bore him a child").

It is argued that surrogacy exploits poor women for the benefit of those who can afford to pay. Are surrogates different from other people who rent their body or mind for work?

People who wish the state to stay out of the private areas of sexuality and reproduction may also oppose surrogate motherhood, but laws regulating surrogacy are government intervention in that arena. Opponents of surrogacy worry about the "sanctity" of motherhood, the relation of the mother to child, and the mental health of such women who give up their babies. Are these the same issues that concern opponents of abortion?

The issue of what happens when the resulting baby is "defective" in some way remains unresolved. If neither the couple nor the mother wants the child, it may be given up for adoption. If the baby can't be adopted, the state (taxpayers) might pay for the care. Should the surrogate mother and potential parents contribute to the cost of care?

If that reasoning were carried into adoption generally, a woman who puts a baby out for adoption might be obligated to pay for the baby's care if unadopted. Since the mother "started" the baby and carried it to term, she's responsible (she could have had an abortion instead). It can be assumed she's benefitted by upholding her personal moral values in not aborting the baby.

Major legal and ethical difficulties surface when the surrogate mother decides to keep the baby. As a result, legislation has been written in several states which bars or restricts contracts for commercial surrogate births. Such laws may forbid surrogate motherhood, or forbid it for pay, or forbid the rights of the people who paid for the care of the woman during pregnancy. In Virginia, prospective parents can present the surrogacy contract to a judge, and obtain court orders declaring the paternity (and maternity?) of the baby to be born. Florida and New Hampshire screen would-be parents and surrogates.

Court Cases on Surrogacy

Some highly publicized court cases have explored the issues of whose the baby is; results have been mixed. The baby has been given to the genetic father and his wife (over the genetic, surrogate mother). Genetic parents have been awarded custody over the surrogate mother who was not related to the baby under the legal theory that intentions matter (not a new idea in law, but not usually applied to a case of this kind). And the baby has been "awarded" to the surrogate mother. Usually some kind of joint custody and visitation rights are given to all parties. It has been suggested that a solution like Solomon's be tried: Faced with two "mothers" arguing over the child, the judge ordered the baby cut in half, one for each woman. The real mother was identified when she asked that the thief be given the baby (to save him). Solomon gave her the child instead.

Attitudes of Couples and Surrogate Mothers

Preliminary studies show that the couples and women involved are happy with the arrangement. They seem to be mentally normal people (as much as can be measured by tests), before and after the event. Several of the surrogate mothers express an altruistic motivation, enjoyment of the pregnant state, and a feeling of giving life. The women studied are mostly Caucasian (there are more babies available to adopt in the black and hispanic populations). Surrogate motherhood—when done for pay—is expensive, and thus the practice tends to occur in the population most prevalent at higher income levels.

The Center for Surrogate Parenting in California has arranged 300 surrogate births since 1980. Lawyer brokers who arrange surrogate contracts may be legally in the same position as private artificial insemination clinics, so they have a duty to screen donors for disease. Such a center may be held liable for injuries to surrogate mothers who are infected with diseases from sperm carrying viruses (see above for possible liability of AI clinics as well).[9]

The people who want a baby, and the woman who bears the baby, both have interests (*bear* means "to suffer" and it also means "to carry"). The baby, too, has an interest in the proceedings. Should this interest be the paramount concern when conflicts arise between the adults?

Adoption and Precedent

The ethical issues and interests of the parties to adoption are similar to those of surrogacy, and the law is developing in similar ways. The courts struggle with a familiar question of the relative importance of "genetics" versus "environment" (the nature-nurture debate). Questions include the "best interests" of babies raised by parents of another race or gay couples, or mothers past menopause who are pregnant with a donated ovum. (An irony: Little question is raised when a man of that age fathers a child by a younger woman.)

Some question whether it is "fair" to babies who at 21 years of age will have a mother who is 80. Some assert that children have a right to parents of a certain age range, and certain attitudes. In contrast, questions usually are not raised when abortions are committed because of mixed-race parentage; or when a lesbian woman has an abortion; or when a 49-year-old aborts a child inconveniently conceived. A lack of controversy on these issues may be revealing. Is the assumption that life with such parents is such a problem, that no life for the child is preferable to life in such situations?

Despite the technical differences, surrogacy and adoption are not new phenomena: Women have given away their babies for millennia. In the Old Testament, Rachel has her handmaiden Bil'hah become pregnant by husband Jacob, and then Rachel "bears" the child when Bil'hah delivers—the sperm is considered the whole child; the female merely carries:

> . . . she [Bil'hah] shall bear upon my knees, that I [Rachel] shall have children by her.
>
> —Genesis 30

In earlier times in the United States, a childless couple might be given a baby to raise by a relative who had several—an arrangement beneficial to both families. But people do not now usually live in small groups and families—technology both separates and unites all. Things that worked informally when people knew each other in small groups (tribes, families) become both complicated and contentious now that they are strangers. Today, people must rely on formal laws, instead of ethics, to make them do the right thing.

RESOURCES

Annas, G.J., "Fairy tales surrogate mothers tell," *Law, Medicine and Health Care*, 1988; 16:27–33.

Callahan, D., "Surrogate Motherhood: A Bad Idea," *New York Times*, 20 January 1987.

Hanafin, H., "Surrogate Parenting: Reassessing Human Bonding," a speech presented at the American Psychological Association (APA) Convention, 28 August, 1987.

In re. Baby M, 537 A.2d 1227 (N.J. 1988).

Contraception and Technology

Ethical and legal questions about contraception continue regarding the use of technology and its effect on attitudes toward children, and about differential fertility (the controversy that some groups have "too many" children relative to others).

Contraception is a shortened form of the two words: *contra* ("against") and *conception*.

Some feminists and others oppose the entire technology of reproduction and believe the "problem" is contraception technology. For others, contraception itself is an ethical issue. The issue is about artificial contraception;

abstinence from sexual intercourse is contra-conception in a "natural" sense. But, as noted earlier, artificial versus natural is an unhelpful distinction.

At first glance it may appear that not much ethical conflict about contraception exists—an impression soon dispelled.

Under the heading of Eugenics—a movement to improve the human race—questions abound regarding contraception and fertility. In a political context, people worry whether the "lower" classes (poor, disadvantaged, underclass are some labels) are overpopulating—historically a common worry of early promoters of contraceptive freedom for women, including Margaret Sanger, the founder of Planned Parenthood. Her intent was to provide contraception freedom for poor women, to reduce the numbers of babies born to that (assumed inferior) class.

Overpopulation seems of less concern in the United States and other developed countries, since market forces and better economic conditions have resulted in a natural voluntary decrease in the birth rate. The theory is that as people get richer and more secure, they have less need to have babies to work to support them in their old age.

Many countries in the world continue to experience birth rates far in excess of the developed countries. Population control or fertility decrease may be desired in those countries. When working on aggregate fertility (of whole populations), however, one is confronted by problems of differential fertility (one or some groups more fertile than others). This consideration may be unstated, but it often underlies political decisions made about contraception, population policy, and control of fertility.

Some examples of differential fertility:[10] Hispanics in the United States have a higher fertility rate than Caucasians; Israelis have a high birth rate, perhaps because the Arab birth rate is high; Serbs excused killing Muslims in Bosnia, some say, on grounds that the Muslims are outbreeding them; in the Kosovo, Albanians do have a higher birth rate than the Serbs; Christians in Lebanon are said to fear their country has a Muslim majority (so they won't allow a census to confirm it); Nigeria has problems with censuses (fear of the results?) because of differential growth of different groups; Singapore's initial eugenics policy in 1984 failed, it is stated, because of the resentment of less educated and poorer groups (the majority Malay).

Pronatalist (pro-birth) policies have existed in France, East Germany, Russia, Japan, and countries with below replacement fertility (about 2.1 offspring per woman). The opposition party in India (the BJP, which may one day rule the second most-populous country in the world) worries that Muslim populations are growing faster than Hindus (Hindus practice family planning). In the United States, the population control organization Zero Population Growth (ZPG) has addressed the problem of differential fertility.[11]

Is there a "human right" to reproduce? Yes, according to the United Nations Universal Declaration of Human Rights (1948), Articles 16 I and

16 III. Others say there is no right, at least not without some concomitant duties and responsibilities.[12]

In seeking differential fertility control, poor and non-Caucasian women are often targeted. The birth control movement in the United States before WWII coincided with the Eugenics movement. Contraception for poor and minority women was cited as way to improve the "quality" of the population. Differential population control by the Germans under its National Socialist government made people in other countries wary of such policy—applicable as well to the issue of euthanasia.

Norplant as Contraceptive

A new form of contraception resulted in controversy. Norplant (on the market since 1990), a new way to deliver a long-term contraceptive, eliminated the daily choice to take a daily contraceptive pill. The implant contains six rods or capsules filled with the hormone levonorgestrel; as of 1993, 780,000 American women had the drug implanted.

With devices such as Norplant, new methods open doors to governmental policy. Judges in California and Texas have made the implanting of Norplant a condition of probation for women convicted of child abuse. Several states have considered legislation mandating the use of Norplant by women convicted of certain crimes, or have considered incentives to get poor women to use it (to cut costs of welfare and Medicaid).

But a California court overturned a judge's use of Norplant as condition of probation. The higher court said the probation condition (insertion of Norplant) was unrelated to the underlying offense (child abuse). Courts in Kansas, Florida, and Ohio have ruled against similar probation agreements. The California court said the Norplant order impinged on fundamental reproductive rights. The Center for Reproductive Law and Policy (a spin off of the American Civil Liberties Union), believes "gender, race and class bias" come into play in such cases.[13]

Complaints about Norplant were also about its cost to buy initially, with need to also pay for insertion and removal five years later (but the cost was half that of equivalent oral contraceptives for five years).[14]

Another problem: Some social-planning technology to prevent conception (such as Norplant) will not prevent AIDS/STD, as condoms are promoted to do. Teenagers are not likely to use condoms if they have Norplant to prevent pregnancy.[15]

The use of Norplant in India's family planning program has been criticized.[16] The country's leaders desire to decrease the fertility rate from 5.4 to 4.0 births per 100 women per year, and to increase contraception use from 35 percent to 50 percent of families. But family planning is unpopular in India's four *Bimaru* states (Hindu slang for "sick/poor"). Forced surgical sterilizations were done there during India's population control "National Emergency" in 1976 and 1977.

Women's groups in India were against the USAID proposal to include Norplant as a fertility control. They said the contraceptive was "untested and harmful" and that unfit U.S. drugs were dumped on India and other countries in the second world.

DEFINING "THIRD WORLD"

"Third world" may be an outdated phrase: The developed/Western countries were considered the first world, the Communist countries the second world, and the rest, the third world. Since the collapse of the Communist bloc, terminology is shifting to two "worlds"—the first world (still the developed West) and second world countries (former Communist and less developed nations).

Another implication of such long-term and effective contraception is this finding: Childlessness, or having a child after 30, increases the risk of breast cancer. Women in such groups have a 50 to 100 percent greater-than-expected risk of dying from breast cancer. This situation has recently been noted in women managers and professionals—but it has been known since the eighteenth and nineteenth centuries, when scholars observed an excess of breast cancer among Italian nuns.[17]

Fear of Technology

Technology allows both birth control and abortion to be done safely and relatively easily for the woman. The technologies of contraception, AI, in vitro sterilization, and abortion may cause a money value to be put on children, however. Technology allows having children when and in numbers one can "afford." That power raises the issues of whether it is fair that "the rich" are able to have more children than "the poor," and whether it is fair for some to be able to have fewer.

People who oppose *all* technology echo long-existent feelings that technology is both wonderful and threatening.

"Luddite . . . One of a band of workmen who (1811–16) tried to prevent the use of labor-saving machinery by breaking it, burning factories, etc.—said to have been so called after Ned Lud, a half-witted man who about 1779 broke up stocking frames."[18]

Ancient peoples' ambivalence toward technology is symbolized in the Greek myth of Icarus, who invented wings made of feathers and wax (high tech). He then flew too high (another lesson), melting the wax and crashed.

Some feminists worry that contraceptive technology separates sex from procreation and allows choice about when and if to have children; thus they echo the Catholic Church's opposition to contraception.

The argument of some feminists is that a woman using the technology of IVF cannot be certain that the baby is really *hers* (was there a mixup, accidental or deliberate?). By creating the same uncertainty about paternity (maternity) that men have always endured, it is asserted that women will, like men, develop the need to dominate. Such an argument assumes, first, that men *do* intentionally dominate (and that women do not); and, second, that this reproductive uncertainty is the cause of it.

Another feminist argument against technology in reproduction is that separating a woman from procreation separates her from her "original" and "elemental" power of life. That separation gives men the power to reproduce, which, it is argued, men have always wanted. Technology in reproduction makes children into products, with different prices and different values to society. Is this true now of abortion, especially of disabled babies?

Abortion

> Abortion has become more an ethical and legal issue since improved technology made the procedure cheaper, safer for the woman, and more accessible.
>
> Abortion ethics and law illustrate that the law is a minimum and not the highest ethic; the procedure is legal, but many believe it is not ethical.
>
> Nurses who assist with abortion should have engaged in assessment of their personal values.
>
> In a democracy (and in most other systems of government) attitudes of the people determine the ethics of abortion (and eventually the law).
>
> The labels used in the abortion debate are used for both their emotional *and* non-emotional effect.

Abortion is the technical word used for expulsion of a fetus, either spontaneously (naturally) or induced (artificially). The controversy about abortion is over *induced* abortion, made more possible by improved technology. Here is another area of ethics and law in which controversy arises from practice: The ability to do abortions as a practice—easily and safely. Before technology made abortion safe, cheap, and accessible, the issue was less intense. Few women had abortions because they were dangerous and costly and difficult to obtain (not only because they were illegal) as a practical matter.

Within the abortion issue is most clearly seen the overlap of law with ethics, and the movement of the law from a higher to a lower ethical standard. The law of the United States allowing abortion is seen as unethical by many—but so are laws restricting abortion.

The issue of abortion centers around the value of life, of the child; also involved is the value of freedom (autonomy) of the woman. Doing good (beneficence) may be invoked as a value (no "bad" life for an unwanted child). The value of not harming (the baby/fetus) may be invoked. Finally the value of being true (loyalty) may be involved—loyalty to the tribal norm (whatever the norm or custom of this tribe).

The values of a people are explicit in what they do. And some believe that people demonstrate what they value by what they protect.

> In our time, the intellectual and moral norm is to regard a baby seal as of infinitely more worth than a human fetus.[19]

Nursing Considerations in Abortion

Nurses whose practice is performing or assisting with abortions will have already done intense thinking about their work in the context of the values in this book. Other nurses, too, will have thought about their attitudes toward the morality of abortion, as well as their position on its legality.[20] Any nurse may have as a patient a woman who has had an abortion, and who may have a need to resolve feelings about the event, even years later. Nursing as a profession should address abortion in the context of the values in this book: valuing life, valuing freedom, being fair, being true, doing good, and not harming.

Abortion is reflective of issues surrounding women and their sexuality and its expression. Even at the height of the sexual revolution some realized there was a down side:

> The freedom of women to be involved (sexually) hasn't always been accompanied by the capacity to protect themselves when they are.[21]

Research in 1982 said that men and women differ on the reasons they give for engaging in sex. Women give as motives for sex: love, commitment, and emotion; men more often say their motives are pleasure, fun, and physical reasons.[22]

In another time (1946 nursing ethics book), *lack* of sexual freedom was seen as a problem. Sexual repression was thought to cause abortions (because women didn't know how to prevent pregnancy), and to cause failed marriages (because girls and boys were often segregated and didn't "know" about each other).

> "Deaths, ill health, and lowering of racial stock . . . are only part of the bad effects of our [unfree] attitude toward sex." [MATERIAL IN BRACKETS ADDED].[23]
>
> Note the reference to eugenics prevalent at the time in the phrase "lowering of racial stock."

Too much sexual freedom, or too little, depending on the time and the problems. Unless one adopts a "present perfect attitude," one might wonder what a nurse of the year 2046 will think of the problems and philosophy addressed in *this* book.

Data About Abortions

A 1936 source estimated that 400,000 illegal abortions were performed that year in the United States, with "several" thousand deaths. Married women were estimated to comprise 90 percent of the women who aborted illegally.[24]

In some states abortions were legal in the United States before 1973. After *Roe v. Wade*, when the U.S. Supreme Court ruled that abortion could not be restricted by state law during the first three months of pregnancy, the numbers of abortions increased. But before that decision, in 1973, 744,600 *legal* abortions were reported in the United States[25]; in 1985, there were 1,588,600. In 1973, 19 percent of pregnancies ended in abortion; in 1985, 30 percent of pregnancies were aborted. The rate of abortion has decreased in recent years.

In a democracy, attitudes of the people will eventually determine the ethics and thus the legality of abortion. Among black people, 45 percent believe abortion on demand should be legal (as now); 42 percent believe it should be legal in some circumstances, but with more restrictions than at present; 13 percent believe it should be totally illegal.

Among white people, 49 percent think abortion on demand should be legal as now; 42 percent think that it should be legal but with more restrictions, and nine percent think totally illegal. (People are not actually white or black; but more brown or more pink.)

Among women, 47 percent want to keep abortion on demand legal (as now); 40 percent want it more restricted; 11 percent want it to be illegal. Among men: 51 percent want unrestricted; 38 percent more restricted; 8 percent illegal.

Percentage of the public approving abortion under various circumstances: *Over* 50 percent approve abortion for maternal health, fetal defect, rape. *Under* 50 percent approve abortion for financial problems, unmarried status, family size.

About 50 percent of abortions are done in the first eight weeks of pregnancy; 90 percent are done by the first 12 weeks, and fewer than one percent after 20 weeks. This one percent is the percentage of pregnancies that the Missouri statute required be tested for viability (ability to survive outside the womb), that statute being upheld by the Supreme Court in the *Webster* case.[26]

Twelve percent of abortions done in 1985 were funded by the taxpayer. Who pays for abortion has become an emotional and political issue in the 1990s. Many private health plans fund abortions. Some who oppose abortion object to being made to help pay for it—but people who oppose war must help pay for it; and for IVF; and for heart surgery for 90-year-olds.

The law is a minimal, agreed-on compromise about an ethical issue. Thus, while it is law for all, of necessity it does not encompass all behavior that is ethical; in every case, some people will find some law (or the absence of it) to be unethical. The current law which prohibits states from restricting abortion in the first trimester is a good example.

People who believe this law to be unethical, wish to make the law conform to their ethics. When and if they do, the law will then seem unethical to other people who favor keeping the law as it is.

Abortion for any reason is legal during the first three months of pregnancy, everywhere in the United States. A majority of people believe the law should be different (see survey above). Men are the only subgroup in which a majority (51 percent) wish to keep the law as it is now, abortion on demand during the first three months.

Words Used for Effect

As noted above, the words for the human cells before fertilization are *ovum* (oocyte) and *sperm* (spermatocyte), and the word for both is *gametes*. After they unite, the result is a *zygote*. When implanted in the uterus, the result is an *embryo*. When the practitioner can see with ultrasound at eight weeks, or hear heartbeat with a doppler stethoscope at ten weeks, the term used is *fetus*, until the time of delivery.[27] In lay speech, people talk about the baby in utero, but the word *baby* is loaded with connotations, such as person and human being.

Some people insist that the only correct word to use at any time before birth is *fetus*. Other people insist that *baby* is the only correct word. Fetus has been a less–emotionally loaded word than baby, but as *fetus* becomes the correct word to use for an unborn baby, the word comes to carry all the emotions attached in the past to "baby"—the "thing" referred *to* has not changed.

In abortion discussions, the word *woman* is often used in place of *mother*, which also has many connotations. Traditionally, "mothers" do not kill their "babies" (but—see History and Law, below—some have).

The terms that proponents and opponents of abortion use are examples of using words for political and emotional impact. Pro-abortion, anti-abortion, pro-choice, pro-life—"anti"-anything sounds negative; "pro"-anything sounds positive. The people against abortion have adopted the term "pre-born child" to remind (or convince) others that the fetus is a child before birth.

Words are especially important in law. Under the U.S. Constitution, live human beings (whether called fetuses or babies) have no rights unless they are deemed persons. The fetus does not become a person under the Supreme Court's decisions until somewhere between viability and birth.

Other kinds of law recognize some earlier personhood, and thus provide remedies for injury to the fetus. For example, lawsuits can be brought for manslaughter, damages, and criminal acts to "viable" fetuses (see Legal History below).

History and Law of Abortion

> Some induced abortions have been performed throughout human history (as has infanticide).
>
> English common law punished aborting a "quick" child (from the time the mother felt its movement).
>
> U.S. state statutes from the mid-1800s prohibited abortions in order to protect women from the dangers of abortions.
>
> Several states in the early 1970s were in process of changing statutes to allow for abortions under some conditions.
>
> The U.S. Supreme Court, in 1973, declared a fundamental right of privacy that prohibited states from interfering with abortion during the first trimester; that allowed states to regulate abortions during the second trimester to protect the woman, and to regulate abortions during the third trimester to protect the fetus.
>
> In later decisions the Supreme Court let stand a Missouri statute that prohibited abortions after viability, and the Court rejected the "rigid trimester framework" while still holding to the essential holding of *Roe* (that states cannot completely prohibit abortions).
>
> A symmetric definition of death, and life, would have life begin and end with the same criterion: either brain activity, or higher brain activity.

Termination of pregnancy before delivery has been going on since women first got pregnant. Spontaneous abortions, occurring without intentional human action (also called miscarriage), have always existed. And there have always been some abortions induced by human action, using drugs, violent falls, or other physical interventions like insertion of various materials through the cervix into the uterus.

Ancient Persian herbalists knew of abortifacients, and they also punished abortions under the criminal law. Abortions were aided by some doctors in ancient Greece because part of the Hippocratic oath of that time promised that ethical doctors would *not* do it:

> "I will not give to a woman a pessary to produce abortion; I will not give to a woman an abortive remedy."

Both Plato and Aristotle discussed and approved of abortion. The Greek Pythagoreans, who were also against suicide, opposed abortion because they believed the embryo was "animate" beginning at conception.

St. Augustine (Roman Catholic bishop 396–430 A.D.) distinguished between *embryo inanimatus* and *animatus*. He wrote that the embryo was formed and alive at 40 days for a male, at 80 days for females. Aborting an *embryo inanimatus* presumably would not have been a sin.

Infanticide, also a reality of history, is sometimes cited to justify the present practice of abortion. Plato recommended killing infants born defective (born disabled) to a greater degree than would fit into his ideal world, and societies have controlled birth rates by killing children of the wrong sex, characteristic, or handicap, at birth.

In Roman times, a baby market existed in which unwanted newborns were left at a place commonly understood to be where one could get a child. The word for that practice, *exposition*, may have been wrongly interpreted as being that these children were left exposed to the elements; instead it may be that such babies were on *exhibition*. Children left there might be taken and raised by slaves or the poor or others who didn't have a child.

Children were wanted at one time in history for economic reasons. They were a source of free labor and thus added to the family's wealth more than their cost. This was true in the rural United States into the twentieth century. Exposition in Rome may have been infanticide, but it also may have functioned as an adoption agency when demand for infants was present.

During the Middle Ages some babies (who usually slept with their nursing mothers) were suffocated when the mother "overlay" them (accidentally or deliberately). The poor or people with too many children also had the option of putting children in the local monastery or church.

Another incidence of infanticide, closer in time than the Middle Ages: The Chinese, whose aim is to control their population, order abortions for women pregnant with the second baby. It is also relatively common in that country (which values boy babies for many social reasons) to kill the girl baby at birth. In a report on China's "missing girls," ultrasound was said to be available widely for sex selection, and female infanticide still practiced; producing a ratio of 114 boys to 100 girl babies born.[28]

China plans a policy "to avoid new births of inferior quality and heighten the standards of the whole population." People with congenital illnesses or defects which are inheritable are candidates for abortions, sterilizations and marriage bans. They do not promise to do euthanasia (infanticide) on handicapped babies, but do observe that "more than 10 million disabled persons who could have been prevented through better controls." They warn that 300,000 to 460,000 disabled children are born annually in China, and this could be disastrous economically and to the "quality standards of the population."[29]

Infanticide is not just a Chinese practice.[30] Is the practice of aborting female fetuses when a boy is wanted (or vice versa) and aborting fetuses identified as genetically defective, using the same rationale, but earlier?

Legal History.   Most of the states in the United States inherited the common law of England as their first laws, in the early 1800s. Texas, whose state abortion law was struck down by the U.S. Supreme Court in *Roe v. Wade*, established English common law principles in that state in 1840. Under that English-originated law, aborting a "quick" child was a capital offense. Abortion before quickening was not indictable. Quickening occurred when the mother could recognize movement, between 16 and 18 weeks. The concept of "quickening" is related to the use of "viability" in American law.[31]

In the United States, the laws criminalizing abortion were passed in mid- and later 1800s with the purposes of discouraging illicit sex, protecting maternal life from the usually septic techniques used to abort, and protecting prenatal life. The statute that was struck down in *Roe v. Wade* was passed by the Texas Legislature in 1854.

By the 1950s all U.S. states prohibited abortions unless to save the life of the mother; Alabama and the District of Columbia allowed abortions for danger to the mother's health.

Then, a trend in the state legislatures toward liberalizing their abortion statutes resulted in 14 states changing their abortion laws by 1973, to allow abortions under some conditions. (See the numbers of abortions performed legally in 1973, above.)

In 1973, the *Roe* decision struck down the Texas statute by saying it violated personal, marital, familial, and sexual privacy.[32] The Supreme Court found a right of privacy in the U.S. Constitution; the right, not written specifically in that document, was found to exist in the "penumbra" (poor light of a shadow) of all the rights written in the Bill of Rights.

The *Roe* decision did not find an unqualified right to abortion in the Constitution. It did say that privacy, which includes abortion, is a "fundamental right." That means that a state would have to have a compelling interest in order to pass a law restricting abortion in the first trimester (first three months).

The state would have to prove that it passed such a restriction only because there was *no* less-restrictive way to achieve its compelling interest. In constitution talk, this means that the state can't pass a law restricting abortion in the first three months because there is virtually no state interest that compelling. And if there were, almost always *some* less-restrictive way could be found to achieve whatever was the state's interest.

In the second trimester (second three months), the state could regulate abortions in the interest of the mother's health. That is, the state can require abortions be done by a doctor, in a hospital.

In the final trimester, the state could consider the fetus or baby's interest. In shorthand:

First trimester: No state interest.

Second trimester: State can protect mother's [health] interest (require standards for the procedure).

Third trimester: State can protect fetus or baby's interest.

In 1979, the *Webster* case, cited above in Data About Abortions, upheld a Missouri statute that required doctors to assess for "viability" before performing an abortion, if the pregnancy was in its twentieth week or later (normal gestation period is 40 weeks). As of this writing, the earlier limit of survival outside the womb—and therefore "viability"—is 24 weeks.

The rationale for the 20-week restriction is that, if the date of the last period date is mistaken, the estimate of gestation can be off by four weeks—that the baby might really be 24 weeks old and thus viable when a 20-week abortion is done.

At 24 weeks gestation, about 25 percent of fetuses survive; at 25 weeks, 60 percent live; at 26 weeks gestation, 80 percent live. By gestational age of 29 to 30 weeks, about 90 percent will live.[33]

The U.S. Supreme Court has *not* said when life begins, or even when a fetus becomes a person (which could result in a constitutional protection of fetal life at some point). The Court did come close to such a definition in the *Webster* decision, upholding a bar on abortions after "viability" (at 24 weeks).

An informed discussion on the time of beginning of life, or even person-hood, is beyond the scope of this book. However, the fetus is *alive* according to any meaning of the word. (Some pro-choice advocates point out that cancer cells are alive, too.) The real question is whether the killing of the fetus is to be equated with killing a person.

Symmetry is a word for a theory in which the same test of life is applied at both extremes of life: Death of the organism (and of the person) occurs when the brain stem is dead. That's the current legal definition of death in most states—total brain death.

At the other end (that's the symmetry), the life of the organism and life of the person might be defined as starting when brain stem function starts. Brain stem function in the fetus starts 8 to 12 weeks after the last menstrual period (6 to 10 weeks postconception). Abortion done after that time could be considered murder, and made illegal.

But if the definition of death is moved back to the time when the *cortex* of the brain is not functioning ("higher" brain death), then [symmetrically] the "life" and personhood of the baby would begin later, when the cortex of the fetus's brain starts to function.[34] (See also the discussions of "new" definitions of death under A Time to Die, the latter half of this chapter.)

If one's next question is about *which week* of pregnancy starts cortical function, one is assessing this theory by the result (by what the result of its application will be) rather than whether the concept is a logical one. One is looking to the practical ends (At what week will abortion be forbidden?) rather than the means or the principle to use (What logical test will decide when life begins?).

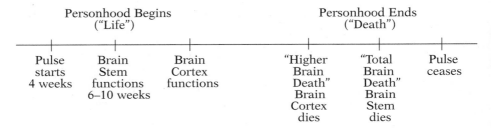

Personhood Begins ("Life")			Personhood Ends ("Death")		
Pulse starts 4 weeks	Brain Stem functions 6–10 weeks	Brain Cortex functions	"Higher Brain Death" Brain Cortex dies	"Total Brain Death" Brain Stem dies	Pulse ceases

Another definition of "viability" is developing (a definition other than the accepted one of "ability of the fetus to survive outside the womb"): A Catholic newsletter notes the assertion that "the anencephalic fetus, though living from the moment of conception, will never achieve viability." By that it might be assumed that viability meant survival for a certain length of time outside the womb, or survival in certain neurological health.[35]

In 1992, in *Planned Parenthood v. Casey*,[36] the U.S. Supreme Court reaffirmed the "essential holding" of Roe: There is some limit on the states' powers to prohibit abortions. But the Court also said "we reject the rigid trimester framework." A state may encourage a woman to know that there are arguments in favor of continuing a pregnancy, and may assure that she knows "the consequences for the fetus" of abortion; and that her right to an abortion may be "burdened" but not "unduly" by the state's restrictions. What constitutes an "undue burden" (a "substantial obstacle" to the woman's choosing of abortion) will be decided by the Court in future cases.

In 1993 the U.S. Supreme Court let stand the Mississippi abortion law, passed in 1986 but not applied because it had been challenged in court since its passage. Like the Massachusetts and North Dakota laws, girls in Mississippi who are under 18 now must get consent from both parents before an abortion can be done. Twenty other states require that at least one parent give permission or be notified.

Under the now-applied Mississippi law, a judge can waive the consent requirement *if* the minor proves she is mature, informed about the abortion, or proves her parents shouldn't be told because they are abusive. If the judge refuses, the minor can request a state Supreme Court review. She needs only one parent's permission, if they are separated or divorced, or if one parent is "unavailable."[37]

U.S. Supreme Court Justice Ruth Bader Ginsburg has said she supports "choice," but she once wrote that the Roe decision

> . . . fashion[ed] a regime blanketing the subject, a set of rules that displaced virtually every state law then in force. . . . A less encompassing *Roe*, I believe, might have served to reduce rather than to fuel controversy.[38]

Through the years, decisions on laws subsequent to *Roe* have changed the prohibitions outlined in that case. Some state statutes have restricted where abortions can be done, required procedures to notify parents and husbands, required some delays, and required explanations of the development of the fetus and alternatives to abortion. Some states have passed laws restricting abortion to cases of rape or incest. These will be considered by the Supreme Court, too, unless *Roe* is expressly overturned. If that is done, any restrictions on abortion will be determined by vote of each state legislature. This is being done now, with *Roe* still in effect but not "rigidly" so.[39]

Abortion Law Outside the United States

Most industrialized countries do not prohibit abortion, but do regulate the practice. Ireland is an exception, along with some of the eastern European countries, which have returned to more restrictions on abortion after having a system of abortion on demand under Communism. Many of those countries are Catholic; the religion and its expression, including feelings against abortion, were repressed under Communism.

In 1993, Germany's highest court ruled that country's new abortion law unconstitutional because it does not protect the fetus. The legislature must rewrite the law it wrote in 1992, establishing a compromise between the laws of what were formerly East (abortion on demand) and West Germany (abortion only in restricted circumstances). The 1992 law permitted abortion during the first 12 weeks of pregnancy, but it required counseling at least three days before.

The German court said a pregnant woman must be counseled that she has an entitlement to government-provided support if she continues the pregnancy. *West* Germany formerly had one of the more conservative abortion laws in Europe; more permissive laws were in effect in France, Britain, Italy, Austria, Belgium, Netherlands, and Scandinavia. As noted, Ireland bans abortion entirely, and laws protecting the fetus to some extent are in effect in Spain, Portugal, and Switzerland.[40]

In 1993, the Polish Senate approved strict limits for abortion. This was seen as a defeat for the Catholic Church, which had supported a total ban. Divisive debate about the prior abortion on demand law began in 1989 when the Communists were toppled. The new law allows abortion when the mother's life or health is seriously threatened, when the fetus is badly deformed, or when pregnancy results from rape. This law, one of strictest in Europe, will virtually end abortion as commonly practiced under Communism.[41]

Among the industrialized countries, only the United States allows abortion on demand during the first trimester. Most countries require physician certification that the abortion is for a reason other than birth control. Some countries forbid abortion after the first trimester. Some require delay and furnishing information to the woman seeking the abortion—like the Pennsylvania law considered in 1992 by the Supreme Court (*Casey*, above).

The United States has another abortion distinction: It is the only country in which abortion on demand was made legal by judicial decision. The current law permitting abortion on demand during the first trimester, was not established in the United States by legislative vote and the usual legislative process of compromise.

After *Casey* the U.S. Supreme Court seemed unlikely to outright overturn *Roe v. Wade*. Some states were enacting further limits on abortion, and some were not. The process of legislation, halted in 1973, began anew and will continue.

A problem seen by some abortion proponents is that state laws vary, so women will be able to get abortions freely in some states, not in others. People who are unable to get an abortion in their own state, may not be able to afford travel to another state. Court decisions will not change that situation; even now women in some states have little or no access to abortion, because few clinics in their state do the procedure.

No matter what the outcome at the Supreme Court level, people will still disagree about the abortion issue. The *Roe* decision did not stop the disagreement, and the continued reducing of its scope or even its overturn will not stop the disagreement either. The issues must be debated, and compromise reached, if any law is to be accepted.

The law is a minimum ethic, and not the full text of ethical behavior. People *could* agree that abortion is wrong ethically, but the law might not punish abortion at some early stages of pregnancy, and/or for some reasons such as rape or incest. People who believe that it is unethical to abort at any stage for any reason could still believe that, since ethics is always about how people *should* behave, not how they *must* behave. More focus could be placed on the immorality of abortion, leaving it legal at some stages and for some reasons. To equate immoral behavior exactly with illegal behavior is dangerous, because then behavior that is legal will be seen as moral behavior also.

Realizing that law is the minimum, and ethics is the ideal, and compromising on what is to be the law, is the difficult, painful, unsatisfying, democratic process. Nobody gets to win it all (as they do in court). Everybody gets to win a little (as they do when they don't go to court). They can agree on a solution even if it's not exactly what each side wants.

Who Aborts and Why

> The reason for the abortion is important in some countries, where laws permit abortion only for specific reasons. In the United States, virtually no restriction is placed on the reason for abortion; abortion may be done for disability, sexual preference, or convenience.

As noted, in some countries the reason for aborting is a factor in whether abortion is allowed. Through amniocentesis and other sometimes easier tests, much can be known early about the pregnancy—early enough to choose an abortion if the news is bad.

What is bad news? Bad news might be that the baby will be developmental disabled, or anencephalic, or with a genetic defect that will cause pain, or a defect that she may transmit, or that she has a gene for homosexuality, or that she's a she.

Sonograms can tell the sex of the baby; studies show that they are overused and usually make no difference in health, and that *not* doing them on every pregnant uterus might save $1 billion a year.[42] In one sense, sonograms are "baby's first picture." Some businesses are even doing the video/sonograms in studios, without any medical interpretation—they zoom in on testicles in utero and add a caption for home viewing: "the family jewels."[43]

The sonogram estimates the age of fetus; and that could make abortion safer for the woman. Since the sonogram tells the sex of the baby, if a girl is wanted and not seen, there is time to abort. If the logic for allowing abortion is to protect the woman's choice, does the logic extend to choice to abort for sex selection?

Amniocentesis (examination of the amniotic fluid in the pregnant uterus) detects conditions of the fetus during pregnancy. This information may influence the decision to abort for some conditions (producing controversy about those reasons). Prenatal diagnosis was used as early as the 1960s, to detect fetuses with gross chromosomal defects.

Couples can routinely have amniocentesis and genetic testing to determine whether they or the fetus carry genetic problems likely to be passed on to their children. A project is underway to map the entire human genome structure; this may make possible diagnosis of many other problems in utero or before pregnancy, in the parents of potential babies.

Genetic reasons given to abort are many now, and they are increasing. Tests are available to the woman who is pregnant, to determine whether her baby has Down's syndrome, or fragile X, both of which cause mental retardation; or another genetic condition that might be undesired in her child. In most cases the results are available early enough to abort.

Amniocentesis is necessary to make determinations in many of these conditions; amniocentesis is available only if the practitioner will do it. Practitioners vary on their willingness to do amniocentesis, depending on the age of the mother and the reason she wants the test. Usually practitioners limit amniocentesis to mothers of age 35 and over, since they are the group most likely to have Down's syndrome babies. Limiting such services is an ethical issue for both practitioners and patients. (The subject of patient demand and practitioner autonomy was discussed in Chapter Four.)

In the late 1980s, a survey of doctors in various countries revealed that 78 percent of doctors said they would do amniocentesis on a 25-year-old who was anxious, with no other medical indication for the amniocentesis. In a mother that young, there is a 0.50 percent risk of losing the baby as a result of the amniocentesis, but only a 0.13 percent risk of having a Down's syndrome baby.[44]

As more is known about genetics, chromosomes, diseases, and babies before birth, the numbers multiply of conditions that can be "prevented." Is the *condition* actually prevented—or, is the birth of the baby with the condition?

In a study of almost 27,000 pregnancies, 84 percent of the amniocenteses studied were indicated, due to risk of a chromosomal disorder. The median maternal age was 36 years. Of amniocenteses done, 1.5 percent revealed chromosomal abnormality; 73 percent of those pregnancies were terminated. Severity of the genetic disorder affected the decision; autosomal abnormalities (mental retardation) caused termination in 92 to 95 percent of cases. Of babies identified as having sex chromosomal abnormalities, half or fewer were aborted. A high proportion of couples finding abnormalities terminate the pregnancy. The degree of clinical severity predictably influences parental decisions.[45]

Amniocentesis and other tests for genetic abnormalities are available; abortion for those abnormalities (or for normality) is legal. Social planners wishing to reduce costs might encourage or suggest mandates for women to have such tests and abortions if the test is positive.

The issue: Is it right to allow a handicapped child to be born, if it can be aborted (is it right for the child who may suffer, right for the society that might have to pay for its care)? A related question: Is it right to have children who carry chromosomes that will in the future present a risk of genetic defect? In 1930s Germany, under the National Socialist government, people possibly possessed of a genetic defect were forcefully sterilized, so the issue of aborting their children never arose.[46] (See discussion of sterilization, below.)

Society might admit that abortion is for the parent's own good, that the energy and strength and money cost of a handicapped child are more than some people can bear. (Is it more than the society can bear?) If so, perhaps that should be said, and *not* clothed with the insistence that the "interests" and "rights" of the child-to-be are being protected.

Under current U.S. law, economic/cosmetic/purely personal reasons for abortion are enough. Women who have abortions cite all as reasons. Unlike a century ago, children are no longer seen as economic assets, contributing wealth to a family; they are enormous economic costs—almost luxuries.

There are sexual reasons given to abort. In India (and in other countries), some pregnant women who have an amniocentesis choose to abort when they find the baby is a girl/female. The feminists of India are particularly offended by this, as are others; they call for a ban on abortion when done for that reason. Infanticide of female babies is widespread, and ultrasound is available, even in remote villages, for use in identifying female fetuses so they may be aborted.

In India a baby girl is a liability, the dowry needed to marry her successfully a big expense. Boys are needed to do physical work on the land; and having a son, in India, is a form of "social security" for his parents.

Doctors offering selective abortion are assumed to believe that antenatal diagnosis of sex, and selective abortion, is preferable to allowing the pregnancy to continue if there is the risk that the infant will be killed or mistreated. (On the other hand, is "risk" preferable to certain death by abortion?)

An observer comments that it is curious that Westerners condemn abortion of female fetuses in India, which is done to save the family enormous expense; yet the abortion of babies of either sex for relatively "trivial economic difficulty, psychological strain, or social inconvenience" is not condemned in the West.[47]

In the survey mentioned earlier, of doctors about amniocentesis, 34 percent of U.S. doctors said they would test for the sex of a fetus. The hypothetical conditions given to the doctor were that the couple wishing amniocentesis had four daughters, and planned to abort if the fetus turned out to be the fifth daughter instead of a desired son.[48] Should the prohibition of sex discrimination be extended to fetuses?

Discrimination is prohibited against the disabled (who *have* been born); and selectively aborting disabled fetuses might be considered discrimination as well.

How to Abort and When

The technology of the procedure affects the ethics and law of abortion (for example, whether the procedure is done early or late, whether perceived to cause pain to the fetus, or whether done with a "morning-after" pill that makes it difficult to regulate).

The physical techniques of abortion limit the timing of abortion. The technique used early in pregnancy is dilating the cervix and suctioning out the contents; later abortion must be done by dilatation and curettage (French for using a curette to scrape out the contents of the uterus).

Still later, when the fetus is too large to dissect with the instrument and remove through the minimally dilated cervix, a solution is injected into the uterus through the cervix. Labor is induced, causing the baby (fetus) to be delivered vaginally. Or the fetus is extracted except for the head, which is decompressed by suction and then delivered. All these require some anesthesia, sterile equipment, and skilled practitioners.

States laws that require an abortion to be done in a hospital have the effect of limiting the availability of abortions. Fewer places for abortion would be available, with the result being fewer abortions done; advocates of such laws say that women deserve the protection of abortion procedures done under strict standards of care.

The contraception method of intrauterine devices (IUDs) is thought to work by causing the fertilized egg to fail to implant after entering the uterus from the fallopian tube. Some abortion opponents oppose to this method of contraception for that reason, while others oppose all contraception, except abstinence, on religious grounds.

Still others oppose abortion, but not contraception. As in labeling any diverse group of people, it is hard to characterize all anti-abortion or pro-choice people. Pro-choice leaders do fear that losing the abortion right at the constitutional level would encourage opponents of birth control to mount forces against that technology as well.

More Technology. A drug has been developed and used in Europe to accomplish early abortion without the necessity of the above techniques. Called RU486, the drug is given orally; and then, 24 hours later, pro-staglandin is administered to cause uterine contractions and expulsion of the contents of the uterus. The drug must be given under supervision, as complications are possible (but not usual).

RU486 can be used during the first weeks of pregnancy. It was developed in France by Roussel-Uclaf SA (majority owned by Hoechst AG of Germany). The company sought FDA approval to market the drug in the United States, where a boycott of its considerable other business might result, by people who are pro-life, anti-abortion.

The drug is 99 percent effective; a system using oral prostaglandin results in reduced risk of failure and simpler administration. With the drug alone, three percent abort; with prostaglandin given 48 hours later, 61 percent abort within four hours and 33 percent later (added together, about 97 percent effective). In another study, a second smaller dose of prostaglandin is given if the patient has not aborted within four hours of the initial dose. That whole procedure results in abortion in 99 percent of pregnant women. Likely the two-dose process will be used in the United States.[49]

If opponents of abortion conduct a boycott, ethical questions will arise regarding whether it is ethical for people to enforce their own moral vision of keeping a drug off the market, by a boycott or threatened boycott. The same issue arises regarding whether one should enforce moral attitudes by boycotting lettuce because it was picked by nonunion people, or try to influence the pro-life owner of a pizza chain by boycotting the pizza, or seek to change the alleged sexist attitude of a brewery management by boycotting its beer.

Pharmacists may face ethical problems in filling a prescription for a drug to be used as an abortifacient (the same issue faced in filling prescriptions for drugs prescribed for suicide in Oregon, discussed in the next half of this chapter). The issue is whether druggists have the right to refuse to fill prescriptions that patients will use to commit suicide, or that might be used to poison another person, or to commit an abortion.[50] Are pharmacists who refuse imposing their personal values on the patient, or upholding personal ethics in not participating in what is believed to be killing?

State statutes provide "conscience clauses" in abortion law that prevent job discrimination against nurses who refuse to assist in abortions. Some have suggested these clauses must be extended to cover nurses who refuse to assist patients to suicide, and to cover nurses who refuse to assist in dehydrating patients who are not dying. (Legislatures have generally not written such clauses for those situations.) Perhaps pharmacists will seek legislation to protect those whose conscience exceeds the minimum ethic of the law.

Another controversy in the abortion debate is over late abortions. Of the 1.5 million abortions per year, about one percent (about 15,000) are done after the twentieth week. If they are not killed in the procedure, these babies may still be born alive—and, if they breathe spontaneously, the practitioner must make the decision whether to support them or allow them to die.

As noted at the beginning of this value, the nurse who works in this field must do some "values clarification" about her role, whether her patient be the woman who does not want a live baby, or whether responsibility extends to the child. Other nurses who may care for patients who have had an abortion must examine their own attitudes also. Law may require minimum responsibilities, but law—in this and many other issues—does not solve the problem of the practitioner's ethical choice.

INTERESTS

> The interests of various parties to the abortion decision must be considered; the practitioners right/duty to inform of alternatives to pregnancy and abortion, the woman's interest in not having a child, the father's interest in protecting his child, the child's interest in life (or in not being born into danger or a "bad" life).

The Practitioner's Interest

Regulations of the Republican administration under President George Bush required health professionals to tell any pregnant woman requesting information on abortion that abortion was not considered a method of family planning.

Some state statutes, which mandated what practitioners must say to women before abortion, had been struck down on grounds that they violated the privacy right; the privacy within the practitioner/patient relationship was upheld. In these the Supreme Court found, by narrow majorities, a privacy right in the Bill of Rights (although it is not specifically written there).

When the Bush regulation was challenged, the Supreme Court upheld it in *Rust v. Sullivan*.[51] The Court did not find a privacy interest in that case (nor in *Webster*, cited earlier). The lack of a fundamental privacy interest meant the federal government did not have to show a *compelling* need for the regulation (only a reasonable need). And, it meant the government did not have to show that there was no other possible way to achieve its goal.[52]

Some practitioners felt that the confidential relationship of practitioners to patients was jeopardized by this decision: that the freedom and responsibility to give women information about abortion when indicated was jeopardized. Contrary arguments were made: That this was not an unusual exercise of employer control over policy; that such regulations about what patients are told or what treatment is to be provided, are necessary to the agency's interest.

The Bush administration changed its regulation again, in March of 1992, *allowing* physicians (but no other practitioners) to counsel patients in such clinics about abortion. This distinction between professionals raised further ethical issues, such as whether professional autonomy is more important for physicians (whether the patient-practitioner relationship more important in that profession than others).

The regulation was changed again in 1993 by the Clinton administration, allowing *all* practitioners to counsel abortion in federally funded family planning clinics. The *Rust* decision could still cause ethical problems, for example if some future administration wrote a rule instructing practitioners to advocate abortion as a birth control measure to patients.

Abortions actually do control (prohibit) birth. They are not contra or against conception, because they do not prohibit conception; instead they deal with its consequences. Some women use abortion instead of contraception as birth control (only 43 percent of women seeking abortion had been using birth control prior to the pregnancy).[53]

The Father's Interest

The value discussed here, under the father's interest, is fairness (justice). His interest is in fair treatment under the law (fair, relative to treatment of the mother). The issue is how much weight will be given to the father's interest (when, if ever, his interest takes precedence over the mother's interest in being free from pregnancy and a child). The father also has an interest and some legal remedies when his child is placed for adoption. He has some interests in visitation and contact with the child, if the child is not aborted (and, he has some financial responsibility).

An unmarried father's interest was not given much weight by the U.S. Supreme Court in *Michael H. v. Gerald D.* Justice Scalia wrote a plurality opinion (meaning that not all of the majority of justices who voted against the father, joined exactly in Scalia's reasons). The Court upheld a California court in its decision to refuse to grant a paternity hearing to a man who had a daughter with a woman married to another man (the child of a married woman is presumed to be the child of the husband). Justice Scalia said that the only Fourteenth Amendment liberty interests to be upheld were those "traditionally protected" and that states had not given such protections to an "adulterous natural father."[54]

The Woman's Interest

U.S. society values greatly the right of the individual because it is a pluralistic society, compared to others. U.S. citizens are not of one tribe—their individuality therefore is inevitable, a product of that plurality (not a choice arbitrarily made). Individuality is the philosophical base of the value placed on freedom (autonomy). The value most important for the pregnant woman in the abortion issue is also the value of autonomy (the freedom to be pregnant, or not to be, after conception).

In extreme negations of their autonomy, women and men have been forced to undergo sterilization—in 1930s Germany, because they carried undesirable genes; in the United States, as recently as the 1970s, because they were mentally "defective." Earlier in the twentieth century, and prior to the awful example of the Germans under the National Socialists, the laws of 29 states of the United States allowed forced sterilization of "feeble-minded persons."

> A respected nursing ethics book, published in 1946, stated: "Many people are ignorant of this danger to our social stock and the expense to the state in supporting defectives whether in or out of institutions."[55]

Between 1907 and the early 1960s, 60,000 "mental defectives" (including people considered retarded, criminals, prostitutes, rapists, epileptics, inebriates, the insane) were sterilized in the United States. Blacks, immigrants, and poor people were special targets.[56] Even a nominee for U.S. Surgeon General, Dr. Henry Foster, performed such sterilization as late as the 1970s.

Other violations of the interests and autonomy of women: Women have been forced to undergo cesarean sections because the life of the baby they were carrying was in danger, even though that surgery put their own lives in danger. But some courts refused to order surgery in such situations.[57] Women have been kept on life support for weeks, although seemingly brain dead, so that their babies could develop longer. In such a situation the woman was literally a life support system for a baby.[58]

In history there is a tradition of "fetal rescue," sometimes at the woman's expense. It is told that the Greek god of medicine, Asklepios, was cut alive from the womb of his dead mother. Six hundred years before Christ, the Roman *Lex Regia* (law of the king) mandated that, when a pregnant woman died, the infant be delivered abdominally. After the Caesars (emperors) came to power in Rome, the title of the law became *Lex Caesarea* (hence the word for "cesarean" delivery).

Although more dangerous for the woman, cesarean sections are common in some groups: White women have more babies by C-section. Hospitals get more money for them. But the doctor delivering a Medicaid mother gets little more for a cesarean than for a vaginal delivery. The surgery is more convenient (most are done during business hours on weekdays). Sometimes this is for the convenience of the doctor; at other times, for the woman.

The C-section rate for whites is higher than for blacks, higher for college-educated women, and increasing.

The woman's right to work in certain jobs, even one that potentially could damage her child if she conceived, has been upheld by the U.S. Supreme Court in the *Johnson* case.[59] Critics of the company said that its policy was an excuse to keep women out of higher-paying jobs for which they were qualified. It was said that the real purpose of the policy was to minimize the risk to the company of lawsuit. The Supreme Court said that to exclude pregnant or potentially pregnant women from jobs that might harm their baby was discrimination because of their possible or actual pregnancy—and that is against federal law, the Pregnancy Discrimination Act of 1978.

The closer to full development and birth, the more the interests of the baby increase.

The Child's Interest

The child has a major interest—in *living*. However, the child's interest is not self-expressed. Whose interests "win" depends on how much society values the interests of the woman, versus the interests of the baby. The decision may rest on how much adults are valued, versus how much children are valued.[60]

The fetus also has an "interest" in being born healthy. That interest obviously may conflict with those of a pregnant woman addicted to drugs she wants, or feels she needs. Some drug-taking pregnant women have been prosecuted for child abuse, and jailed to prevent their drug use, especially if they've had treatment available, offered, and refused.

Criminal Liability. The fetus also has an "interest" in not being born with damage from alcohol. A Missouri woman was charged with second degree assault and child endangerment, when her son was born with blood alcohol content reported to be in excess of 0.10, the legal level for intoxication. Doctors reported the blood alcohol level to police.[61] Could the mother have sued for breach of confidentiality? (See Chapter Six for the defense theory.)

This case was similar to more widely-reported occurrences of mothers prosecuted when their babies were born addicted to crack cocaine or other drugs; several of these cases have been brought in Florida. Delivery of cocaine (through the umbilical cord) and contributing to the dependence of a minor are the usual charges. Pensacola authorities began arresting mothers who use cocaine in an effort to encourage pregnant women to seek drug treatment before giving birth.

Many in the medical community believe that such prosecutions will drive pregnant mothers away from seeking treatment for themselves or their babies. Such cases publicize the dangers of crack addiction in babies or fetal alcohol syndrome when the mother drinks to excess, but social welfare workers fear that publicity about prosecution will deter the mothers from getting help.

The trend of the law at the appellate level is moving the other way: The conviction of a mother for delivering cocaine to her child through the umbilical cord was overturned by the Florida Supreme Court; and the Connecticut Supreme Court said that doing a cocaine injection before labor doesn't justify taking the addict's child.[62]

Addicted mothers still present problems. If they are unable to help themselves (to choose), some people say the society must choose for them to protect their children. This is based both on a need to reduce harm to the child, and a need to protect society from increased costs of birth of a damaged child.

Related to this, new technology in contraception allows the government to do a "forced sterilization" that is reversible. That is, a judge can (and some have) ordered a woman implanted with a time-release birth control drug (see discussion of Norplant, above). In the particular case, the woman was found guilty of child abuse; and the judge's motive was to protect a potential child.

Recent cases allow lawsuits by children against parents. In former times, the family was seen as a unit, so no individual could assert a claim against another, particularly a child against a parent.

Many states now allow suit for harm in civil liability or for criminal prosecution for an act done to a "viable" fetus. In a state like Missouri, where a statute declares that the life of each human being begins at conception, the question of viability has resulted in litigation.[63]

In Missouri and most states, prosecutors will only prosecute for criminal activity directed against a live "person." Personhood has generally been held to occur at the age of viability, when the child can survive outside the uterus. But contrasted to that, civil liability (money damages) might be assessed for injury to a non-viable fetus later born damaged. That could mean liability for *injury* to a non-viable fetus that survived past the injury; but *no* liability if the injury killed the child (in that situation, a killer would have no liability but an injurer would).[64] Thirty-eight states have established civil liability for the wrongful death of a *viable* fetus.

Contrasted with the right to abort non-viable fetuses, even the non-viable unborn have "rights" that arise under state criminal and civil laws. These include property rights, rights to inherit, and personal rights, which are sometimes recognized by the appointment of a guardian *ad litem* (Latin for a guardian appointed for the duration of the *lit*igation or court case).

A Missouri court held that a child can sue for malpractice occurring even before he was conceived. The negligence was the failure to record the mother's positive Rh factor and subsequent failure to administer RhoGAM after the first baby, which failure caused injury in the second son. That foreseeable harm created a duty to a child not yet conceived.[65]

A similar ruling, in Oklahoma, is significant because it is establishes criminal liability instead of civil liability. Oklahoma's highest criminal court ruled that killing a fetus in a womb when the fetus has developed enough to live outside (at the point of "viability" [23 to 24 weeks]) is homicide.[66] Three other states (Kansas, Massachusetts, and South Carolina) have also abandoned the legal rule once followed across the nation (and in England since the 1300s) and now their law is that a child can be a victim of murder or manslaughter even without being carried to term and born alive.

The Oklahoma court pointed out that the crime did not apply to abortions, but did declare, "A viable human fetus is nothing less than human life." A drunk driver had run into the mother four days from her due date, fatally injuring the baby. The driver was convicted of killing the fetus and she was sentenced to eight years in prison. If it had been her own fetus and she had aborted it under different circumstances, it might not have been a crime.

The baby has an interest in not being exposed to harmful chemicals in utero merely because the mother chose to work in a dangerous place or felt she had to. But a company cannot discriminate against a woman to protect her baby; (see the *Johnson* case, above, under The Woman's Interest.) In the *Johnson* case, the interests of the women were valued over the potential interests of the children.

In some states children can sue parents for negligent or intentional harm; for physical abuse, failure to safeguard, and—in the drug-abusing mother— for negligent or intentional exposure to harmful drugs. Many of such mothers have no money, so the damage awards won't come up very often, but it is increasingly possible. Some suits have been instituted for alleged child abuse "remembered" many years later, increasingly a controversial issue.

A child could sue a drug manufacturer who supplied a defective drug to her mother that caused an injury; by the same reasoning, a child could sue a mother who exposed the child in utero to drugs or alcohol, thereby causing damage. Assault, battery, and outrageous conduct are possible claims; and some courts have held parents responsible for negligence in supervision of their children.

With advances in technology permitting treatment in utero and (in future) genetic correction of problems, the unborn child has an interest in obtaining treatment needed in utero. If the mother refuses, again a conflict of interests between the mother and child arises. The same issue arises if the practitioner recommends during labor a cesarean for a compromised fetus. Cases and practitioners are split on whether surgery may be done to protect the fetus without the woman's permission.

The baby has an interest in being born with the best possible chance to live, whether white or black. African-American babies have lower birth weight than white babies, and the difference is not erased by the social status of the mother or the amount of prenatal care given. Several researchers believe that the numbers used to assess low birth weight should be determined differently for blacks than for whites. Research is needed to determine the cause of low birth weight, since lower birth weight is associated with higher infant mortality.

This racial difference accounts for most of the reason that the United States has relatively worse infant mortality rates than European countries with white/homogeneous populations. In turn, this explains the somewhat lower life expectancy in the United States than in Europe.[67] The infant mortality rate directly affects life expectancy numbers. Studies continue to show that prenatal care does decrease the incidence and cost of neonatal intensive care admissions.[68]

One-third of infant deaths are associated with very low birth weights. The rate of death among low birth weight (LBW) black babies is less than among white LBW babies; but African-American mothers have LBW babies much more frequently than white mothers. Black women who receive no prenatal care have a LBW rate of ten percent (with prenatal care, the rate is two to three percent).

> "Perinatal, neonatal, and infant mortality rates [in the United States] for high-risk pregnancies and for very low birth weight infants are now as low as anywhere in the world. It is only incidence rates that remain unacceptably high."[69]

Contrasted, hispanic women who receive no prenatal care have a LBW rate of 1.4 percent; with prenatal care, the rate is one percent. Differences in genetics and/or behavior within the population of the groups of women must account for this difference.[70]

Infant mortality statistics are interpreted in light of current medical thinking, which regards pregnancy as a pathological condition requiring medical care. To contrast this with another view of pregnancy:

Mexican-American women are the fastest growing minority population in the United States. Comparatively more impoverished than black women, they have even less access to medical care—but the infant mortality in their group is the same as, or lower than, the rates for "privileged European-American women." Good prenatal care is vital, but mothers who do not get it now, may still not get it if it is even more available. Whether genetics or behavior, the question must be answered as to whether the women who don't get prenatal care are different from those who do.

In the Mexican-American culture, the pregnant woman is helped by the community. Other women who have experience in pregnancy and birth gather round, embrace, and support the pregnant female. The African-American mother-to-be, in contrast, is said to be often isolated from "nourishing social relationships."[71] Great technology in the delivery room is not enough, and professional prenatal care is not enough. Support from the community—from the family—can't be bought with tax dollars.

Related to the fact that some women do not get prenatal care—even if it is available and paid for—is that even the well-insured fail to get care that is available; cost is not the impediment. In a study of 1,500 of one company's employees, less than half the employees' two-year-olds had been vaccinated as recommended—although their company's insurance covered all or most of the cost. These findings are about the same as those of HMOs.[72]

Is it wasteful to keep increasing money for prenatal care to solve the problem of low birth weight babies, when evidence shows that *availability* of care is not the problem?

Neonates

The issues about neonates (at the beginning of their lives) are similar to those about very old people (at the end of theirs):

Whether they are fully human (with full rights in the society).

Whether they should have expensive illness care, which may or may not save their lives (considering the "quality" of their lives).

Whether mathematical models that apply to an average (a group of individuals) can be used to predict outcomes or limit or justify care to individuals.

Whether life as a person not "normal" is worth living.

Whether statues should be used to protect individuals at risk of neglect or discrimination from abuse.

More than ever, smaller and younger babies can be saved, and most of them end up healthy and "normal." But some don't. Caring for tiny babies costs a lot, money that some say would be better spent on prenatal care, well babies, preventing low birth weight, and doing immunizations. If it were documented that more money for prenatal care worked, and if the care and money could be transferred from the neonate in the Neonatal Intensive Care Unit (NICU) over to the prenatal clinic—*should* it be?

CPR in the NICU

One study[73] concludes that CPR is not useful for very low birth weight (<1,500-gram) infants. None of the babies that underwent resuscitation in their first three days survived; and only four of 11 lived more than 72 hours after CPR. Three of the four that survived had residual neurologic deficits (one seizures; one residual hypertonicity after meningitis; and one intraventricular hemorrhage). The unspoken question is whether those who survived were better off dead.

Of 49 babies in the study, all but three were already on ventilation, so CPR amounted to epinephrine and chest massage (not very expensive intervention). But the authors suggested from this evidence that infants less than 1,500 grams be given an automatic status of DNR, unless the situation demands otherwise. Critics of the study pointed out the defects in methodology and sweeping generalizations made from inadequate populations.

Predictors of CPR futility in the NICU have been found to include previous CPR in delivery, prolonged hypotension unresponsive to vasopressors, and irreversible septic shock (predictable predictors of mortality/futility).[74]

Ethical Decisions by the Numbers

Assessing survival probability in neonates (much less projecting quality of life for them) is risky business, as neonatal ICU nurses know.[75]

Mathematical models are being developed which will be used to predict mortality risk for newborns. One model, based on admission data for infants weighing 501 to 1,500 grams at birth, used the data to identify neonatal ICUs where the observed mortality rate differs significantly from the predicted rate.

Statistical adjustment methods should be used only with caution (if at all) to rank the performance of neonatal ICUs; predictive models are not validated, and relationships between care and outcomes are not understood.

Mortality risk prediction models do not assess effectiveness or quality of care. Mortality may not be the best indicator of quality; decreased *mortality* may actually increase *morbidity*. Predictive models do not contain all the determinants of mortality risk. "Excess" mortality may reflect risks that the study did not measure, instead of ineffective care. Finally, mortality predictions may not be accurate enough to identify centers with better or worse than average performance.[76] Extreme caution is advised in using predictive models, like APACHE (Acute Physical Assessment and Chronic Health Evaluation), developed at George Washington University in 1985.

> "The performance of these scores does not allow clinicians to apply them to decisions on individual patients. . . ."[77]

APACHE has a sensitivity of 0.5. The sensitivity is the number of "abnormal tests in abnormal populations"; here it is the percentage of times that patients, predicted to die, actually died. Using that test for predicting which patients will die was exactly as predictive as flipping a coin— 50 percent of the time, when APACHE predicted the patient would die, he did.

The specificity of the model is 0.9. Specificity indicates the normal tests in a normal population; here it is the percentage of times patients predicted *not* to die actually do not die. Out of 100 patients predicted by APACHE *not* to die in the ICU, 90 do not. As can be seen, APACHE as a "predictor" may not help with individual patients.

Of babies smaller than 750 grams (22 weeks gestational age), fewer than 20 percent survive and one-third of survivors have clinically important cognitive, sensory, or motor handicaps.[78]

As costs are cut in the illness care industry, it is asked whether newborn intensive care is cost-effective. NICUs are proven to improve the infant mortality—from 20 deaths per thousand births in 1970, down to eight deaths per thousand in 1992. Diverting money to preventive pediatrics is suggested, but these programs have not been proven to be effective (see data on immunization rates above, even when insurance covered the cost).

Some advocate limiting treatment for low birth weight babies, but point out that it's not the cost (small, relative to other expenditures) but a question of priorities. Some ask whether taxpayers' health care dollars should be used only on those with the potential to repay society for their care. Some advocate that care be given only to people who will live to pay enough taxes to make the care "cost-effective" (to those who will be "worth it" someday).

"Should society decide that eligibility for newborn intensive care is to be governed by the potential for economic payback, software would be developed to assign every newborn, not just the very low birth weight infant, an economic quotient. After measuring weight and gestational age, a data bank of school transcripts and tax statements for the graduates of the nursery would be consulted. The minimum score to qualify for care would be adjusted annually to the budget deficit and gross national product. Of course, only infants born to families with no insurance with large copayments would undergo such economic triage. Families with good insurance will always have access to newborn intensive care. Needless to say this software will find its way to all medical contexts."[79]

"Normal"

Extremely low birth weight is linked to moderate or severe development problems, said a Loyola University Medical Center study.[80] Of such babies, 26 percent tested "normal," 23 percent had severe disabilities, and 51 percent had borderline intelligence and language delays. "Borderline" intelligence is that IQ at or above 70, the mental retardation range. If the average IQ is 100, then half the people are below 100 (100, the average, is considered "normal").

Unless future ethicists decide that only "normal" babies of "average" birth weight should be saved, nurses will work to improve the lives of the LBW babies saved. Studies show that in one program, home visits, child development center visits, and parental group meetings increased the IQs of low birth weight infants. Infants whose parents were better educated and had community resources did well, with or without intervention.

Heavier infants (2,001 to 2,500 grams) had a mean increase of 13.2 IQ points over the control group. Eighteen percent of that group had IQ scores of less than 70 (the mental retardation range) and 50 percent had IQs less than 85. Lighter infants (≤2000 grams) in the intervention group increased their IQs by 6.6 points over the control group. Lighter infants with IQs less than 70 showed no difference with intervention. Conclusion of the researchers: It is impossible to predict which low birth weight baby will have lower or higher IQ.[81] Life is indeed like a box of chocolates.

"Neonates"

Newborn children are increasingly being termed neonates (from the Latin for "newborn"). The term may be an attempt to sound more scientific, but it also has the effect (intended or not) of considering the newborn somewhat different from older children. This attitude may make it easier to deal with children born severely handicapped.

The interest of the newborn is assumed to be in living; but some writers on the subject say that the child has no interest that should be considered. It is asserted that the child has no experience (and no thought process), therefore people "outside" of the child may evaluate its fate.

Some might say a severely disabled newborn, such as an anencephalic, has an interest *not* in living but in dying. But, what of the somewhat disabled newborn? In the *Baby Doe* case of the 1980s, a Down's syndrome baby was born with a birth defect (esophageal atresia), which could easily have been (and always) corrected by surgery if the baby had been mentally "normal." At the parents' request, nurses allowed Baby Doe to starve/dehydrate to death in a hospital nursery.[82]

Some insist that the family and doctor should always be able to decide whether a child is too disabled to live, that the law should *not* intervene; but others disagree:

> Legal immunity can too readily feed the destructive dynamic already visible in some physicians' and families' reaction even to minimally deformed children.[83]

The Baby Doe situation prompted federal law requiring whistle-blowing, the Child Abuse Amendments of 1984.[84] The federal statute mandates that states "establish programs and procedures in child protection services systems to respond to reports of medical neglect." Medical neglect is "withholding of medically indicated treatment from a disabled infant with a life-threatening condition."

MEDICAL NEGLECT DEFINED

". . . failure to respond to the infant's life threatening conditions by providing treatment (including appropriate nutrition, hydration, and medication) which in the treating physician's medical judgment, will be most likely to be effective in ameliorating or correcting all such conditions."[85]

Statute: Treatment *can* be withheld in certain situations:

1. When the infant is chronically and irreversibly comatose;
2. When treatment would merely prolong dying;
3. When the treatment would not correct all life threatening conditions or would otherwise be futile in terms of survival;
4. When treatment would be futile in terms of survival, and when treatment would be inhumane. The law also establishes Infant Care Review Committees to review treatment of children and monitor potential abuse. Regulations implementing the statute authorize the Child Abuse and Neglect Prevention and Treatment Program. The regulations parallel and expand on the statute.[86]

Regulations: Medically indicated treatment can be withheld from infants only if:

1. The infant is chronically ill and irreversibly comatose;
2. The provision of treatment would merely prolong dying, would not be effective in ameliorating or correcting all of the life-threatening conditions, or otherwise would be futile in terms of survival (a good definition of futility); and
3. The provision of treatment would be futile in terms of survival and the treatment under such circumstances would be inhumane.

The regulations specifically provide that appropriate nutrition, hydration, or medication may not be withheld or withdrawn. This law is also enforces the minimum value of being true (fidelity); it mandates blowing the whistle on medical neglect of handicapped kids, when appropriate. The law also enforces the minimum values of not harming such children and doing good to them.

> Evidence exists of prehistoric Americans' attitudes, ethics and values, about children born disabled: An archeological site in Florida (Windover) revealed a burial site with the skeleton of a carefully buried teenager. Examination by experts revealed that the teenager had been born with spina bifida, a condition very difficult to care for, even with the resources of today. The child had been cared for and lived several years.

Attitudes toward disabled newborns is mixed:

In 1992, the parents of an anencephalic baby asked the Florida Supreme Court to allow the baby's organs to be removed for donation, before her death. Anencephaly is not curable and is fatal; but for a time the baby eats, moves, and breathes her own. The Florida court refused, the baby died, and the court later addressed the issue, saying that declaring anencephalics "dead" could not be automatic by virtue of their diagnosis.[87] The American Civil Liberties Union said in the case that any "view of life" is inherently religious and that an attempt to establish a clear line between life and death involves improper "religious judgments" (by that reasoning, legislatures may not define death in statute).

A study of 75 nurses, who gave direct care to anencephalic infants in a program of potential organ donors, revealed that an ethical issue for a majority of the nurses was concern about dignity of the life of the infant. The nurses were also concerned about whether the infants felt pain, and that the infants had physiological responses.[88]

When nurses make moral judgments or values they cannot implement, they feel distress. This happens to nurses who care for premature infants allowed to die without intervention, or when decisions are made not to treat children with disabilities.[89]

Use of Aborted Fetuses in Research

Another issue in this area is experiments on abortuses. (A first question might be why the word *abortus* is used, instead of aborted baby or aborted fetus: Is emotion perhaps averted thereby?)

Research using fetal tissue transplants has expanded possible treatment options for several traumatic and degenerative neurologic disorders. However, the expectations of therapeutic benefit to be gained from these methods have been challenged.

Fundamental viewpoints regarding abortion, physical autonomy, and the principle of harm have been raised against continuing research and the use of fetal tissue transplants. The issues of supply and sources of fetal tissue are unresolved. Nurse must clarify their values and ethical position when working in situations in which fetal tissue transplants are used.[90]

In 1988 the Bush administration (anti-abortion) wrote a rule banning the use of tissue from fetuses for research and transplants as a condition to receiving federal money (the ban was reversed by President Clinton in 1993). Use of fetal tissue from spontaneous abortions and abortions necessary to prevent health risks to the mother, are not at issue; the use of fetuses from elective abortions is.

Pro-life people believe that the use of the tissue is immoral; that to benefit some, from the deliberately-caused death of others, is wrong. If women are informed about the use of their dead fetuses for transplant, they may be more inclined to decide to abort. But if they are not informed of the possible use of the fetus (in order *not* to so influence them toward abortion), then their consent is not truly informed.[91]

Reports of benefits to research on diseases like Parkinson's, Huntington's, and diabetes, caused some members of the U.S. Congress to propose legislation lifting the ban. They cited the benefit to individuals and the whole of society from use of the tissue.

As researchers gain more information about genetic problems in utero, there may be more pressure to have aborted fetuses available for use in transplanting genes. Then, might women become pregnant and abort for economic reasons, to sell genes to rich parents for their own babies? Are the issues the same as prohibiting the sale of organs for transplant (except, the organs are not the woman's)? Is the sale of ova the same?

Scientists are working on the possibility of using ova from fetuses (and from corpses and from women in PVS) to use as donor ova, for women who need ova for use in IVF. Ethical questions have been raised about the effect on children who would later know that their biological mother had never been born, or that they were conceived after she died, or that she was a "vegetable."[92]

The State's Interest

Throughout this examination of issues surrounding the time to be born, many "interests" have been considered. Nurses must also consider their interests, both as members of society and as participants in the state.

The word *state* is used to mean "society" (other people, all individuals as a group). *Society* (like ethics) is a word, a construct, and a concept, and so has meaning only as all agree on its meaning. The interest of the state (all people) is in preserving the lives of people without defenses (the original enforcement of "Do unto others").

The question, always, is where to draw the line—when to have the state intervene in family life. The autonomy of the family, the parents, the child, are not absolute; the law prohibits child abuse, drug abuse, sometimes homosexuality, not many abortions, and not contraception. No interests are absolute. The rights of citizens are whatever the people decide them to be, subject to the innate ethical limits people are born with as humans.

"Rights" are only words. They become reality only if people are willing to tolerate, fight for, or enforce them. But a line needs to be drawn somewhere. The line is redrawn by each new election. Together and individually, people draw it anew, every year, every generation.

Draw the line.

_____→

A Time to Die

_____

> *Who dies? The old, the sick*
> AGE AND DEATH BIAS • LIFE EXPECTANCY, AVERAGES, RISK
> PROBABILITY
>
> *Why do people die? Why should they die?*
> COST OF CARE • QUALITY OF LIFE • COMPETENCY/CAPACITY
>
> *How do people die?*
> CPR/DNR • WITHDRAWING VS. WITHHOLDING, TREAT OR LIMIT
> TREATMENT • DEHYDRATION • CASES/THE "RIGHT" TO DIE

What is death? What is dying?
> PVS • BRAIN DEATH AND HIGHER BRAIN DEATH

When do people die—and who chooses?
> NAZI EUTHANASIA • KILLING: ASSISTED SUICIDE •
> OTHER-KILLING: EUTHANASIA • INTENTIONAL DISTINCTION
> • SELF-KILLING • POSITIONS OF DOCTORS AND NURSES •
> THE HOLLAND EXPERIENCE • PAIN CONTROL

The values implicit in ethics and law about dying and death are those of Life, Freedom (Autonomy), Doing Good, and Doing No Harm.

Because strangers (nurses) now care for patients—instead of families who have more information about the patients' situation—the tendency is to treat all patients the same (fairly, but perhaps in an inappropriately intensive way).

The ethical and legal questions—the who, why, how, what, and when—about death and dying are addressed in this chapter. *Where* death and dying happen is important to both the individual and nurse; the *where* of dying is discussed in the context of the other ethical and legal questions. Assuming that the patient's wishes are honored as much as legally possible, *where* death happens is not often an ethical question for the patient. Depending on the circumstance, it may be a very important issue for the nurse (if the patient is to die while in her care or at her hands).

Dying

The values most often mentioned when death is discussed are the values Life, Freedom, Doing Good, and Doing No Harm. The most important value within the topic of death is the value of life. All else being equal, people *act to preserve life*. What may change that action is the value of the freedom of the patient.

People want to do good (beneficence) and to do no harm (non-maleficence). Sometimes they can agree on the right action; if the patient is competent and doesn't want treatment (here freedom is valued)—if treatment will do no good and will actually prolong pain (here not harming is valued)—then people agree that the patient can refuse treatment. In that case, to die is good (dying is valued).

People don't always agree on what to do if the patient is incompetent, however—or in a coma (or "vegetative"), or if the treatment will keep the patient alive, but won't return to the earlier functional level. Nor do people agree on cost limits, nor if the patient is competent, wants to die, but isn't dying.

Even before ICUs and technology and the money crunch, people questioned whether to treat or to limit treatment for the patient. Treating meant a drain on resources. The drain was more personal, not abstracted to a figure like dollars per day for the ICU bed, or percentage of GNP. The drain was whether the family could or would spend its time and money on someone who was not going to recover, or be a functioning member of the family if she did.

Physically and technically, people in past times couldn't get some of the treatments possible now. Ventilators were invented relatively recently, to prolong breathing for people with lung disease. Tube feedings were not available in times past, to provide nutrition to people who couldn't be fed orally. Now that these technologies can be used, however, the conflict is over whether they should be.

Strangers

The family has turned the care over to strangers, who do the care for money. That means the nurses (the strangers) don't know the patient the way the family does; they may not know that the patient was a happy, busy grandparent until the stroke two days ago. They may not always know that the patient had been lying in a nursing home without family, without cognition, for months before that stroke two days ago.

Nurses don't have all the information that the family would (if there were a family); therefore, they tend to treat all the patients similarly or nearly the same. The value expressed at this level is being fair (just). But treating all patients the same means treating all *intensively*, since strangers can't judge quality of life for another stranger. Trying to be fair, nurses treat them all as extensively as possible, until someone says stop.

Who Dies? The Old, the Sick

Since all people die (and all old people die), the attitudes toward dying and death (thus the ethics and law) are related to attitudes toward old people.

Only about five percent of people over 65 are in nursing homes. Many conditions associated with being old are not the result of aging, but of treatable disease.

Agism is defined as bias against people merely because they are old; numerous examples of the bias are found in life in the United States.

The periods of dying and dying people are avoided or not accepted fully in U.S. society; the term "end of life" is used instead of "dying," possibly because the former implies that people can choose to end their lives when they wish (and avoid the dying process).

Old people die. (No one has ever been proven to have lived beyond about 115 years of age.) Younger sick people and injured people die, too, but much of the worry about death is equated with being old. Not all sick or injured people die; but *all* people who are old eventually die (thus, all people eventually die). The lucky ones live to be old before they die. To understand the ethics and law of dying, the values held about being old should be examined—being "old" and being "dead" are nearly synonymous to some.

People can easily believe that the old go "away" to nursing homes—out of sight and out of mind. They know that the dying go to hospitals (the great majority of people die in the hospital or nursing home, not at home). The undertaker takes them away in the night, they're cremated or embalmed, the casket is closed, and many never confront a dead body. Some people keep their children away from funerals so that they won't be upset by the reality of death.

Nurses should know better than that about the old; they work with the old, the sick, the dying. With any insight, they know that they too will one day be among them, aging, dying, and dead. But nurses' views can be skewed, too; depending on where they work, old people may *all* seem sick, or all sick people may seem old (neither is true).

It is easy for nurses to forget that not all old people are sick, and the population in general forgets that all of the old do not reside in nursing homes (only about five percent of the elderly population do).

Aging is not a disease; people don't get old by being sick. Advertising promotes the idea that people who take care of themselves (for example, who buy certain products) won't get old, implying that people who do get old must have done something wrong. The opposite is true: People live to be old because they do some things (a lot of things) right, or they are lucky. Being young is not the alternative to being old—being *dead* is.

More research is being done on aging, now that a large percentage of the population is reaching middle age and facing old age. The research finds that many conditions associated with being old are not the result of aging itself, but of diseases than can be treated.[93]

Despite the reality that a large segment of the population is old, subtle and overt biases against the old are apparent—defined by Alex Comfort as "agism."

AGISM DEFINED

". . . the notion that people cease to be people, to be the same people or become people of a distinct and inferior kind, by virtue of having lived a specified number of years."[94]

—Alex Comfort

Aging (and illness and death) are realities, but the various media do not express that reality. Old people are not depicted realistically in the ideal media world. A study by researchers at the University of Dayton reported that old people are "no better represented on TV today than they were in the 1970s." They report that only 34 of 1,446 television characters identified were 65 years old or older. Only Andy Griffith, Angela Lansbury, and Estelle Getty portrayed leading characters who were at least 65. Might this be one reason the public thinks "better dead than old"?[95]

Another writer asserts that only two of 100 commercials contain older characters. Of 265 articles on aging in a large midwestern newspaper, none dealt with older people active in communities; all dealt with the "problem" of age. A poll cited found that the majority of Americans believed that "most people over 65" were not very "sexually active, not very open-minded and adaptable," and "not very useful members of their communities."[96]

American Nurse (a nursing newspaper published by the American Nurses association) labels without comment some very negative-sounding data as "facts you should know."[97] This voice for organized nursing said that those over 65 account for one-third of the health care consumption in the United States. It also projected that old people may "consume" (their word) one-half of the total health care dollars by the year 2040. Further, *American Nurse* thought nurses should know: 50 percent of hospital admissions involve the elderly and every person now reaching age 65 has a 36 to 63 percent chance of entering a nursing home at some point in his or her lifetime. (The actual proportion of elderly needing nursing home care is 5.7 percent.[98]) The paper continued that 60 percent of the elderly fail to take medications properly. (One might well ask, what percentage of the younger do so?) This, in a publication that should be relatively pro-elderly; but one can project that bias as present in the whole of society.

Another, different view of aging and dependence are portrayed in a brochure asking for volunteers to help old people. A baby is pictured, with the words:

This person needs love, human contact and food to survive. . . .

A picture of an old lady is next:

. . . eighty years later, nothing has changed!

In Western philosophy of individualism, "independence" is valued so highly that some equate "dependence" with death. (They assume the dependent person might as well be dead, perhaps would rather be dead, or perhaps in some sense is dead.) "Dependence" thus becomes associated with or equated with death.

Death and dying are not popular subjects. Even the actual words, *dying* and *death*, are avoided. The term "end of life" is being used instead; nurses care for "end-of-life" people instead of dying people. Some explain the need for the change by saying that humans cannot define exactly when "dying" occurs, nor when "death" will happen naturally. But if it is termed "end of life," people can then choose when their life will end (with suicide or assisted suicide or euthanasia). As example of use of the term, the Kellogg Foundation has a "Decisions Near the End of Life Program,"[99] and the ANA has a "Task Force on the Nurse's Role in End-of-Life Decisions."

People fear not only death and dying, but they also fear the knowledge that they are going to die (as if they don't learn it early on). Some people (particularly the young) say they want to die quickly (not even to *know* they are dying); they are not fearful of the pain or discomfort of death, nor of being dead, but of the *knowledge* that death is coming, and of living the period of time of knowing and waiting for death to come.

In earlier times, the knowledge of impending death was valued, since one would have time to arrange affairs, say goodbye, perhaps make amends for hurts done to another. In those times people often died very quickly from diseases, especially infectious diseases, and more people died in childhood from accidents. A person could be hale and hearty one day, and dead of an overwhelming infection the next. Today, people are more likely to die of chronic diseases and old age—thus, they are more likely to know they are dying, before they die.

BRETON TALE OF DEATH

An illustration of earlier attitudes is the old tale told by Breton peasants (in the northwest corner of France). In the story, Death comes to a rich man's house in the guise of a beggar. The rich man feeds him (Doing Good), and so Death rewards the rich man. The reward? Not to avoid death—no one can do that. But Death delays taking the rich man for three days, so that the man has time to get his things in order.

This time of dying may be the value of doing CPR on the very old, sick, or even a dying patient (who will not eventually survive to leave the hospital). Perhaps CPR is valued in some patients, even if they will live only a few days, as time for patient and family to get their minds right for the inevitable.

If people so fear death, and they don't experience people who are dying, then perhaps they can convince themselves that nobody has to die (out of sight, out of mind). If people in PVS are not allowed to live, PVS is effectively eliminated as an experience people will never have to worry about. But, eliminating the *disease* by eliminating the *diseased* can apply to a lot of chronic diseases.

Life Expectancy, Averages, Risk Probability

Misconception: Life Expectancy Vs. Life Span

> The differences between "life span" and "life expectancy" are important, since information about the concepts affects the ethics and law of aging and death.
>
> Life expectancy is better called "the present average age at death"; it is determined by averaging the ages at death of people who have died.
>
> Higher infant mortality rates lower the life expectancy number (since more small numbers are averaged in with the numbers of adults that die old).
>
> In times past, when the life expectancy was 50 years, most people either died as infants (more of them) or as old people (fewer of them); but most did not die at 50.

The concepts of life span and life expectancy are related to aging and death, and are important in many ethical discussions. The terms are often misunderstood; this section will make effort to dispel the confusion since the misconceptions that there are too many old people, or that people live to be too old, are dangerous.

If those myths are widely believed, then solutions to the "problem" of old people will (do) create further ethical problems. Where certain people are perceived as a problem, there are always advocates for solving the problem by eliminating the people. This was learned from the German experience with National Socialism under Hitler.

Much of this section about death deals with ethical and legal consequences of attempts to "solve the problem" of "too many, too old" people.

Life expectancy: The common misconception is that this number represents how many years an average baby born this year will live. Conditions will change in the next century; it is obviously impossible to project that number. Life expectancy doesn't really mean "how long a baby born this year can expect to live;" instead it should be called "the present average age at death." The number is determined in general in this way: by writing down the ages of all the people who died *last* year:

> For example: Two people died last year. One was 99, and one other was one year old.

1. Add: 99 + 1 (the baby) = 100.
2. Divide 100 by the number of people who died—two: 100 ÷ 2 = 50.

This number is the life expectancy for a baby born this year: 50 years. Life expectancy is the average age at death of all the people who died last year, including the infants.

Another way of saying life expectancy is the "50 percent survival age." That is the age by which half the newborns will be dead, and half will live beyond.

The life expectancy number depends on how many people die as babies. If the average of 1.5 million abortions each year were counted as "infant deaths," U.S. life expectancy would be a lower number (because the infant mortality rate would be higher). In the year 1850, only a third of newborn children could be expected to live to 60 years old; today 83 of 100 children born will do so—which is why the "life expectancy" has increased.

In 1900, the "life expectancy" was around 50 years, because many people died in infancy. Their young ages at death, averaged into the total, brought down the average age at death to 50. But most people of that time, who survived infancy, lived to far beyond the age of 50. This can be known from mathematics, since the average age at death was 50. To get an average age of 50 at death, many people had to live to be older than 50. The life expectancy (average) is not the maximum age—it is the "middle" age, near the median age of *all* the deaths. To balance many baby deaths (low numbers in the average), there must have been many deaths of old people (high numbers in the average). This is the only way averaging all the ages at death will yield 50 as an average.

Not only does the logic of math show that people who lived past infancy lived to be old, there is empirical evidence. Nurses who visit an old graveyard of that time will notice the ages at death on the tombstones: More dead babies were noted than now, and many people lived to be 90 years old.

Life span represents the actual years lived by people who do not die as infants.

That fewer babies die in infancy is due to better economics (sanitation, housing, food), not due to improvements in illness care.

Because fewer babies die as infants, the life expectancy (average age at death) has lengthened.

More people live to be older than in earlier times, but they do not live much longer than old people did then.

Men whose lifestyles are comparable to women's live as long as women (adjusting for smoking, alcoholism and accidental death).

The percentage of the population who are old is increasing, because more babies live through infancy and, thus, live to *be* old.

The *mis*perception that people are living to older ages contributes to bias against the old (and against care for them).

The average of life span is a more helpful term; it represents the actual years lived by people who do not die as infants. Since 1900, the life span of people who live past infancy has increased by only about two years.

Beware the Average. An average life span, by definition, is the age at which half the people die before, and half die after. (In mathematical terms, that's actually a *median*, but the numbers come out close to the same in this situation.)

The theoretical maximum life span of an individual human appears not to have increased since *homo sapiens sapiens* lived in Africa about 100,000 years ago. (No human lives to be more than 110 to 120 years old.) About that time, however, the maximum life span of humans did dramatically increase (at the same time humans developed bigger brains). The earlier *homo erectus*, discovered in Africa by Robert Leakey, had a maximum life span of about 78 years.[100]

Today, fewer babies die, due to better economic conditions (diet, housing, sanitation, water). Very little of the small increase in life span (and the large increase in life expectancy) is due to "health care," but improved ways of treating illness do make better the years that people survive.

Because fewer babies now die at infancy, more people live to be old—not to be much older than they did before, but more of them survive to become "old." In 1900, most people didn't die at 50; they either died as infants (many) or as old people (fewer); the average was 50. Many politicians, medical experts, and about half the medical texts make this error. The reader now will not.[101]

There are more old people now than before. There will be even more in the future as more babies are saved as infants and more accidents are prevented that kill people at young ages. Those were the ages of deaths that decreased the life expectancy before, because they died with low age numbers. But old people are not older now, than old people ever were.

> "The conditions of life . . . have already changed. The influence of hygiene and measures of sanitation practiced since the beginning of the last half century, together with the wonderful discoveries and inventions employed for the comfort and protection of mankind generally, have unquestionably raised the lifetime of a generation several years . . . now even the octogenarian may hope to spin out a few more years." [WRITTEN IN 1893.][102]

Another myth: women age more slowly than men. Men do die at younger ages than women, of environmental causes developed in this century. When life span is adjusted for smoking, alcoholism, and accidents (all of which were more prevalent among men than women in the last decades), men live to be as old as women do. This is true now in some subgroups, such as among the Amish.

The perception of many can be summarized in a headline: "Elderly Increasing at Rapid Rate." (It might be imagined that they were "breeding" and having old babies.) That misperception is very close to the assertion in *American Nurse:*

> The three million men and women in the United States over age 85 comprise the fastest growing subset of the elderly, with a growth rate nearly three times that of the overall elderly population.[103]

It is true that a higher *percentage* of the population is older than before. Whether that is good news or bad news depends on whether old people are valued or not, whether long lives are good or not, and whether saving babies, who in other times died in infancy, is good or not.

In 1980, 8.5 percent of world's population was aged over 60. By 2025, it is projected that 12.5 percent of the population will be in that age group and that 72 percent of the old will live in developing or developed regions. Development (which saves babies) is the reason more people live to be old in those areas.[104]

Among 65-year-old women, on average half will live *longer* than 18.3 more years (to be older than 83). Among 85-year-old women, half will live beyond seven *more* years (to be older than 92 years old). Of men 85 years old, half will live longer than 5.5 *more* years (longer than 90). The assertion that a patient should be denied treatment because she or he is 80 and has lived a "good life" already, means that perhaps 10 or 20 more years of "good life" is discounted.

The easy bias against age is everywhere: Even a leader in the Clinton administration's health care reform effort "repeatedly cited the example of a 92-year-old man given a quadruple heart bypass . . . she suggests that if the system is changed such surgery will not be performed."[105] The surgeon who performed the surgery considered the 92-year-old an excellent candidate, with the physical condition of a 70-year-old.

Misconception: Risk Probability

Risk probability numbers are used when ethical (and legal) conflicts arise about which groups of people or "disease" should get money.

Risk probability numbers relate to populations and are used by planners and policy makers; they have little relevance to individual patients.

A *group* can have a risk probability (say, that 50 of 100 in a group will have cancer), but an *individual* can't (the individual will either have cancer or not—0 percent or 100 percent "risk").

False information can cause bad decisions about ethics and law, since the decisions do not reflect reality.

"Association" (of two factors) does not mean "causation" (that one caused the other). Meaningless associations are often found when large amounts of data are accessible by computer; associations are virtually certain, rarely informative.

Significant (as in statistical significance) is a mathematical term; it does not automatically mean "important" (neither does it mean useful, helpful, causative, or meaningful).

Using a lower confidence interval decreases the value of a study (for example, a 95 percent confidence interval means 95/100 chances that the finding was not accidental; a 90 percent confidence interval means one in ten chances the finding was an accident and other findings might be the reality).

Another misunderstood number concept is risk probability. Risk probability numbers are used when ethical and legal conflicts arise about which groups of people or "disease" should receive money. When used, they reveal the user's ethical stance; a bias toward one or another value the user has about sick people.

The risk probability concept is about populations, not about individuals. The numbers are properly used only when used by epidemiologists studying large groups. Risk probability has little relevance for individuals and their care.

For example, suppose that one is in a population with a 50 percent risk of having breast cancer during one's lifetime. The *individual* does not have a 50 percent risk. Instead, the *population* (the whole group) of which the individual is a member has a risk, called the class probability. In a 50 percent risk, 50 of 100 in the group are predicted to have breast cancer during their lives. But an individual will either be one of the 50 that *do* get it (100 percent personal risk), or one of the 50 that *don't* (0 percent personal risk). The individual's probability is not 50 percent; the individual's risk is either zero or 100 percent.

The group of 100 can have a percentage of risk—a class probability—because 100 people or pieces can be split into segments (percentages). A group (a mental concept) of 100 can be 50 percent cancerous. But the individual is not a group; she is just one person. She cannot be split into a percentage of herself that will have breast cancer, and a percentage that will not.

The individual's probability of breast cancer can only be 100 percent (that is, she will certainly develop cancer) or 0 percent (she will not). When people "reduce their risk" they join a different group, with a different probability for that group. That knowledge does not mean that individuals should not try to get in a lower risk group; the actions taken to reduce their risk (which means they join a group with lower risk) will perhaps keep them healthy.

A weather forecast analogy is helpful: If there's a 50 percent chance of rain today, that doesn't mean that it will rain 50 percent of the time where one is. It means that rain is likely somewhere in the area. (Consider the forecast area as a "group" of places, and consider the spot where one is standing as personal chance of rain in that spot.) It either will rain where the individual is (a 100 percent chance of rain for that spot/person) and will be known only after the fact (*after* it rains).

Or, it will not rain. Afterward the individual will know there was zero chance of rain (or cancer). There is no way to know *in advance, for certain* whether it will rain at the spot where one is, or whether one will have breast cancer until it occurs (at least not with the science presently available).

The individual doesn't know what the personal "risk" was (meaning what actually happens to her or him) until death—either having had breast cancer during life (100 percent risk) or not (0 percent risk).

Patients should be helped to understand these concepts before having a prophylactic mastectomy for a "50 percent risk of breast cancer."

Data can be misunderstood and even misused in ways that have ethical (and thus legal) implications. The purveyors of false data (intentional or not) may cause laws to be passed that are either unnecessary or outright harmful. The adversarial democratic process in law—whether in the legislative, executive, or judicial branch—should operate to allow and encourage *all* information, especially information in opposition to the accepted dogma.

Nurses should have a basic knowledge of statistics, at least enough to know when to be skeptical of numbers used to justify ethical (and thus legal) positions.

RESOURCES

An excellent, readable review of the possible misuses of statistics in medicine is Michael, M., *et al.*, *Biomedical Bestiary: An Epidemiologic Guide to Flaws and Fallacies in the Medical Literature*, Boston/Toronto: Little, Brown and Company, 1984.

Other good resources are:

Dans, P., "Looking for answers in all the wrong places," *Annals of Internal Medicine*, 1993; 119(8):855–857.

Mills, J., "Data torturing," *New England Journal of Medicine*, 1993; 329:1196–1199.

And the classic: Huff, D., *How to Lie with Statistics*, New York: Free Press, 1965.

Statistics can be interpreted to show unlikely and meaningless associations; it cannot be overstressed that the *association* of two factors does not mean that one factor caused the other. For example, Canadian data[106] show an association of the occupations of the fathers and associated birth-defect risks of their children, but the associations are nearly meaningless.

> "This study has several limitations and the results must be viewed with caution. Nonetheless, the study provides new leads for further evaluation of the role of father's occupation in the etiology of birth defects."[107]

The real role of epidemiology is to direct attention to areas of research in which a hypothesis will be formed, an experiment designed and tested and sought to be disproved. Unfortunately, many times epidemiological studies are reported as "research" that finds causation.

Sample conclusion of causation: A study done by Richard H. Lovely of Battelle Memorial Institute in Seattle, as part of an attempt to link electromagnetic fields (such as power lines) with adverse health effects,[108] suggested that electric razors might be linked to cancer. Men with leukemia are 2.15 times more likely to have used an electric razor (for more than 2.5 minutes per day) than healthy men. Less than 2.5 minutes of shaving was not associated with risk. To compare "increases in risk," note that the smoker's odds of getting cancer are increased only 2.5 times over someone who doesn't smoke (razors might be interpreted as being almost as dangerous as cigarettes).

The authors say there is no proof of causation in this study. They did not recommend that men stop using electric razors; they also found a connection of cancer with hairdryers, black and white TVs, and electric blankets. The problem is not in the statistics themselves, but with the use of the statistics to link electricity to cancer.

Some researchers find statistical significance in their numbers by lowering the "confidence interval" they use. A 90 percent confidence interval means that the chances are nine out of ten that the difference in the numbers is not due to chance (accident). Most reputable epidemiological studies use a 95 percent confidence interval, which means the odds that the results are not an "accident," are 95 percent (19 out of 20). Note that is still not a certainty.

Data have been used to "prove" that passive smoking causes cancer. The problem with the data are, that the researchers used a 90 percent confidence interval. Because of that, it is possible that data about passive smoking may actually prove the opposite of what the researchers wanted to show; the data might prove that passive smoking reduces the risk of lung cancer.

The data could be evidence that people who are exposed to passive smoke, are at *lower* risk of lung cancer, than people who are not exposed to smoke. The use of the lower 90 percent confidence interval means that the real numbers of cancers in people exposed to passive smoke may be even higher than estimated, or may be actually lower than estimated.[109]

Cost of Care

Misconception: "Too Much" Money Is Spent on the Last Year of Life, the Last Illness

The statement—"too much money is spent on last illness, last year of life"—assumes several things:

1. Assumes that the money spent on illness should be distributed evenly across the individual's life span (or even that more money should be spent on the healthier/younger years than on sicker/older years);

> 2. Assumes that if the money were not spent or last year of illness that large savings in illness care costs would result; and
> 3. Assumes that the last illness/last year can be determined in advance of its completion (death).
>
> People express unhappiness with spending significant amounts of money on "last illness/last year" of others, because they are forced to spend (through taxes).

Even well educated and thoughtful people comment disapprovingly, "One-third a person's lifetime expenditure on health care is spent on their last illness." This judgment can only be made with hindsight, when it is known that the patient actually died of (what turned out to be) the last illness. One alternative is to spend no money on care of the patient who is ill, in case it is the last illness and too much money is spent on it.

> "The time of death is usually unpredictable. . . . There is no method to predict months or weeks in advance who will live and who will die . . . it is difficult to know in advance what costs are for care at the end of life and what costs are for saving a life. Only in retrospect, after a patient's death, can we identify the last year or month of life."[110]

The suggestion is that the lifetime expenditure for illness care should somehow be evenly distributed over the lifetime and as much spent for earlier illness (such as self-limiting conditions like tonsillitis) as is spent for the potentially life-threatening or chronic conditions (like breast cancer and diabetes care). The reality is that more care is needed as people age and become sick. The amount and cost of care may normally, usually, rightly, increase as one gets older—although there is data that younger people on average have more episodes of acute illness. But care and its cost are not (probably cannot nor should be) "averaged out" over a lifetime. People are dependent and need care (usually by parents, for free) when very young, and they may be dependent and need care (often by strangers, for pay) when very old.

Exceptions exist, but almost all care is done assuming that this illness is not the "last illness." Only a supernurse could triage a patient, saying, "No treatment for her. This is her last illness." To do so would be a self-fulfilling prophecy; not treating *some* illnesses would in fact make it the last one. A 45-year-old who comes into the ER with a myocardial infarct, collapses, and shows V-fib on the monitor, could be assessed as in the last illness; not treating the condition would *make* it the last illness.

Even if it were somehow possible to determine in advance who is dying now and who will die later, not treating the last illness is a value judgment in the extreme—indicating that people who will not recover from an illness are not valued by society.

Relative to the discussion of DNR orders below, many diagnoses "predict" a finite average number of years of survival. People diagnosed with AIDS, congestive heart failure with coronary artery disease, liver cirrhosis, or lung cancer, all have on average less than five years life expectancy. Once diagnosed, these people could be thought of as "dying" and no money spent on them; a cutoff could be made. The diagnosis of an illness with a predicted life span of five years is then considered "dying," and care will not be given. Or the cutoff could be established at four years (or two months?), depending on the value placed on the time spent dying.

Even if they *could* be identified and all care for dying patients curtailed, one study said this drastic measure would cut health costs by very little—3.3 percent at most.[111] The estimates were based on data that showed that people 65 and over, who died in 1988, spent $29,295 each for all services that year. Those under 65 who died, spent $34,102 (giving terminal care to the old seems cheaper than giving terminal care to the young).

Those figures were then reduced by 27 percent (because giving hospice care alone during the last six months of life has shown to reduce cost by 27 percent.[112] The total potential savings that would be even possible if all the dying care could be identified and curtailed, was 3.3 percent of the total cost of illness care.

Society must evaluate why sickness care is given those over 65 at all: When they recover, they will cost the taxpayer money. Even if they go home healthy, they'll collect Social Security. Care of the sick in a society is not done because it's economically smart; even preventive medicine is not economically efficient. Preventing the fatal heart attack at 45 will let the individual live to collect Social Security and to use Medicare benefits (perhaps even to eventually use nursing home care). Some ethicists admit that preventive care is a bad idea, if the whole reason to give care is to save money. People cost money—all their lives long.

If not about money, why do people give care to others? Back to the ethics, back to the religion, back to the values of Doing Good, Doing No Harm, Fairness, Being True, Freedom, and Life. It is not done because it *pays*. It is done because people want it done to/for them some day (because they too will eventually be sick, dying, dead). At bottom, the ethic is that people should care for others as they want later to be cared for, themselves.

The reason for the belief that too much money is spent for the last year/last illness—and that too much money is spent on illness care in general—may be that the care is paid for by the people who are not receiving it. Taxpayers pay for almost half of care given.

If people pay for their own care, with their own money, then they as individuals can decide how much was "too much"—as is done in buying cars, food, houses (nearly everything else in life except illness care). Would reducing the amount of care paid for by taxpayers begin to stop the complaint that "too much" money is spent on last illness/last year of life?

Quality of Life

> Quality of life is a subjective judgment made by the person experiencing the life, which is contrasted to the imagined condition of being dead.
>
> The Quality Adjusted Life Years (QUALYs) combines expected length of life remaining with a quality of life assessed by one person for another.
>
> The Germans under National Socialism in the 1930s and 40s assessed some people's lives for them, and found them not worth living.
>
> People who are younger and healthier will have higher scores under the QUALYs system and will get more or better treatment whenever that system is used to allot care.
>
> Rating systems like HRQOL and APACHE (used to predict outcomes of ICU treatment) are based on the mythical "average" patient and are useful for planning for groups of patients; they are inappropriately used for care decisions in individual patients.

If the value of life is not absolute (if it is relative) then its value depends on its quality or conditions. When the "quality" of someone's life is discussed, the value of that person's being alive is contrasted to that person's being dead. Quality of life is always subjective; only the individual can decide his or her "quality" of life—how valuable the life personally.

Life may be not valuable to a person (the person may consider that death is better than life) under certain conditions. These conditions are the subject of attempts to make the quality of life a constant number for a particular condition. The Quality Adjusted Life Years (QUALYs) is an attempt to make another person's quality of life objective (numerical, impersonal); it combines the years of life the *average* person is predicted to live, at any given age, with the quality of life of the person (as assessed by another).

In discussion about life, people recognize instinctively that their lives are valuable to them. By projection, they value others' lives. If not, existence would be constant war, with the temporarily strong dominating all others. The self-interest in valuing Life is that it prevents war against all, by all.

National Socialist Quality of Life. People for whom life was not the highest of all values (not "sacred") were the Germans under the National Socialist government. The value of life for other than their own people was relative. The German people, prior to and under their Socialist government, had a term for some lives other than their own people's lives: *Lebensunwertes leben*. Translated: *Leben* ("life") *unwertes* ("unworthy") of *leben* ("living").

Such people were judged, in a cost-benefit analysis, as costing more than they were worth. Under such programs, thousands of children with congenital handicaps, mental retardation, and mental deficits were marked for "treatment" (a euphemism for killing). Next were people termed "incurables" (schizophrenia, epilepsy, syphilis, encephalitis, Huntington's disease). The killing of these people was followed by killing of disabled adults, "asocial" persons (like labor leaders and homosexuals), Jews, Gypsies, Poles, Slavs, and Catholic and Protestant "troublemakers." Even German soldiers returning from battle with disabling injuries were euthanized, a practice considered a cost-effective veterans' "health" policy until the public objected. Estimates of the numbers killed during that time: 6 million Jews and 4 million others.

People who object to withdrawing or withholding treatment from the terminally ill or Persistent Vegetative State (PVS) patients assert that those actions are the same as German Socialist "treatment." Others say it's different because the *motives* are different; it's not being done for cost saving, or because those lives aren't valued—it's done to "help" the patient (in the patient's best interest). The chief medical officer of the National Socialist Third Reich was Dr. Karl Brandt, whose feeling for hopelessly ill patients made him want to find for them "a peaceful end." He defended his compassion (until his death by hanging for war crimes) in giving painless deaths to such people. He designed gas chambers that could kill thousands—"painlessly."[113]

Citizens of our time can forget the National Socialist experience, *if* they believe that—unlike themselves—Germans were particularly unethical people, and if they believe that Hitler was a mad superman, able to cause all the killing by himself. Then such a nightmare could never happen now. It will not happen here again if people continue to remember what happened there, and measure their motives and actions by that experience. The French memorial at Dachau, a German concentration camp outside Munich, says "*Jamais rien*" (never again).

QUALYs: Quality Adjusted Life Years and Other Measurements

The QUALYs could be used to decide who gets what treatment. QUALYs attempts to reduce the quality of life to a number; the patient is assessed by noting age, computing the average life expectancy left after treatment, and factoring in a number for the quality of life the patient will have. People predicted to have more life left (younger), and who are less ill (healthier), will always have a higher QUALYs. They will get better or more treatment under any system that prioritizes care by the numbers, like the Oregon Medicaid Plan.

Proponents of the use of QUALYs agree that the concept is difficult to grasp; they disagree as to how to compute it, lack reliable data to calculate it, and admit they may be attempting the impossible (to reduce the quality of life to a number). Over 50 years ago, investigators said that such an approach led to a serious *loss*, not gain, of information; but present day proponents still say it's better than nothing.[114]

Techniques to measure quality of life include asking *healthy* people to gauge life quality currently, and then to estimate what their quality of life would be if they were in a projected condition, which is anticipated to be a result of treatment. A series of questions may be asked about the healthy person—for example, difficulty with ambulation or toileting. The answers to the questionnaire are computed out to a number. Then the healthy person is asked to *imagine* what difficulty in living there would be, say, with a colostomy as a result of colon cancer. That number is calculated, and subtracted from the former (healthy) quality of life number. The problem is that healthy people are fairly inaccurate when gauging the life quality of sick people.

Another measure, the Health-Related Quality of Life (HRQOL) attempts to measure the patient's quality of life from one time compared to another (a part of the measure of outcomes of therapy).[115]

The assumption in most "objective" assessments is that people who are more independent are happier (have a better quality of life). Most disabled and ill people, however, report that they have a relatively good "quality of life" (they are as happy as people who are totally independent). Suicide rates are not higher in such groups. Is the assumption that dependence equates with poor quality of life based on the valuing of Autonomy more than Life?

To make (subjective) quality of life assessments numerical (and so appear to be objective) several tools have been developed. The Acute Physical Assessment and Chronic Health Evaluation (APACHE), developed at George Washington University in 1985, predicts the rate of survival for the average patient in intensive care. Treatment might be considered futile if the score gets too close to zero probability of survival. Whether treatment be abandoned, if the probability is too low, depends on whether the practitioner believes the scale is perfect, and the computer objective. The practitioner still must make ethical analyses even if the numbers say "quit treating."[116]

Such numbers must be used for the purpose for which they are created—as probabilities for a class of patients. The numbers were determined by averages of past experience with patients who are different from the nurse's individual patient. The nurse's patient is not a class but an individual case; the patient's probability of living to leave the ICU is either zero or 100 percent, no matter what the other patients in the class did, averaged together. If one patient died and one patient lived, the average is 50 percent survival; not very helpful information in caring for *this* patient in the ICU, who has neither survived intensive care nor died yet.

Other "tools" are the SIP (Sickness Impact Profile), PGWB (Psychological General Well Being), the PQOL (Perceived Quality of Life), and the QLIS

(Quality of Life Improvement Scale). All may be useful, but all must be used with caution and not as a substitute for individual practitioner responsibility.

A way to employ such tools is to apply them in a benefit-burden analysis. (The terms "benefit" and "burden" are of religious origin.) An economic analysis using the same concept can be called risk-benefit analysis or cost-benefit ratio. The cost involves more than just money. People have always weighed the "good" against the "bad" consequences when making a decision about action. Now there are names and sophisticated numbers to apply, but it's still about as "accurate" as forecasting the weather. Practitioners will make decisions they want to make, using such tools and the patient's "quality of life" to justify the decision.

Quality of Life for Others

> Quality of life, being subjective, is only assessed for others when they are unable to assess and communicate for themselves. "Burden and benefit analysis" is another term for assessing the patient's quality of life. Such assessments are about as accurate as random chance.

Quality of life is only discussed when the patient is incompetent and cannot personally express wishes. When people can express their wishes they decide for themselves. Some patients decide to live and fight for life in situations that amaze; nurses may project that they personally would have long ago given up in the same situation.

The patient's life and its quality is the patient's decision; nurses recognize that. But when patients are not able to decide, others may decide for them. Assessing the quality of life for someone else as an individual (or as "planners" deciding for a whole group of people who are in effect also unable to speak) is difficult; the decision for someone else that life is more burden than benefit is difficult.

The term "quality of life" has no generally agreed meaning. Three possible definitions have been proposed:

1. The individual's subjective satisfaction with his or her own life (the philosophy of individualism).
2. An outsider's estimate of another's life, either as a reasonable person (used in law) or by a person in a similar situation as to age or illness.
3. The degree of achievement of success valued in society.

In a major study, physicians made decisions whether to intubate or not to intubate a patient described in a hypothetical situation. Of the doctors who decided *not to intubate*, more than 80 percent said *their* decision was supported by quality of life factors given for the patient. Of the doctors who decided *to intubate* the patient (same hypothetical), more than 80 percent said *their* decision was supported by quality of life factors.[117]

These doctors saw the patient's quality of life differently; some decided to intubate based on that perceived quality, and some decided not to intubate based on the same information. The criterion for quality of life is personal. The doctors used their own values (nurses do, too). Nurses in the newborn ICU admitted their surprise when they realized they were wrong in their assessment of the probability of their newborn patients' survival. The babies they expected to flourish didn't, while the baby they felt sure wouldn't make it, did. They had not put their projections into operation; so the baby with a "poor" chance still got her chance, and made it. The prognosis of survival/quality of life was subjective.[118]

Nurses must know and be able to identify when their own values are working. A values assessment tool and process for making decisions about ethics is described in the first chapter, Ethics and Law. The values history described there may help nurses ascertain their own feelings about life and death—feelings they will inevitably project onto their patients.

Assessing the quality of life for another person is often no more accurate than flipping a coin (the assessment is actually a guess). In one study, 100 percent of doctors thought their patients treated for hypertension had improved; only 48 percent of the patients thought they were better (eight percent said worse), and 100 percent of the relatives thought the patient was *worse*.[119]

Competency/Capacity

Ethical conflicts about dying are invariably about incompetent or incapacitated people; it is assumed that competent people make decisions in their own best interest, either choosing life or not as it is best for them.

Freedom is not absolute for any person; and for incompetent/incapacitated people, it is much more restricted.

Some distinguish between legal incompetency and functional incompetency (incapacity); and some state statutes have changed the state of being "incompetent" (legally) to being "incapacitated" (the same legal condition) in order to decrease the stigma attached to the condition.

Being declared legally incompetent is the ultimate loss of freedom (autonomy) short of death.

Ethical conflicts that arise in the process of dying rarely involve competent people. Caregivers (almost) always honor the wishes (value the freedom) of a competent person. They assume the person is acting in his or her own best interest. (Best interest and its equivalent, substituted judgment, are discussed below.) Plato even questioned whether one *could* act in any other fashion than in one's best interest. The person will always choose what is best for himself, even if choosing to die for another. Most people will choose life as in their best interest, in most cases. They want as much treatment as possible, if they believe the treatment will return them to their life as it was before their illness, or at least to some lower but acceptable level of life.

Patients do fear the worst case scenario: Becoming incompetent, being treated intensively, and lingering on as a "vegetable" for years, because the people doing the treating do not know their wishes. The people helping are strangers.

This worst case scenario, however, is a very unlikely occurrence. Only five percent of people over 65 years old are in nursing homes. Of those in nursing homes, most have some meaningful life experience. Only about two percent of the five percent minority of people in nursing homes are classed as "vegetative." That is, of 1,000 people over 65 years of age, only 50 are in a nursing home. And only one of those has a life envisioned as the worst case scenario.

An exercise in exorcising prejudice: Nurses who don't already work in a nursing home should visit one, leaving their "young person" bias at home. Some healthy, young people believe they "wouldn't want to live" at 90, needing a wheelchair. When most people were 20, they thought being 40 years old would be living death. "Who would want to live like that, being 40 years old?"

When people look at others' lives from their own vantage point (as seeing, walking, talking, thinking) they must use care; perhaps they personally "wouldn't want to *be* like that" (not seeing or walking), but if they actually found themselves in that condition, they might not want to die.

The Germans under National Socialism believed they were doing the Jews a favor—the Jews couldn't have wanted to live like that (being Jewish).

Freedom—for Competent People

Only *competent* people have the freedom that Americans and others value so much. Freedom is not absolute; autonomy is not always the highest value. Freedom is limited in many ways.

People don't have complete freedom (power) over their own bodies; in many states, people don't have the freedom to neglect their health to the point that they are "dangerous" to themselves (self-neglectful). If that happens, the person may be taken into custody and forced to get medical treatment.

People are not free to take just any drug wanted, nor to drink alcohol to intoxication and walk on the street—much less drive. Freedom has limits. Freedom is often the highest value, but the patient's freedom to make decisions about care will be honored only if the patient is competent. The decision to respect the patient's freedom (grant autonomy) is based on *competence* or *incapacity*; these words are legal terms, but they must be defined in the context of experience.

Competence or Incapacity

If one is not "competent," the law says that person can be made a ward— some other person (the guardian) or the court (the state) will have complete power over the individual. The individual loses freedom (power over self). Personal decisions about any and everything can be made by the guardian. The guardian "becomes" the incompetent for almost all purposes.

The word *incompetent* has become stigmatized, not surprisingly. It is used to characterize someone who cannot carry out business or tasks with ability—as in "the TV repairman is incompetent." At the legal level, it expressly states that the person designated incompetent cannot carry out business or make decisions for self in any way.

Incompetency is the ultimate losing of control over self, short of death. It is a more limiting condition even than going to prison. The person declared legally incompetent may lose control over the most basic activities of life; where to live, what to wear, what (and whether) to eat.

People fear being incompetent and may hope to ward off this loss of control by signing living wills and durable powers of attorney. The signing won't prevent the loss of control; but some project they would rather die than to live as an incompetent person, even if not sick. Many people say so, and *Cruzan* and other cases like it advance precisely that idea. People assume that other people who can't function as they used to, or as they themselves function, would rather die. Sometimes even families and nurses would rather that the patient die than live "like that" (which says nothing about how the patient would rather live).

In an attempt to dissolve the stigma about incompetency, the word has been changed in some laws to *incapacitated*. (The word *incompetent* was once considered an improvement on the earlier [also] stigmatized term, "unsound mind.") The social stigma attached has not gone away. Similarly, the stigma of the word *graveyard* was not dissolved by changing it to *cemetery*, and then to "memorial park." There are still dead people buried there.

Calling people incapacitated will not make others think of them differently than when they were called incompetent. Since 1817, Missouri law (and similar laws in other states) has provided for a procedure to deal with (or for) people with what was called then "unsound mind"; possibly it is time to return to that usage.

Nurses Decide Competency

Nurses must decide competency with clinical assessment; the shorthand test is whether the nurse would allow the patient to sign a consent for a procedure. If so, the patient may be considered competent (capacitated).

The longer formal test for decisional capacity is whether the patient can (1) understand information and alternatives, (2) consider and make a decision and communicate the decision, and (3) understand the consequences of the decision.

Practitioners should be careful of considering patients incompetent on the criterion that the decision is different from what the practitioner's would be, but the starting point for assessing the patient's decision is whether it would cause death or apparent detriment.

Patients determined incompetent or incapacitated by a court will become wards of a guardian who exercises the patient's autonomy. Many state advance directive statutes require that patients be incompetent (but not necessarily legally so) before the documents are used formally.

Without a legal proceeding, nurses must often decide if their patient is competent. For example, such determination must be made when the patient is asked to give consent to surgery or to a procedure. If the nurse believes the patient is not able to give consent, a decision has been made that the patient is not competent.

Decisional Capacity. Another phrase for "competent" is "decisional (decision-making) capacity." (Note the use again of the word *capacity* as a preferred term for competent.) Even if the patient does not have formal legal capacity to decide (for example, if the patient is a minor and the parent has legal authority to decide), the informal decisional capacity of the patient should be considered. The steps come down to some commonsense questions:

1. Is the patient able to receive and understand information about condition and treatment necessary to make a decision?
2. Is the patient able to consider (feel, reason about) the information, make the decision, and communicate the decision?
3. Does the patient know the consequences of the decision?

If the patient can't understand what the nurse is saying (the number one criterion), the patient doesn't have capacity to decide. If the patient can't consider and decide and tell the nurse of the decision somehow, there may not be decisional capacity. For example, if the patient "just can't decide," and denies that indecision will be fatal (and if it appears probable that indecision *will* be fatal), the patient may lack capacity. But in some cases, not to decide is to choose (to choose the status quo).

If the patient doesn't know the consequences of the decision or denies the consequences after being told of what might happen, the patient isn't competent to decide. For example, if the patient won't eat, but says that refusing food won't cause death, the patient is not competent.

Questions about the consequences of the decision are tricky—sometimes practitioners are mistakenly sure that the patient will die without treatment. A better assessment is whether the patient understands that lack of treatment *might* cause death. Nurses probably can't be sure that any decision will cause any other specific outcome, except that refusing or denying the patient food and water will cause death.

Consent = Competent?

Patients are assumed to be competent when they consent to treatment or refuse treatment that produces the outcome that practitioners want—or when they make a decision that practitioners would, if practitioners were in their place. Nurses are much more critical of, and look harder at, those patient decisions considered to be irrational (different from what the nurse would decide).

In defense of that attitude, the only standard people have for assessment is themselves (their own experience). That subjective assessment is needed as an initial standard—look for incompetence in people who decide something that will cause their death or detriment. It is assumed that rational (competent, capacitated) people want the best—usually, at least life—for themselves. When they make a decision that will result in harm to themselves, it is right to examine whether they are able to understand that the decision will result in harm or death.

Legal Consequences of Incapacity

As noted, a determination by a court that the patient is incompetent will result in appointment of a guardian; nurses then can look to the guardian to make decisions. The guardian's (and the nurse's) ultimate responsibility is for the best interest of the patient. As long as the guardian's decisions seem to meet that standard, the guardian can decide for the patient.

The nurse may also be involved—before a living will or durable power of attorney for health care can be implemented—in application of the informal (but legal) process of determining capacity. All state statutes require that the living will and durable power of attorney be used only if the patient is unable to make decisions. In most statutes, the physician (or two) must certify that incapacity before the directives in those documents operate. Some statutes mandate that such assessment and certification be made in the patient's chart. Regardless of the law, it is good medical and nursing practice to assess and document the patient's mental status.

The nurse's assessment and documentation are important, whether alerting the physician to the need to make the certification of incapacity or whether the nurse disagrees (believing that the patient is capable of making decisions). Regardless of the legal status of the patient, the patient should be consulted and involved in care to the degree possible. Nurses need no law nor ethics text to tell them that.

How Do People Die?

CPR/DNR

CPR originally was to be used with witnessed arrests, sudden death in the young, drowning, and predictable arrests, such as in anesthesia and cardioversion.

> The value underlying CPR is Life; the value underlying the refusal of CPR (the DNR decision) is Autonomy.
>
> Slow codes or partial codes are fraudulent to the extent that they are used to mislead the family; partial codes are acceptable if their use and limits are communicated.
>
> CPR is much less likely to succeed than patients and family believe, especially on very old or very sick patients.
>
> The ambulance crew may be (and probably should be) expected to resuscitate first and look at limits later—their primary task is to revive—and they may assume that, if they were called, their full services were requested and consented to.

Cardiopulmonary resuscitation (CPR) was first suggested as useful for witnessed arrests, sudden death in young people, drowning, and arrests of known etiology, like anesthesia. Instead, almost all hospitals and nursing homes in the United States have policies that CPR be done on all patients who die—for any reason, of any age, with any condition. Unless there are specific orders written to the contrary, CPR is automatic.

"Slow codes" or "partial codes"—or any actions being done to mislead the patient's family into believing a full intensive code is being done when it is not—are unethical and could have legal implications. To the extent the family is deceived and injured, such action might also be illegal under a civil or criminal action for fraud. Limited codes such as "chemical codes" may be justified, if treatment is appropriate and no deceit is intended (the patient and family should be made aware of the limit).[120]

In New York, a state law written in 1988 mandates that consent to CPR be presumed. In effect, that law requires doctors to get consent before ordering the patient *not* be resuscitated.[121]

In a VA hospital it was found that CPR is seldom successful when performed on patients aged over 70, patients ill with sepsis (blood infection), or with cancer. Of arrests outside of the hospital, two of 244 survived. Of unwitnessed arrests, one of 116 survived. Of asystole or EMD (electromechanical dissociation, a lethal heart arrhythmia), one of 237 survived. CPR is rarely effective for hospitalized patients over 70 who have multiple problems. Of 503 arrests with CPR, 112 patients were resuscitated and only 19 lived to discharge. When CPR was needed for over 15 minutes, only one of 360 survived.[122]

When CPR is done in noncardiac ICUs, many patients have an acute illness superimposed on a chronic condition. When those patients arrest and require CPR, 44 percent are initially resuscitated, and five percent survive to discharge. Only two patients of the 114 in the study were alive one year after discharge.[123] That implies there should be a "cure time" for CPR—that survival might better be measured like cancer survival (five years survival means cure/success). How long must the patient survive CPR to make it worth doing?

CPR is done automatically for every patient, even if not appropriate in a given case. Physicians and hospitals may fear that if they do not do CPR on all patients they face losing a lawsuit; not true. Caregivers are never required legally to do procedures that are clearly useless. The reverse is true: They might be sued for performing CPR without consent on certain patients when the medical literature now clearly indicates the futility of the procedure in those certain patients.

But in Ohio, after a no-code order, the patient was coded and sustained a stroke as a result. He sued for two years of "wrongful life." The Ohio court said there was no law in Ohio giving the right to refuse treatment when one is not in a coma nor terminally ill. The court based its reasoning on Ohio's living will law. The court said that being alive is not a harm, and dismissed the case. The court also was concerned that making caregivers liable for doing CPR would discourage hospitals from doing CPR on other patients, without permission.[124]

The situation of calling the paramedics for the hospice or other no-code patient outside the hospital is problematic; frequently the caregiver panics and wants someone to do something when the patient actually dies. Some people wear DNR tags as bracelets, and half-joking suggestions are made to tattoo "DNR" on the chest. The paramedic doesn't have time to be reading living wills and DNR orders—he or she must resuscitate first and discontinue later.

The states of Montana and New York (and in 1995, Texas) have put into statute, provision for community and nonhospital DNR orders. There are required forms, bracelets, and the obligatory nonliability for the paramedic who honors the DNR in good faith.[125]

DNR Orders

The presence of DNR orders varies; the order is not consistent with expected life span in specific diseases.

DNR does not mean DNT—do not treat; but such an order gives rise to that presumption. Future trends may be not to admit patients who are DNR to intensive care, or even to acute care.

A living will does not justify an automatic DNR; a DNR should be written when either (1) the patient refuses CPR or (2) the practitioner assesses that CPR will be futile (informing the patient and/or family).

The DNR order is suspended (along with all other orders) when the patient goes to the operating room in most facilities. The trend is to educate the patient to this policy and allow more autonomy about this situation.

A broad "no-CPR" policy would be as unpersonalized as is an "all-CPR" policy; but CPR could be discussed with the patient, consented to and ordered by the doctor in all but emergency cases.

With a policy of automatic CPR for all, the DNR order becomes very important. DNR is likely to be written for certain conditions, regardless of patient preferences and prognoses. In patients with a five-year prognosis of survival

(AIDS patients), 52 percent have DNR orders. Also with a five-year prognosis, patients with unresectable nonsmall cell lung cancer have 47 percent DNR orders. Patients with esophageal varices and cirrhosis also have only a five-year prognosis, but only 16 percent of them have DNR orders. The five-year prognosis of death in patients with severe congestive heart failure with coronary artery disease prompted DNR orders in only five percent of those patients.[126]

The American Medical Association says CPR does not need consent because it is an emergency—but many nurses will disagree that a code is always *un*anticipated.

As noted in the section under advance directives (Chapter Four), often the mere presence of an advance directive on the chart will give rise to a presumption that the patient does not want resuscitation. Even if the patient refuses resuscitation, experts agree that "no code" does not mean "no treatment." But refusing resuscitation is sometimes presumed to amount to not wanting any treatment at all. The advance directive document and resulting assumptions may provide an easy out for practitioners confronted with burdensome care of a difficult patient with complicated disease.

Nurses who work in intensive care may have ethical and practice difficulties in caring for patients who are ordered DNR;[127] it seems to some that the ICU be a place where all lifesaving measures are attempted. In future, a patient who is DNR may not be admitted to the ICU, or even to an acute care hospital.

The AMA (not the law) says that patients and family must be consulted before a DNR order is written.[128] Individual state statutes may require this, but there is no national standard. Other writers believe that family consent is not needed if the DNR is a reasonable order in the situation, and the likelihood of lawsuit is low.[129]

One case arose out of a DNR written without consulting the patient (who was later asserted to be competent). The patient's estate countersued for this "malpractice," after the doctor sued the estate for the his bill.

Futility. No CPR (or any other treatment) is mandated when it is considered to be futile (also discussed in Chapter Four, Practitioner Autonomy). But not all people use the word *futile* as medical futility (that the treatment won't work). Some use the issue of futility to question whether the patient will be returned to a "meaningful" life; Is that a question the doctor or nurse can answer for the patient? Theoretically, a DNR order made when CPR would be futile, does not need the patients consent. The order should always be discussed with patient or surrogate, however, since they expect that CPR will be done in the event of arrest, and they also expect that it will probably be successful.

In an emergency, consent is not needed; by definition, the occasion for CPR is an emergency. Some writers believe that CPR that is judged to be futile should not be offered to patients. Thus a DNR can be written without consent if resuscitation is believed to be "futile."[130]

One review article concluded that DNR is a medical decision if the patient's death is anticipated. It is a *patient* decision if the patient, in advance, refuses CPR. The article cited data that indicate that CPR results in a 15 percent long-term survival rate (not a bad outcome, considering that the condition before CPR was death).[131]

DNR in the OR

Many agencies routinely suspend DNR orders during surgery. Several reasons are given: The death is likely to be due to anesthesia or drugs administered and thus the arrest is reversible. The OR and the anesthesiologist or anesthetist don't want the investigation and negative record which a death in the OR would bring. And traditionally, all orders of the primary physician are superseded by the OR team during surgery.

A person who does not want resuscitation in a nonsurgery situation, possibly would not want it during surgery either. The patient who does not want CPR, but who does consent to surgery, should be questioned as to full understanding of the outcomes possible in either procedure. The OR exception to the DNR order should be discussed with patient and family; they should be made aware of the hospital's policy and the possibility, likelihood, or certainty of resuscitation being performed if arrest happens in the OR.

OR teams routinely resuscitate patients in the OR until they know patient's wishes—even if the patient has had a DNR written before surgery. As noted above, the policy should reflect discussion and possible reconsideration by the patient of his refusal of CPR in light of the new situation of surgery. New or continued attitudes toward CPR should be noted.

The OR team should communicate with the patient's family and pre-and post-operative caregivers. No blanket policy should be operative which mandates DNR in the OR; nor should there be an automatic "no-DNR" policy.[132]

Proposed CPR/DNR Policy

The policy of agencies should *not* be that no CPR be used on any patient over 70, or with sepsis, or with any form of cancer; the problem with present policy is that it applies to all, and that would be the problem with a broad DNR policy as well. CPR, as any other extraordinary invasive procedure, should be done if ordered by the physician and consented to by the patient in advance.[133]

If selectively-ordered CPR were hospital policy, then no DNR order would ever need be discussed, or written. Patients would assume they would not be resuscitated unless they requested it. An order for CPR would be written and consented to, as orders for surgery are discussed and consented to.

If for some reason the patient cannot communicate, the same rules apply as in other invasive procedures. CPR will be done automatically if arrest happens before the patient's orders have been written. Otherwise, the physician will consult with the family or guardian before ordering CPR be done in the event of arrest (death).

Withdrawing Vs. Withholding—to Treat or Limit Treatment

**GENERAL CONSERVATIVE RULES FOR WITHHOLDING OR
WITHDRAWING TREATMENT**

If the course to follow is not clear, be conservative.

Follow ethical instincts.

If there's any doubt, treat:

Treatment can be withdrawn later but

Treating later won't help if the patient is dead.

The nurse has a duty of allegiance to and protection of the patient, not to the system.

If initial error is to be made, err on the side of life.

Most people in the United States die in a hospital or nursing home; at least 70 percent of those deaths occur without CPR being done. When the experts say that people are allowed to die without extraordinary efforts they do not mean that death is caused by withholding water and food, but that patients die without CPR (with a DNR order). Withholding or withdrawing, giving or limiting treatment to patients, concerns every nurse and potential patient. The reader is both.

In law, withholding is not different from withdrawing, but people doing it report a real emotional (a very fast logical) difference. The practical difference is that withholding treatment usually causes or allows death before analysis can be made, while withdrawing may be done after a decision process.

The distinction is not between withholding and withdrawing, but between treating fully and limiting treatment.

The distinction between nursing and medicine in this situation is that medicine at some point has no more to offer a dying patient, while nursing's ability and responsibility to care continues.

Some ethicists argue that, in theory, there should be no difference between withholding treatment in the first place, and withdrawing treatment later. They say that to withhold the first tube feeding is the same act, logically, as withholding the next tube feeding and the next, after feeding is started. They say that removing the ventilator and allowing the patient to breathe unaided if possible is logically the same act, as is not aiding that breath in the first place.

That is the situation in *theory*; in practice it feels very different. This is a situation similar to the emotional instinct felt when discontinuing a ventilator on a brain dead patient. In reality, in practice, withdrawing is *very* different from withholding.

Logic is contradicted by emotion. Some say emotion is just very quick logic, done at computer speed; human intuition says that not *starting* treatment is much easier than *stopping* it once it has started.

In the law, there should be no theoretical difference between withholding and withdrawing treatment; there is a practical difference. A case about *withdrawing* leaves time for discussion, reaching consensus, and if not, time to go to court—all while the patient stays alive until the conclusion of the conflict. In contrast, a conflict about *withholding* treatment may not have time for much discussion, much less court action. If the treatment is withheld in the first place, the patient may die before any court could act.

Nurses have the technology. Dramatic results can be seen from its use. If there is any doubt about possible benefit, treating first is initially a good plan of action. Treatment can be withdrawn later if response is not good, but the nurse must be prepared—despite what the nonparticipant "experts" write—that withdrawing feels very different from withholding.

The distinction between withholding and withdrawing is similar to that between passive and active, and killing versus letting die. These are often not helpful distinctions. Withdrawing treatment *sounds* passive, like "letting die." But putting the hand down and pulling on a ventilator plug, or turning the dial to "off," is an *act*—just as is starting the machine (active not passive). Passive and active are not helpful distinctions.

The distinction is not really between withdraw and withhold, nor active and passive action. The question is whether providers will treat as fully as they are able to treat, or whether they will *limit* treatment. There is no option for nurses of not treating at all (at minimum, providing comfort care); there is only an option to limit some nursing treatment.

That is one difference between nursing and medicine on the care continuum. Almost all the interventions that doctors are able to do are at an end when at last the patient is dying. But almost all actions that nurses do well still continue as the patient dies. The nurse's job is to do for the patient what can no longer be done for self, until death.

Nurses could never condone "not treating," if that means not nursing patients who need care; positioning, turning, cleaning, giving pain medication. Deliberate absence of all care might require lethal injection (by someone) to prevent suffering.

LIMITS OF MEDICINE, NOT NURSING

Purpose of medicine:

"In general terms, it is to do away with sufferings of the sick, to lessen the violence of their diseases, and to refuse to treat those who are overmastered by their diseases, realizing that in such cases, medicine is powerless."[134]

—Hippocrates

The difference between medicine and nursing is clear here. Nurses do not ever refuse to treat those who are overmastered by their diseases; nurses are not powerless in such cases. (Indeed, such people need nurses more than ever.) When medicine "fails" or at least can do no more to cure, the nurse's job to care continues until death.

The difference between medicine and nursing is the difference between removing a ventilator (medical treatment—permissible to remove) and removing a feeding tube (nursing care—permissible to remove only if that would benefit the patient). A feeding tube may be considered "medical treatment," but this does not change the nurse duty to provide nutrition as long as it benefits the patient (assuming it is also the patient's wish).

There is usually no issue about treating competent people; medically-indicated treatment is given unless the patient refuses. Discontinuing a ventilator from a competent patient who couldn't breathe without it, who had not ask it be discontinued, would not be done.

There are issues about what is medically indicated, but the participation in cosmetic surgery by doctors and nurses has removed any objection that medicine and nursing could have, against doing something not "medically indicated." Much cosmetic surgery is medically unnecessary, but the patient gets what the patient wants.

The ethical conflicts about limiting treatment concern incompetent patients. The competent patient decides for self, but someone else decides for the incompetent patient. How those decisions are made is discussed next.

Myths About Terminating Life Support

CORRECT STATEMENTS OF THE LAW

An act that is not specifically *permitted* by law, is *not* necessarily *prohibited*.

Terminating life support is not necessarily murder or suicide, if the patient is dying and the life support is not medically indicated.

Patients needn't be terminally ill in order for treatment to be terminated; again, the criterion is whether treatment is medically indicated (giving food and water *is* indicated if the patient is not dying, unless it causes harm to the patient).

Ordinary treatment may be terminated (as well as extraordinary) when it is not medically indicated.

Legally, withholding may be the same as withdrawing treatment (but it does feel different in reality). Tube feedings are no different legally (they may be withdrawn if they're not indicated), but ethical concerns are raised if food and water is withdrawn from a patient who is not dying to cause the patient's death.

A court order is not necessary to terminate life support, when the treatment is not indicated.

Some *legal* myths are not myths on the *ethical* level, which is exemplified in the situation of abortion on demand for any reason (for many, the minimum ethic of the law is much different from the higher ethical behavior). Such abortion is *legal*, but much *ethical* concern is in evidence. All the myths below are false, *legally*—but some have ethical validity. It is fundamental to remember that an action may be minimally legal but not fully ethical (permissible but not desirable).

1. *True or false*: Whatever the law or authority does *not* specifically permit, is prohibited.
   False. This strange idea of the law would have people carry immense volumes of law books permitting specifically all the things people do. The opposite is true: Whatever is not prohibited, is assumed permitted (ask forgiveness after rather than permission before).
2. *True or false*: Terminating life support is either murder or suicide.
   False. Usually it is just the death of the patient who is dying. People who are dying will die, whether treated or not.
3. *True or false*: Patient must be terminally ill to terminate life support.
   False. That's the specification for using the living will in some statutes, but the advance directive statute is not the only way people can be allowed to die (most of the statutes say so). Many of the statutes are probably unconstitutional after *Cruzan*.
   Caveat: Although it has been held *legal* in some court cases to cause death by withdrawing food and water from an incompetent patient, the ethical issue for nurses continues (an analogy to the abortion issue—abortion on demand for any reason is *legal* but questionably ethical).
4. *True or false*: It's acceptable to terminate extraordinary (but not ordinary) treatment.
   False. That is from old Roman Catholic terminology—and it depends on what is "extraordinary," which can change day to day. *Extraordinary* is sometimes defined as treatment in which the burden outweighs the benefit (cost-benefit analysis). But there is no requirement to treat if even "ordinary" treatment does more harm (perhaps pain) than benefit. "Extraordinary" is the person who can decide for another person whether treatment is more of a burden than life is a benefit.
5. *True or false*: Withholding treatment may be right, but withdrawing is not.
   False. They are theoretically the same, and if one action is appropriate, the other will be too. If withholding is right in a situation, then withdrawing is legal too. If withholding is not right, neither is withdrawing—legally.
   Ethically and emotionally, the two actions do not provoke the same feelings. People use more than logic; the life of the law (and people) is not logic but emotion (apologies to Oliver Wendell Holmes, Jr., who said the life of the law is *experience*).
6. *True or false*: Tube feedings are different from other treatment.
   False. The Supreme Court has said they are not different—legally. Nor are they are different ethically, if a competent patient who is dying refuses the feeding. When removing a tube feeding from an incompetent, nondying patient is to "allow the patient to die" (of dehydration)—to cause death deliberately—ethical issues for nurses arise.

7. *True or false*: In order to terminate life support, a court order is necessary. False. Avoiding court action is the whole point of having living wills, powers of attorney, and all advance directives—and the point of good nursing practice: talking to the patient, family, colleagues.

RESOURCES

Academy of Critical Care Physicians/Society of Critical Care Medicine Consensus Panel, "Ethical and moral guidelines for the initiation, continuation and withdrawal of intensive care," *Chest*, 1990; 97:949.

Hastings Center, *Guidelines on the Termination of Life-Sustaining Treatment*, Briarcliff Manor, NY: The Hastings Center, 1987.

President's Commission for the Study of Ethical Problems in Medicine and Biomedical and Behavioral Research, *Decisions to Forego Life-Sustaining Treatment*, Washington, DC: Government Printing Office, 1983; pp. 236–239.

Dehydration

Dehydration (at their request) of patients who are dying may be considered medically appropriate and ethical.

Research shows that up to one-half of patients on tube feedings may be retrained to eat orally.

Feeding tubes have been placed in patients because of economic factors (higher reimbursement, lower labor cost).

Some material in this section, and under Definition of Death as Persistent Vegetative State later in this chapter, is adapted from the article "Caring for Corpses or Killing Patients" by the author, with permission from *Nursing Management*, 1994; 25(10):81-89.

A controversial subdivision of the ethical issue of withdrawing/limiting treatment is the dehydration of patients who are dying. The question sometimes asked: "Is it ever acceptable to withhold or withdraw specialized nutritional support from the dying adult patient?" In the opinion of many, the answer to this question is yes, but for only a small number of patients. Provision of nutrition through artificial means is considered by some to be an invasive medical intervention.

Providing nutrition and hydration artificially imposes burdens as well as benefits. In some situations the treatment can be limited. But the needs of the vast majority of dying patients will best be served by providing specialized nutritional support.[135]

Percutaneous endoscopic gastrostomy tubes (PEGs) have enabled the prolongation of the life of some patients who would otherwise die of malnutrition. More factors than merely medical need, influence the decision to use a PEG tube. (See below for economic factors.) Love for the patient by the family is one issue, but there are more universal impacts.[136]

New research[137] creates a new standard for nursing practice to be performed before dehydrating patients with feeding tubes. Data indicate that about half of patients on feeding tubes can be successfully retrained to oral feeding over a ten-week period. Before tubes are discontinued and the patient is allowed to dehydrate with no nursing intervention, a trial of retraining to natural oral feeding may be the standard of care.

Several factors militate in favor of placing feeding tubes in patients who may not require them: The reimbursement from the government for patients with a feeding tube is higher, and the care is less costly than natural oral feeding (such hand feeding takes about 40 minutes per meal). Weaning a patient from tube feeding may disqualify the patient from Medicare reimbursement for skilled care. Taken together, the system rewards the placement of feeding tubes in the first place.

> "We have a reimbursement system that rewards tube feeding over handfeeding, despite the increased cost associated with [handfeeding] and the increased burden to the resident associated with [tube feeding]."[138]

The researchers report that several benefits accrue to the patient (but not to the system nor to the home's reimbursement) from retraining tube fed patients to natural oral feeding. The time the patient spent with the person feeding had a "positive impact on resident socialization and may play a role in the language improvement occasionally seen after weaning a resident from a tube."

In addition (and unexpectedly), all Foley catheters were discontinued in the residents retrained to natural oral feeding.

> "The association between successful weaning and the Foley may reflect an excessive reliance on medical technology in lieu of basic nursing care. . . . "(O)ur experience suggests that all tube-fed nursing home residents should receive an extended trail of oral feeding to allow weaning of the feeding tube."[139]

Since retraining is possible, should all patients on tube feedings who are proposed to be dehydrated to death receive such a trial?

Nondying Patients (NDPs)

> Dehydrating nondying patients to cause them to die raises ethical issues for nurses, whose responsibility is to help patients meet needs they cannot meet for themselves such as nutrition and hydration.
>
> Nurses have complied with orders and requests to dehydrate to death patients who were not dying in several highly publicized cases and others not public.

Nurses worry that prolonged dying is detrimental to the patient as well. Allowing nurses to cause death in patients by dehydrating them allows the doctor to escape the responsibility of euthanizing the patient more quickly by injection or other means.

An analogous situation of "passive death" obtained in Germany in the 1930s and 40s; nurses injected retarded children with drugs to make them sleep unturned for days (the children died of pneumonia).

Some would extend the practice of dehydrating dying patients to patients who are *not* dying, in order to cause their death. Nutrition and hydration have traditionally been nursing acts, so dehydration as a method of causing death, is particularly troublesome to nurses (whose primary function is to help the patient meet needs she is unable to meet without help). Obtaining nutrition and hydration are basic needs, in all patients.

In addition, the history and development of the profession of nursing is inextricably linked to providing nutrition and hydration for people. (See any dictionary for the striking inseparability of the origins and definitions of the words *nurse, nourish, nurture.*)

Under court order, nurses have dehydrated to death their patients diagnosed by some as in persistent vegetative state (PVS) in three very public cases: *Cruzan*,[140] *Busalacchi*,[141] *Bland*.[142]

Nurses in the United Kingdom are concerned also over the ethics of using nurses to cause death in patients not dying. Specifically, some are concerned about the Tony Bland case, in which a young man said to be in a persistent vegetative state was dehydrated to death by nurses, on the order of a court in 1992.[143]

In addition to allowing Tony Bland to be dehydrated, the law lords (the British "supreme court") ordered review of all PVS patients that are to be dehydrated to death, in order to "allay public concern." That order was criticized by some, who said that public concern should be directed to the length of time elapsed before withdrawing "medical treatment that was clearly not in the patient's best interests." That is, that Tony Bland should have been dehydrated to death earlier than he was.[144]

Nurses are on the front line in the unsettled area of ethics and law, in which biologic life can be supported after full cognitive function has ceased.[145] This is not a new situation. People have for millennia lived past their physical and mental peak or even minimal function.

Nurses also worry about the opposite of *not* dehydrating nondying patients. In some articles, they worry that technology can prolonging dying, dehumanize the patient, and produce an unfair allocation of resources under the concept of social justice.

Nurses promise to care, to cure, to treat with dignity and individuality, and to stand by in death. If the nurse cannot restore the patient to the condition before illness (if the nurse cannot prevent the patient from dying), then a duty of loyalty is still owed to the patient. That fidelity to the patient is made visible in the nurse's action of being present as the patient dies.[146]

Several cases have been taken to court; in some cases dehydration by nurses was allowed, and in some cases not.[147] (See further, below, in Cases: The "Right" to Die.)

Some nurses may see their dehydration of nondying patients in the same way some doctors see the issue of what Jack Kevorkian does. Perhaps doctors "allow patients to die" by letting nurses dehydrate them, because doctors don't want to be responsible for killing the patient quickly with lethal injection or carbon monoxide. If so, doctors are ducking the issue and nurses are doing the dirty work for them (an old story).

The patient dies on the nurse's watch—the death is on the nurse's hands. This was done in the same way by German nurses under the National Socialist government—who killed patients actively, independently, and also passively on doctors' orders. One author who supports this interpretation of the current situation is Megan-Jane Johnstone.[148]

Patient Christine Busalacchi was reported to be able to eat from a spoon. In this and other cases where nurses are able to feed their patient sufficient food and water by mouth to sustain life, nurses have been asked and have complied, to deliberately deny the nursing care of food and water that they are able to give, with the intent and result of causing death in their patient. Christine Busalacchi's cause of death was not listed as dehydration but as "complication of persistent vegetative state caused by head injuries" due an automobile accident which caused her head injury years before.[149]

Many nurses have strong personal and religious values. Nurses with religious convictions are requested to violate the commandment against killing when they deny food and water to a person with severe disabilities who is otherwise healthy.[150] Nurses who are not formally religious are no less spiritual, and may find killing a patient violates their personal ethic.

THE ETHICS

The values in this situation (dehydrating nondying patients) are doing good, doing no harm, and respecting autonomy.

Nurses should follow patient's wishes if possible; if not, the surrogate's wishes as long as they are in the best interest of the patient. If the surrogate's desire will result in the death of a nondying patient, the nurse has an ethical problem.

Several guides in the nursing ethics literature assist in the nurse's ethical dilemma when asked to dehydrate a nondying patient.

The first value in nursing care is caring. The law, as is always the case, echoes that minimum. Nurses must not neglect to do what good can be done for the patient. The law that flows from the ethical value of caring mandates the minimal ethic, the duty of doing for that patient what a reasonable and prudent nurse would do.

The value of doing no harm applies also, and the law enforces the minimum standard of "first, do no harm." Nurses must not intentionally harm a patient. Intentionally not feeding a patient, who was determined to need food and water, would violate this ethical standard and law. (But neither must the nurse feed the patient if the feeding actually harms.)

The patient's autonomy (the value is the patient's freedom) is harder to respect in such patients. Here nurses encounter the potential conflict between doing good/caring, versus following the patient's wishes (possibly not to be receive care). Nurses should (ethics) and must (law) respect the patient's wishes as much as can be determined. Since the permanently unconscious person (PUP) is incompetent or incapacitated (depending on the word used in state law), the patient is presently incapable of assessing, deciding, understanding consequences of choice.

Determining the patient's wishes, so that nurses can respect their freedom (autonomy), may be difficult in patients in PVS (and in other patients incompetent and not dying). Even if the patient has a written or spoken living will, it may not cover this situation; living wills do not automatically mean the patient wants to die, especially if some chance of recovery exists as in PVS (see that section below for data). And in many states, living wills are not effective until the patient is declared to be terminal (though they may still be used as guides to the patient's wishes).

If the patient's wishes are unknown, the ethical (and legal) duty of the nurse is to give care. *Without evidence to the contrary*, one may assume the wish is to have treatment, if that treatment maintains life. The ethic is doing good (beneficence). The law is, do what a reasonable nurse would do. That reasonable nurse would care for the patient until ordered to stop, by the patient or by a person with authority to speak for her.

If stopping care will result in the patient's death, the person ordering the care stopped must have legal authority. The research noted earlier will mean that stopping hydration and nutrition must be done with a trial of natural oral feeding; this establishes a new standard of nursing practice. The nurse has an ethical problem (and possibly a legal one) if ordered to cause death in a nondying patient by denying nursing care—as has happened in the cases cited above.

The maintenance of the ethical integrity of the profession is one of the primary interests the state weighs in cases involving withdrawal of food and water.[151] The ethical integrity of the nursing profession is at risk in cases in which courts allow nurses to be used to cause death in nondying patients.

The following is addressed to the prohibition against nurse participation in executions; it also encompasses the rationale against nurses causing death in their nondying patients by denying the nursing care of nutrition and hydration:

> The goals of nursing are the promotion, maintenance, and restoration of health, the prevention of illness, and the alleviation of suffering. The social contract between nursing and society to meet these goals is based upon a code of ethics that is grounded in the basic ethical principles of respect for persons, the noninfliction of harm, and fidelity to recipients of nursing care. *These principles command that nurses protect or preserve life, avoid doing harm, and create a relationship of trust and loyalty with recipients of nursing actions.* Regardless of the personal opinion of the nurse on the moral appropriateness of capital punishment, either generally or specifically, *it is a breach of the ethical tradition of nursing, and its Code for Nurses, to participate in taking human life,* even through a legally authorized civil or military execution. [EMPHASES ADDED].[152]

It could be added, "or through a legally authorized civil order to deny food and water to a nondying patient."

Further ethical guides:

> The nurse acts to safeguard the client and the public when health care and safety are affected by incompetent, unethical, or illegal practice of *any person.* [EMPHASIS ADDED].[153]

Does "any person" exclude surrogates with authority to make decisions for patients?

And:

> Nurses . . . must take all reasonable means to protect and preserve human life when there is hope of recovery or reasonable hope of benefit from *life-prolonging treatment.* The nurse does not deliberately act to terminate the life of any person. Nursing care is directed toward the prevention and relief of the suffering commonly associated with the dying process and the nurse may provide interventions to relieve symptoms in the *dying client* even when the interventions entail substantial risks of hastening death. [EMPHASES ADDED].[154]

Patients in persistent vegetative state, those with Alzheimer's and senile dementia, and those who are merely incompetent (all of which have been conditions of patients dehydrated to death), are not dying.

"There really isn't an ethical conflict in withdrawing nutrition and hydration from someone who is terminally ill [and requests that action] but the PVS is a slippery concept. You're withdrawing treatment from someone who isn't dying."[155]

The ANA committee on ethics has addressed the ethical problem of nurses who withhold food and fluids in some patients who are incompetent.

According to the ANA committee, nurses may participate ethically in withholding food and fluids from incompetent patients, if the following criteria are met:

> If the patient's feeding is futile because of underlying, incorrectable absorption problems,
>
> When it is severely burdensome to the patient, or
>
> When it sustains life only long enough to die of other more painful causes.[156]

None of these situations fits the situation of the patient in PVS, Alzheimer's, or senile dementia, or the patient who is merely old and incompetent. Nurses who are asked to cause death in their patient (who is not dying) because the family and/or society believe the patient to be better off dead, have ethical problems (and possibly legal danger, see below).

As noted earlier and evidenced in the statement below, nurses do not seek to maintain life at all costs in dying patients:

> Increasing titration of medication to achieve adequate symptom control, even at the expense of maintaining life or hastening death secondarily, is ethically justified.[157]

A statement by the American Nurses Association maintains that it is morally as well as legally permissible for nurses to honor the refusal of food and fluid, by competent patients in their care. The statement also suggests that nurses may honor the refusal of food and fluid made by a surrogate on the patient's behalf.[158]

LAW OF DEHYDRATION

The law of dehydration of nondying patients is in a state of change; some court orders have allowed it, some have not.

Nurses who participate in causing death by this method are potentially liable for licensure violations and malpractice, and the existence of a conscience clause in state statute may mean the participating nurse has no excuse (defense).

If society wishes to allow such patients to die, is a better solution than jeopardizing public trust in the profession (having nurses cause the death), to allow the families to do the care, which then will result in earlier death from infection, malnutrition, or some other complication? Would asking families to pay for the care achieve this result?

Legal authority to speak for the patient may have been granted to a surrogate (by an advance directive, the consent statute, or the court who has appointed a guardian). Even so, nurses still have ethical (see above) and legal responsibility to protect a patient from someone who does not act in the patient's best interest. The ethical value of doing no harm is enforced in state statutes punishing abuse (including neglect).

Some states have "conscience clauses" that may allow nurses to refuse to cause death in nondying patients (they may apply only to abortion, however). Some state laws on the subject have to do with life-sustaining treatment of competent patients who have expressed preferences for future treatment, when those patients are dying. Most state legislatures have not considered the situation of nurses causing death by dehydration in incompetent, nondying patients.

Conscience clauses, if they exist, may create more of a legal liability to nurses who do participate in causing death. Such nurses then have no exculpation in an assertion that they did not have a choice (though they may have been pressured in other ways to participate). Conscience clauses are helpful to examine, however, in that they express the concern of the legislatures that nurses should at least not be forced to assist in denying food and water to dying patients.

In those statutes, the legislatures often protect nurses from forced participation in causing death, even in patients who *voluntarily* request that food and water be withheld, and who are dying from other causes. Evidence of a legislature's concern for nurse ethics and personal morals is the "conscience clause" in Missouri's Elder Abuse Act:

> No physician, nurse, or other individual who is a health care provider or an employee of a health care facility shall be discharged or otherwise discriminated against in his employment or employment application for refusing to honor a health care decision withholding or withdrawing life-sustaining treatment if such refusal is based upon the individual's religious beliefs, or sincerely held moral convictions.[159]

The Missouri Legislature here expressed its concern that nurses not be required to participate in denying treatment to patients, which will cause the death of the patient. Note the wording assumes a voluntary "decision."

Denying food and water to a person with severe disabilities, who is not dying, may constitute neglect and abuse. Criminal penalties are provided under several state statutes. There is no statutory protection for nurses who intentionally cause such abuse. In addition, nurses are required to report such neglect and abuse when they observe it, and may be prosecuted for failure to report. Certainly the nurse could be held liable for money damages for such neglect and abuse in a civil malpractice lawsuit The wish of a surrogate for the patient's death in no way guarantees that another family member cannot sue or complain to the licensure board.

The Missouri living will statute is similar to other states' laws in that it protects health care professionals from being forced to participate in withholding or withdrawal of death-prolonging procedures.[160] Giving food and water, however, cannot be stretched to be considered death-prolonging, in a patient who is not dying. Denying food and water in a nondying patient will not fall under this section, and the nurse has no protection from criminal or civil liability.

Neither are nurses insulated from prosecution under their licensure law, which allows license revocation for conduct that can be characterized as incompetency or misconduct. Allowing death by dehydration and starvation in a nondying patient could be characterized as incompetency. Causing death by dehydration and starvation could be characterized as misconduct. Nor are nurses protected from discipline if their licensure law considers violation of any professional trust or confidence as grounds for discipline.

Other courts have expressed concern for nurses asked to cause death in their patients by denying nursing care.

> "I find it difficult to understand how we can order nursing professionals with an abiding respect for their patients to cease to furnish the most basic of human needs to a patient in their care. [Such an order] may impinge on the privacy rights of those nursing professionals."[161]

And:

> " . . . for almost all concerned the adoption of the proposed course [dehydration of the patient] will be a merciful relief, [but] this will not be so for the nursing staff, who will be called on to act in a way which must be contrary to all their instincts, training and conditions. They will encounter the ethical problems, not in a court or in a lecture room, but face to face."[162]

When causing death by denying nursing care such as food and water, it is the nurse who is ordered to perform the act that violates the statute. The physician is not at risk, nor the guardian nor the judge, if one issues the order. Even when "humane" methods of death are administered to persons condemned to die as punishment for crime, physicians are not asked nor allowed to administer death.

Nurses who deny care to patients who are not dying, in order to cause their deaths, are subject to several potential legal risks.

Solution?

Patients like Nancy Cruzan, Christine Busalacchi, and Tony Bland survived their initial trauma as a result of medical technology, and the luck not to be killed instantly. They survived the years after their accidents not because of medical care, but because of nursing care. Their deaths were caused by the denial of that nursing care.

If the nurse will follow the surrogate's order to deny nutrition to a nondying patient in order to cause death, it must be asked if the nurse will follow the surrogate's order to deny other nursing care (such as turning the patient every two hours). If so, the patient will develop pneumonia and perhaps die a quicker death than 14 days of starving and thirst.

In such a case, the worse the nurse, the better for the patient; the better the nurse, the worse for the patient (the longer it takes to kill the patient). This situation stands nursing ethic and theory on its head. Further, if nurses will follow orders that result in death to nondying patients, it must be assumed they will give lethal injections on physicians' orders, or on orders of surrogates.

If the professional nursing care had not been paid for by the government, these patients with impaired cognition would have been cared for by their families and might have died earlier from complications. In these cases professional nurses are paid to care, and then later asked to dehydrate their patient to death. Perhaps taxpayers should not provide free care (for anyone, not just cognitively impaired patients) in the first place; if the care were not free, the family would be caring for the patient. If the families believed the patient wanted to die, the patient would die. Is death from less-than-ideal care at the hands of a loving family member to be preferred to deliberate death at the hands of a professional nurse—for both the patient and for the profession?

Cases: The "Right" to Die

ROLE OF LAW IN "WITHHOLDING/WITH-DRAWING/LIMITING" CONFLICTS

Relatively few cases about the "right to die" (withdrawing treatment from nondying patients) have been decided; literally millions of people have died without obtaining permission from a court.

The designation of dying with "treatment limited" is largely the group of people who die with DNR orders, not those who die as result of withdrawal of ventilator or tube feeding.

Cases are designated as "refusal of treatment," although virtually all such cases are refusal by a surrogate and not by the patient personally.

The test of what is in the *best interest* of the patient is the same test as what is the *substituted judgment* for the patient; the reasoning being that the patient would have always made the judgment (so does the substitute) in his or her own best interest.

The substitute decision maker is preferably a family member or loved one; not because they know better what the patient wanted, but because they love the patient (want the patient's best interest) and because the patient's life or death affects the decision maker too.

Surrogates are allowed to make decisions only for patients on whom practitioners have agreed no further improvement is likely (either the patient's life is considered not valuable, or the life is considered a burden to the patient). (Families are not allowed to decide the fate of patients whose lives are considered valuable—for instance, healthy children).

The law is the minimum ethic of the people. The cases described here (and some cited above) reflect the lack of settled ethics in the area of treatment of people who are dying or who are neurologically impaired. The lack of consensus about law is a result of the lack of ethical consensus about nontreatment of dying and of nondying people. The ethics are still being "made"; so the law is being "made" too.

More than 60 cases on the right to withdraw treatment from nondying patients have been reported at the appellate level in this country. (It is not the "right to die," as it is sometimes characterized.) A case doesn't get reported, thus is not recorded as law, unless and until:

1. It is decided by a lower trial court; and
2. the decision is appealed to higher court, and *that* decision is reported in official records.

At that point the case becomes law, binding on lower courts in that jurisdiction and used as an example in other jurisdictions.

As noted above, the American Hospital Association says that 1.3 million people die yearly as a result of "limiting treatment." Almost all those are people who die merely with a DNR order ("limiting" the "treatment" of CPR). A few people die as a result of removal of ventilators, which then allows them to die of underlying lung disease. Relatively few nondying patients are being deliberately dehydrated to death, but that situation may change.

Since the 1976 *Quinlan* case (see below), some 20 million people have died, without getting full intensive treatment. Very few decisions to limit treatment go to court and make law.

The few cases that go to court are sometimes brought to force decisions in opposition to family wishes. Some are brought to force decisions in opposition to nurse wishes (like *Cruzan*). Some, including the *Wanglie* case, seem to be brought out of fear of lawsuit or fear of responsibility.

Some doctors, hospital attorneys, guardians, and families seek official paternal court sanction rather than accept responsibility for what they want to do. That so few cases are seen is tribute to the fact that most practitioners, attorneys, guardians, and families are acting responsibly.

Several cases that are now law, about ethical conflict, deserve specific mention for their lessons and their notoriety.

Karen Ann Quinlan was a 22-year-old woman in a coma as a result of presumed alcohol and drug ingestion. The court used a substituted judgment test (see below) to allow her to be removed from advanced life support (a ventilator).[163] She breathed on her own, living ten more years with a feeding tube. Her mother said she would never have requested the feeding tube be removed.

One problem in analyzing such cases: Decisions made by third parties for incompetents are characterized as "refusal of treatment"—as though the incompetent personally refused treatment. For example, in one article about "refusing treatment," every case cited is one in which the *surrogate* refused treatment. Not one case used by the author in support of the patient's "right" to refuse treatment, is a case of the patient personally refusing treatment.[164]

One writer asserted that Nancy Cruzan (who had been in PVS or a coma for years) herself wished to have her feeding tube removed because she personally wanted to die.[165]

Best Interest—Substituted Judgment

In deciding these few cases, the courts use at least two tests to measure whether the patient's treatment can be limited. Many legal and ethical cases make a distinction between "best interest" of the patient and the patient's "substituted judgment." (These tests are used only if the patient is incapacitated or incompetent; the competent patient judges best interest personally. There's no difference between best interest and the competent patient's own not substituted judgment).

If the patient is not competent, a "substituted judgment" test may be used. The substitute (surrogate) makes a judgment as though the surrogate were the patient, choosing (judging) what the patient would judge. The patient would, if possible, choose (judge) the treatment that is in their best interest. So "substituted judgment" is *at the same time* judgment of the "best interest" of the patient. The two concepts are identical for the incompetent patient, just as they are in the competent patient.

The important next question is *who* gets to make this substituted judgment–best interest decision. Only because it is assumed that the decision maker is influenced by personal values, is it important who makes the decision. A person biased by relationship to the patient is needed; otherwise the data could be analyzed by computer or committee of strangers and an "objective" decision reached.

Someone who knows the patient needs to make decisions, *not* because they will know how the patient would decide (surrogate decisions are about as likely to mirror the patient's as flipping a coin) but because they love the patient, and they are affected by what happens to her. Surrogates will exercise their *own* interest too; at that point, for that patient, that interest is accepted. The surrogate wouldn't be allowed to decide if the practitioners hadn't already accepted that the value of the patient's life is in question.

By the time a surrogate is allowed to make a decision for an incompetent patient, the practitioners have already decided it's acceptable to let the patient die; either because the patient's life is not valuable, or because it appears the life is burdened by treatment. The trend in recent court cases (seen in the last *Cruzan* case and in *Wanglie*) is that the family can decide. They know the patient and the assumption is, they love her. By letting them decide, the wishes and comfort of the healthy, competent family are put above what is considered a less valuable life or condition the patient now has.

Note that families are not allowed to decide the fate of people who are still valued; for example, people who follow Christian Science are not allowed to withhold medical treatment from their otherwise healthy children. If the parents refuse care and cause harm to the child, they are punished. The family is allowed to decide for the patient only if the decision is already made that the patient's worth is less than the family's wishes.

CRUZAN

The *Cruzan* case is the most important bioethics case yet decided by the U.S. Supreme Court; the Court upheld the right of a state to set its own standard of evidence that a nondying patient would want to be dehydrated to death (in Missouri, it is clear and convincing evidence).

Evidence "beyond a reasonable doubt" is the standard that must be met in order to take a life or liberty (as in criminal law).

Evidence that is "clear and convincing" is a lesser standard, but higher than that for civil lawsuits, which is the evidentiary standard of "preponderance of the evidence."

The Supreme Court's ruling established a constitutional right to refuse treatment under the Fourteenth Amendment's guarantee of Liberty (before the case, the right to refuse could be changed by state statute or case law).

Cruzan is the most important bioethical legal case in U.S. history so far—the first case of its kind to be decided by the U.S. Supreme Court.[166] The case has been characterized as being about the "right to die"; but it is really about the right to refuse treatment.[167] At issue in the case was the state's right to set evidentiary standards in such situations. Also decided in the case was the competent person's right to refuse treatment, in advance.

The details: Nancy Cruzan was injured in a car wreck in 1980. Paramedics and practitioners worked to save her life and did. Eventually a feeding tube was inserted to make it easier for her to eat. She was diagnosed as PVS (see below) in 1988.

Her family wanted her feeding stopped, but the nurses and the institution refused. Conflict, no compromise, and recourse to the courts. Note that if no recourse to the court were possible, one "side" or the other would have had the absolute power to make the decision about treatment (or if they couldn't go to court, they could go to war as people used to do).

The rule: In Missouri (and in other states, including New York, New Jersey, Maryland), before withdrawing treatment that would kill the patient, clear and convincing evidence is needed to show that the patient, while competent, indicated a wish to refuse treatment in such a situation. It is not a best interest–substituted judgment test, as in *Quinlan*; and not a family's decision. It is an expression of absolute freedom (autonomy) of the patient. The patient must decide in advance and clear and convincing evidence of the decision must be presented.

But in accord with the trend to leave the lives of less-valuable people, or people with burdensome treatment, in the hands of their family, the family's wish to have their daughter dehydrated *was* granted by a lower court in Missouri, after the U.S. Supreme Court ruling.

Standards of Evidence

There are three levels (standards) of evidence in court cases: beyond a reasonable doubt, clear and convincing, and preponderance of the evidence.

Beyond a Reasonable Doubt. The highest level of evidence, most difficult to attain or prove, is evidence that convinces *beyond a reasonable doubt*; this is the level of evidence needed to convict in criminal trials. That standard of evidence must exist before the person's life or liberty is taken. It was not the test of the evidence in *Cruzan* (though her life was at stake).

Clear and Convincing. A second and lower level, *clear and convincing*, is the standard for various kinds of cases. This standard of evidence must be met in some states before punitive (punishing) damages can be awarded in a liability case. The clear and convincing standard is used in Missouri and several other states as a level of evidence that must exist before a person's life support—including food and water—can be withheld. There must be enough conflict about the withholding to take it to court; life support is withheld every day, and if there is no conflict between doctor and nurses and patient or family, there is no court case.

If there is no clear and convincing evidence, made in advance of incompetence, that the patient would refuse treatment—food and water included—then the ruling will be that there is no refusal (a judge will decide if the evidence is clear and convincing). Under that standard of evidence, if there's no refusal, there will be no termination of treatment.

Preponderance of the Evidence. The lowest standard of evidence is preponderance of the evidence. That level is used in civil court cases—for example, to establish liability in a malpractice lawsuit. The nurse testifies that the bedrails were up, and the patient testifies they were down. If there is a little more evidence for the nurse (perhaps the chart reflects that fact too), then that's a preponderance. Anything over 50 percent, and the trial court decision will stand up on appeal.

In *Cruzan* the U.S. Supreme Court found that Missouri could use the clear and convincing standard of what a patient wanted, before withdrawing her food and water—or the state could adopt a lower standard, if it wished. The people of Missouri could, through their legislature, establish some other standard of evidence in such cases.

An important reason to use the mid-level or clear and convincing standard of evidence is that the highest standard of evidence, beyond reasonable doubt, is necessary to convict a guilty person before execution for the crime. Even if guilty, the convicted would not be executed if incompetent. Requiring at least the middle standard, clear and convincing, would not be considered excessive before taking an innocent person's life (a person who is incompetent and arguably has not asked to die). Causing death by the method of dehydration instead of lethal injection, and using nurses instead of prison employees to cause the death, causes even more ethical conflict and reason to use a higher evidentiary standard than the lowest.

The Fourteenth Amendment and the Right to Refuse Treatment

After *Cruzan*, a constitutional right to refuse treatment exists based on the Fourteenth Amendment to the U.S. Constitution, which states that no state can deny life, liberty, or property without due process of law. The liberty interest (freedom/autonomy value), so dear in the United States and its Constitution, protects individuals from state courts, legislatures, and majorities that would limit their right to refuse or consent to treatment. (But it does not give patients a right to demand treatment.)

Before *Cruzan* there was a right to refuse treatment established by judge-made law (common law), state by state—not a national constitutional right. New York case law had been the standard for many years, and had been adopted in all other states in some form:

> Every human being of adult years and sound mind has a right to determine what shall be done with his own body. . . .[168]

That case established the right to sue for battery when unauthorized surgery was done.

As long as the right to refuse treatment was a common law right established by state judges, or state legislature-made law, states could interfere with and restrict the right as they chose. For example, many "advance directive" laws operate only when patients are terminally ill, and don't allow patients to refuse food and water in their advance directives. Now that the Supreme Court in *Cruzan* has recognized a constitutional right, states may not be able to restrict that right of competent patients to refuse whatever treatment they specify and under whatever conditions they choose, through advance directives.

The U.S. Supreme Court did not differentiate between levels of treatment. Food and water can be withheld if the advanced directive requires it. And the Court indicated that advance directives would constitute clear and convincing evidence in a case such as Cruzan's (living wills can be spoken).

After the Supreme Court decision, witnesses were found who then testified that Cruzan had stated (or didn't disagree with someone's statement) that she "wouldn't want to live like that" (about a situation similar to the one she came to). The same trial court judge who originally ordered the feedings stopped, found this evidence to be clear and convincing evidence of Nancy's wishes. He again ordered the feedings stopped. This time the state institution (in the person of the attorney general of Missouri) did not appeal the decision. Nancy Cruzan's gastrostomy tube was removed and she died 14 days later.[169]

Research cited earlier (that perhaps half of patients on feeding tubes can be retrained to eat orally with assistance) creates a new standard in such cases. A trial period off the feeding tube, with retraining, could be required; just as trials off the ventilator are done only after weaning the patient off the paralytic agent, and hyperoxygenation.

BUSALACCHI—INCOMPETENT PATIENT, NO ADVANCE DIRECTIVE

In the case of Christine Busalachi (follow-on and related case to *Cruzan*), a girl who was questionably in PVS was dehydrated to death. Her nurses raised the issues that dehydration is an inhumane method of causing death and that nurses should not be asked or allowed to cause death by denial of nursing care.

In another state that required clear and convincing evidence of wishes to refuse treatment, the guardian of a woman who was senile sought her death by dehydration. The court refused.

Evidence exists that some patients in PVS "wake up," but these are not given much publicity.

A competent quadriplegic sought and was granted permission to receive nursing care while starving herself to death; she did not carry out the permitted starvation.

Many state constitutions have a written right of privacy, which has been used to strike restrictive abortion laws as well as to grant guardians the right to remove feeding tubes from their wards.

One court delegated the decision about dehydration of a senile patient to her guardian and a court-appointed ombudsman.

A Canadian case held that withdrawing care from a dying patient was not murder, but revealed that the family was not as unanimous about the withdrawal as the doctor believed.

A later Missouri case is that of Christine Busalacchi, a patient similar to Nancy Cruzan—except that she had not expressed any earlier statement about her treatment in the event of such a condition. And, her nurses and some doctors disagreed that she was in a persistent vegetative state (see below for discussion). Busalacchi's father wanted to move her to Minnesota for diagnosis of PVS by neurologist Dr. Ronald Cranford (an advocate of dehydrating patients in PVS) and subsequent removal of her feeding tube.

Several nurse groups, especially nurses who had cared for the patient for several years in the same hospital with Nancy Cruzan, protested the method of causing death in the patient.[170] They believed it to be inhumane to cause death in a person by a method that is illegal to use in animals and that is never chosen as a method for suicide by people who are competent (nor is it a method of executing criminals).

Further, they objected to the use of nurses as agents to cause death by withdrawing nursing care. They asserted that the provision of nutrition is an indispensable function in the nursing of patients able to take such nutrition, and who are not dying. The nurses objected that few nurses were consulted (or apparently believed) when they asserted their assessment of the condition of the patient (as not being in PVS). The court relied instead on the statements of neurologists who had spent little time with the patient. The nurses and other employees of Mt. Vernon Rehabilitation Center consistently asserted that this patient was able to take fluids by mouth, able to express emotion appropriately, to make purposeful movements, and to feel pain.

The case had been appealed to the Supreme Court of Missouri, whose newly elected state attorney general had run on a platform of not denying patients the "right to die" in such cases. Predictably, the day he was sworn into office, he withdrew the state's objections to dehydration. Christine Busalacchi was dehydrated to death by nurses at Barnes Hospital in St. Louis, Missouri, dying finally on 11 March 1993.[171]

MRS. O'CONNOR—
ANOTHER CLEAR AND CONVINCING

In New York, the guardian of Mrs. O'Connor, diagnosed with senile dementia, sought to have her dehydrated (she was not asserted to be in PVS). Note that efforts to dehydrate patients are not limited only to patients in a persistent vegetative state. The New York court said she should keep the feeding tube when there is no *clear and convincing evidence* of the patient's wishes.[172]

Reason for the Clear and Convincing Standard

These conditions are sometimes reversible. Examples are not uncommon of patients comatose for long periods, "awakening." Such examples confuse the wish to believe that such people want to, and should be, dehydrated.[173]

COMPETENT PATIENT, CURRENT DIRECTIVE

Very few cases considered by the courts have been about competent patients who personally wish to be dehydrated to death. The following are such cases: Elizabeth Bouvia, a young woman with cerebral palsy and a quadriplegic, but not terminally ill, sought the right to refuse food and water in order to be allowed to die with hospital care (nursing care).[174] She was granted that right by a court, but now lives on a liquid diet in another hospital.

Hector Rojas, another quadriplegic, also petitioned a court to allow him to dehydrate while under hospital care. The court granted his wish, and he died after 14 days, having requested and been administered morphine for the discomfort of dehydration.[175]

A publicized Canadian case held that withdrawing the ventilator at the request of a competent patient with Guillain-Barré syndrome does not violate the criminal code.[176]

State Constitutional Right of Privacy

The U.S. Supreme Court in *Cruzan* found the right to refuse treatment in the liberty interest of the Fourteenth Amendment. They did not discuss the case under an "unwritten right of privacy" in the U.S. Constitution. But many state constitutions have a written right of privacy. Surrogates who wish to stop treatment of their wards may find relief from state laws requiring feeding tubes, in their state constitutions.

Florida's living will law prompted regulators to rule that nursing home residents who don't eat, must get a feeding tube or be discharged. But Florida's right of privacy in the state constitution allowed a resident's guardian to authorize feeding tube removal.[177]

Nurses can find out if their state's constitution has a written right of privacy by looking at (the first article) the state constitution, found in the front of the first volume of the set of state statute books (almost every branch library has a set).

State Requires Ombudsman

Claire Conroy, 84, was a nursing home patient with senile dementia (the diagnosis before Alzheimer's was extended to old people). Again, note that dehydration is not limited to patients with PVS. The court decided that the substituted judgment or best interest standard should be used to decide if the her tube should be removed. The court also ordered a state ombudsman, plus a guardian, be appointed to decide the fate of such people.[178]

Withdrawing Care Is Not Murder

In another case, the worst fears of physicians were realized. Care was withdrawn from a comatose patient, with the consent and desire of the family—or so the doctor thought. A complaint led to a murder charge filed by the prosecutor, but later withdrawn. But testimony revealed that the family was not so clearly commited to the patient's death as the doctor had thought or wished. Lesson? Know the patient and family well enough to ascertain their wishes, even if delay in terminating treatment is necessary.[179]

What Is Death? What Is Dying?

Definition of Death

Defining or redefining death in law (as is done with any law) is done for a reason. The change from the thousand-year-old definition of death as "cessation of pulse and respiration" to "brain" death was done so that harvesting organs would not result in a charge of murder.

Some experts have called for another redefinition of death—higher brain death—which would declare as dead, patients in persistent vegetative state (PVS), and possibly Alzheimer's and senile dementia.

PVS is a relatively newly coined term, used to describe patients who have severe neurological damage and are not conscious, but who seem to have sleep-wake periods and other evidence of higher brain activity.

The diagnosis of brain dead is made in patients in order to harvest organs; patients in such conditions will die, even if ventilated, in a few hours or days.

Depending on the etiology of PVS, the patient is more likely to recover (young, trauma etiology) or not (old, not trauma etiology).

In times past, other diseased people were labeled as dead (lepers), but the diagnosis did not cause them to be actually killed (as the PVS diagnosis has done).

Instead of changing the definition of death to higher brain death the definition might be returned to "cessation of pulse and respiration" (since technological advances promise organ retrieval from cadavers).

The theory of symmetry, applied to life's beginning and ending, would apply similar neurological tests both to when personhood begins (a fetus becomes a baby) and when a personhood ends (the person becomes a "vegetable").

People who do not breathe, whose hearts do not beat, are dead—human beings know when someone is dead. So why change the definition of death established in law for centuries? Changing the definition of death must be for some purpose; either to evade the consequences of some law or the ethical consequence of treating a live "person" in some way.

The "brain death" legal definition of death was originally made in order that surgeons harvesting organs from living bodies would not feel guilty nor be guilty of murder. That 20-year-old new definition has not succeeded—doctors and nurses can diagnose brain death, but they do not consider those patients dead (nor do they pronounce them dead).

Some people now call for extending the definition of death to still more lively people—people with PVS, Alzheimer's, senile dementia, and perhaps to people who are merely incompetent. The change in the definition of death again is made for a reason. Defining people with these diagnoses as "dead" would allow escape from the ethical (and legal) dilemma of killing them.

If people are legally classed as dead, then whatever is done to them is not killing them (a person who is "dead" already, can't be killed). Their bodies can be dehydrated; no ethical nor legal consequences.

Definition of Death as Persistent Vegetative State (PVS)

Diagnosis. "Persistent vegetative state" was the label suggested for a condition first described in 1972 in a British medical journal.[180] PVS is not a specific disease but a collection of symptoms. It is variously described as wakefulness without awareness—the patient is unaware of self or surrounding environment. There is no voluntary movement, emotion, or cognition. Some patients gag or cough, or their eyes move. They seem to have periods of sleeping and waking. The condition is in some cases reversible and cannot be diagnosed with certainty, or permanently. The condition is not found in standard lists of mental health diagnoses.

This is said to be a new disease that came about as a result of the technologies: IV or enteral feeding, IV antibiotics for infections, and good systematic nursing care. All these factors allow these patients to survive various insults, which formerly would have killed them.

There is no published set of accepted criteria for this set of symptoms, although a task force has set forth proposals. No lab tests will diagnose it, and no diagnosis may be made from x-ray, although x-rays and blood flow studies may show damage to the central cortex. The EEGs are often normal.

Causes of the condition are said to be variable, mechanical, and are not understood. The symptoms overlap with other neurological symptoms (coma, dementia, irreversible coma, and "locked-in" syndrome). Patients in "locked-in" syndrome are but one step removed from PVS, in that they have almost no motor function left. They do experience sensations and think, as *may* patients in PVS.

Experts caution that the term "vegetative" is not the same as "persistent vegetative" and neither condition is permanent nor irreversible. Making the diagnosis is not the same as forecasting the prognosis. To predict the future course of the patient, one needs to know the etiology of the injury, the duration of the condition, and the age of the patient.

A very old patient, in a persistent vegetative state for a long time after a cardiac or respiratory arrest, has a poor average prognosis. A young person, with a short time on average in PVS after head trauma, has a good chance of recovery.[181]

The literature on the ethics of treating PVS patients is extensive.[182]

Recent studies on this syndrome or collection of symptoms suggest that these patients (an estimated 10,000 of them in the United States) are capable of prolonged survival with good care.

Of 1,611 nursing home patients examined in one study, three percent (62 patients) were identified by staff to be in PVS; 11 of the 62 were subsequently determined by the investigators to have been misdiagnosed. That is, these patients had some awareness, volitional movement, and two of them improved after admission.

Of those finally diagnosed "correctly," 53 percent had CPR status ordered, about the same as for general hospital patients. All patients were on daily meds. Seventy-eight percent had pressure sores; 27 percent were on antipsychotic medications, although behavior of any kind should not have been a problem for such patients. During the course of the study, 60 percent were hospitalized for some reason, usually acute infection, and 29 percent had surgery (for example, for fracture repair or pacemaker replacement).[183]

Always mentioned is the high cost of nursing care for such patients—upwards of $100,000 per year per patient—although many could be cared for in nursing homes or at home more cheaply.

Patients discharged from hospitals in a so-called vegetative state frequently recover; a 1991 report found that 58 percent did so. Significantly, six percent of those recoveries were in patients who had been "vegetative" for more than two years. An analysis of demographic and neurologic features failed to identify any useful prognostic indicators of recovery from the vegetative state.[184]

The condition is frequently misdiagnosed—some 37 percent of patients diagnosed as "PVS" were not in PVS. Errors in diagnosis resulted from confusion in terminology, lack of extended observation of patients, and lack of skill or training in the assessment of neurologically devastated patients.[185] This information is particularly troubling when considered with the consequences that a diagnosis of PVS may have for the patient.

The consequences of the diagnosis (possible deliberate dehydration and death) raise the question of why the diagnosis is being created and made. Does the physician, with the help of nurses, make such a diagnosis to give better care, or to justify giving less or no care?

In several writers' opinions, patients diagnosed in PVS should have no treatment (not even nursing care of hydration and nutrition), because they are already dead. Diagnosing patients as PVS and having nurses dehydrate them to death, comes to the same result as declaring PVS patients to be dead; the diagnosis results in death.

Nurses and neurologists are not disinterested scientists and caregivers on this issue; neurologists and nurses who define PVS, specify criteria for diagnosis, and make such diagnoses, are responsible for the consequences of their use.[186] In the 1930s, psychiatrists and nurses in Germany under the National Socialists assessed mentally ill and mentally retarded as "hopeless," knowing that the consequence of their assessment was death for those patients.

Some writers assert that it is a lie to give families the right to decide to refuse treatment for their loved one in PVS; the clear and convincing evidence standard is excused only in PVS cases. In those cases, even a little evidence is enough to prove the patient wanted to die. Families are given this right to decide to terminate treatment for PVS patients—not in other cases.

For example, when non-PVS children are the subject, families are not given the decision about their loved child's fate. Prosecutions of Christian Scientist parents have been made when their children were harmed by lack of medical treatment. In those non-PVS, nondisabled child cases, the parents were not allowed to make decisions for the children. That is only done in PVS and disabled children, and only when the parents decide what society agrees is the right decision.

One writer asks that decisions about PVS patients not be left to their families—he believes the honest action is to declare the patients dead.[187]

Another writer believes that suffering *is* relieved by mercy killing—the suffering of the *relatives*. He advocates that the honest, accurate, and truthful course of action is to admit that real motive for diagnosing and dehydrating PVS.[188]

If PVS patients were considered legally dead, then the diagnosis of PVS would have even more important consequences.

Declaring diseased people to be dead is not a new human phenomenon. In the early 1200s, persons diagnosed with leprosy were officially declared dead in a ceremony. They lost rights as citizens (for example, to inherit or bequeath property). The leper was brought from home to the church, mass was read, and extreme unction given as though the person had died. Warning was given never to go to church, market, tavern or bathhouse, never to work bare-handed, drink from a well, touch anything bare-handed, and to warn all people of the leprous condition. The leper was then taken to the cemetery to an open grave, where the priest three times threw earth on the leper; and lastly, the leper was conducted to the leprosarium (when available).[189]

If people in PVS are declared dead, treatment must be discontinued and their bodies killed. (Declaring them dead might be seen as more honest and compassionate than inventing the fiction that they would refuse treatment if they could, resulting in death by dehydration.) After the PVS diagnosis is done and feeding is stopped, should some lethal injection would be administered? Do prohibitions against "animal cruelty" proscribe death by dehydration? The bodies could serve some useful purposes for experimentation or transplant, as aborted fetuses might.[190]

Proposals for Changes

Since suggestions have been made that PVS and some other incompetent patients are dead already, proponents say the law should be changed to reflect the reality. They advocate that the loss of upper brain function, which seems to be lost in PVS and senile dementia of the Alzheimer's type, should be the legal definition of death.[191]

Several years ago pressure for organ transplant caused a change in the definition of death to brain death—loss of total brain function, including the brain stem. Brain death need not be declared unless the patient's organs are sought for another patient; the brain dead patient will die within (at most) a few hours or days.

Subsequently, most state legislatures adopted the brain death definition as law, so that a surgeon removing organs will not be considered legally to have killed the patient.

Practitioners can now diagnose irreversible loss of brainstem function with a high degree of certainty. But they don't all diagnose that condition as death. Many years after the adoption of "brain death" as legal death, practitioners still do not declare patients as brain dead for organ retrieval. A study indicates that experts *can* identify patients with a permanent loss of all brain function. However, three-fourths of a group of all practitioners, and one-third of a group of experts, did not agree that permanent loss of all brain function meant the patient was *dead*.[192]

ICU nurses in particular face ethical issues around dying patients. On the one hand, nurses believe that death is natural, not forever the enemy—an inevitable end of life. On the other hand, the death of some patients is seen as a defeat, and the nurse works intensively to preserve the patient's life.

People (nurses are people) seem to recognize instinctively that people with beating hearts are not dead (this is more evidence of disagreement over the present definition of death as loss of total brain function).

Do human beings have ethical instincts that rationalization for a desired result cannot educate away? Even during the time of wild euthanasia in Nazi Germany (when doctors and nurses were encouraged to go through the wards and pick out victims), most nurses and doctors did not participate.[193]

At a time when practitioners still disagree over that "whole brain" definition of death, further requests have appeared to redefine death to a still more "alive" level. Instead of changing the definition to "higher brain death" might the definition of death be returned to "cessation of pulse and respiration"? Organ retrieval from cadavers is increasingly possible, in future removing the need for total brain death as a definition.

As noted earlier, most state law defines death as loss of the total brain. New definitions of death would be loss of function in just the higher levels of thinking and awareness. These people breathe on their own, have heartbeats, have brain stem function, feel pain, and many think cognitively at some level.

Some ethicists' advice has been heeded; PVS patients have been treated as dead (dehydrating them to death). If patients are declared dead before they are killed by dehydration, the result will be breathing bodies that are declared dead.

Organ retrieval from potential donors among the PVS is mentioned as a beneficial outcome of declaring them dead.[194]

The people declared dead could be used for research; the fertile young women could be used as surrogate mothers. Brain-dead mothers have already been kept alive to allow their infants time to develop to term.[195] (These women were not actually *brain dead*; if they were really brainstem dead by the criteria established, they would live only a few hours or days.) Or, patients declared dead could be buried (or sent directly to the undertaker). If not, someone must "kill" the patient declared dead. In several cases, treating the PVS patient as dead has resulted in nurses causing death by the method of withholding nursing care.

Brain Death and Higher Brain Death

Deciding when to stop treating and deciding when a human being is dead, are not new issues. People have always had to decide whether to care for dying or injured people, and when to stop. But treatment of dying or ill or unconscious people has become more sophisticated; and as their treatment has been removed from the family and given to strangers, it has become more difficult to decide when to quit treating. (Treatment can certainly stop when the patient is dead, unless organs are to be obtained). *When* death occurs is important to nurses, not least because nurses are increasingly responsible for legally declaring patients dead.[196]

For millennia, death was considered to have occurred when the heart stopped beating (usually secondary to respiration ceasing). But today, with ventilators, bodies can be kept going for a while after the brain is dead (for a few hours or days at most).

The terminology "brain death" has since arisen—to facilitate recovery of organs for transplant. Subsequently, state legislatures have debated that definition and adopted it with variations, as law. Such law has made it possible to cut into a breathing, heart-beating body and remove the organs, without having that act considered unethical or illegal. But even many years later, practitioners do not all agree on what is death, nor can they diagnose total brain death.

Doctors and nurses have had specific, concrete lists of criteria for brain death for many years.[197]

CLINICAL CRITERIA FOR BRAIN DEATH

No response to external stimuli.
No reflex activity except of spinal cord origin.
No pupillary response to light.
No corneal reflexes.
No eye movement with caloric testing or "doll's eyes" maneuver.
No gag reflex.
No cough reflex.
Apnea in presence of adequate carbon dioxide stimulation.

The criteria are not applied uniformly and extensively, perhaps because the conclusions of their use violate the instinctive human response that people whose hearts beat, who breathe, whose skin is warm—are not dead.[198] More recent proposals define death as loss of function in still higher levels of thinking and awareness.[199]

The utilitarian who defines death considers not what is right, but instead considers what will accomplish the result desired outcome. That approach results at least in keeping the definition of death as "death of the whole brain," a middle ground between cardiopulmonary death and "higher" brain death. Utilitarians would say that death occurs whenever people decide that death occurs; they assert that death can be defined any way people want.[200]

Another theory, that of symmetry, would apply to *death* the same criteria as the start of life—either when the lower brain starts to function or when the higher brain starts to function. This has implications for the ethics and law of abortion.

When Do People Die—and Who Chooses?

The causation of death can be divided into unintentionally caused death (natural causes, act of God, or disease) and intentionally caused death (suicide by the patient, euthanasia by the practitioner, murder).

Euthanasia has had a negative image since the German National Socialists of the 1930s and 40s used it—a period that culminated in what is now termed the holocaust.

Nurses and their organizations were actively involved in the euthanasia and subsequent killing in that era.

A sizeable number of people consistently believe that "incurable" or people disabled to some degree, would be better off dead.

People die either unintentionally (of a disease or by someone who did *not* intend to cause the death), or intentionally (either by their own hand or by someone else who *did* intend to kill them). Unintentional death by disease is considered to be "God's will" or "natural causes"; it is not an ethical issue in this book. Unintended death caused by a person could be negligence, in which case it is covered by the ethics and law of malpractice.

Intentionally-caused death done by the patient is suicide. Intentionally-caused death done by the patient with help is assisted suicide. Intentionally-caused death with consent is euthanasia; without the patient's consent is termed "involuntary euthanasia" or "nonvoluntary euthanasia," or murder.

National Socialism/the Nazis

The most "successful" use of euthanasia (involuntary killing) in the history of the world was that of the Germans under National Socialism. The euthanasia program was "successful" in that it accomplished many of its goals: from eliminating many "lives not worth living" to virtually eliminating Jews from German society.

Much evidence has accumulated about the participation of the German medical profession in the euthanasia program of the National Socialists. The medical and nursing professions had full knowledge and cooperated. Those who assert an analogy between Nazi and U.S. society would do well to study that evidence.

For those who do *not* worry that euthanasia is a "slippery slope" to what happened in Germany:

> This same psychological dynamic [avoiding the work and pain of dealing with difficult different people] can feed the impulse that leads from authorizing the death of comatose people to retarded people already suffering from terminal physical illness to retarded people suffering only from retardation. It can lead from old people who have become too burdensome to sustain to anomalous newborns whose sustenance is too burdensome to anticipate.[201]

Below are references for any nurse who cares to pursue reading about the euthanasia program in 1930s Germany.

RESOURCES

Annas, G.J., and Grodin, M.A., Eds., *The Nazi Doctors and the Nuremberg Code: Human Rights in Human Experimentation*, New York: Oxford University Press, 1992.

Caplan, A.L., Ed., *Medicine Betrayed: The Participation of Doctors in Human Rights Abuses*, London: Zed Books, 1992.

Hoedeman, P., *Hitler or Hippocrates: Medical Experiments and Euthanasia in the Third Reich*, Sussex, England: Book Guild, 1992.

Kater, M., *Doctors under Hitler*, Chapel Hill, NC: University of North Carolina Press, 1989.

Lifton, R., *The Nazi Doctors*, New York: Basic Books, 1986.

Weindling, P., *Health, Race and German Politics Between National Unification and Nazism, 1870–1945*, Cambridge: Cambridge University Press, 1991.

Perhaps mercifully, nurses have not merited a separate book on their participation in the holocaust. Nurses are liberally mentioned in the above references, almost as an afterthought. Of course, Nazi doctors could not have done all that they did without nurses, who did more than collaborate with physicians. Nurses took an active, assertive, independent role in selecting and euthanizing their patients. Doctors are still engaged in torture in countries around the world—and they must still have help.[202]

Nurses and their organizations cooperated fully with the National Socialists in killing patients under that government. Few nursing texts acknowledge the active role that nurses took in Nazi euthanasia; some research is ongoing, and more knowledge about the role of nurses in active euthanasia is seen in the written literature.

Hilde Steppe (a German nurse working in the Department of Nursing of the Ministry of Youth, Family, and Health in Wiesbaden, Germany) has researched the original files and collated data about the participation of nurses in euthanasia. She concludes that German nursing changed during the National Socialist period. Some of the changes were positive for nursing: an improved social status, unification of professional nursing organizations, "improved" (tighter) nurse licensure laws, and increased politicization of the profession. These improvements were of course gained as a result of collaboration with and support of the National Socialists.

Steppe does identify some real nurse heroes of the time: Sister M. Restituta (Helene Kafka), an Austrian nun, who worked in an operating room in a town near Vienna. She fought National Socialism, continuing to hang the Holy Cross in patient rooms after being forbidden to do so, and distributing a soldier's poem that suggested desertion. In 1942 she was arrested in her OR. Few spoke up on her behalf after she was sentenced to death. She was executed in March 1943, at the age of 49.

Nurse Emmy Dörfel was a Communist, arrested in Germany in 1935. She left for France; worked with the Spanish Communists during Spain's Civil War; interned in France, and later returned to Germany. Then she was taken to the concentration camp at Ravensbruck, escaping in 1945—she lives today in Berlin.

In articles written by nurses at the time, and in interviews with nurses who lived through the era, Steppe found that many of the German nurses accepted the National Socialist's rewrite of society's and nursing's ethics. The nurses assumed that through their obedience they were doing good, remaining true to their professional ethics, unaffected by the social change around them. This "apolitical professional consciousness" made it possible for the profession to be made a part of the larger political system. Steppe, believing there are lessons in that experience for contemporary nurses, said:

> I believe that we must be clear that nursing never takes place in a value-free, neutral context; it is always a socially significant force. This means that we cannot simply observe what is taking place around us but must take a stand and get involved, helping to shape sociopolitical developments.

> I also believe that we must deal with the history of our profession, especially its darkest hours, so that we may remain sensitive to any signs of inhumanity. We

must call into question traditional principles, such as obedience, and replace them with professional competence, professionalism, and creative self-consciousness.

And not least, we have a moral obligation to the millions of victims of National Socialism, even if it only means that, through historical research, we assure that they are not forgotten. By taking responsibility for this part of our history, we can become more sensitive for the future, with eyes and ears open for all social injustices.[203]

Hilde Steppe presented a paper in 1993 in which she detailed the research: Of the nurses who had participated in the killing under the National Socialists, a few were condemned to death and a number were sentenced to prison. Others continued to work, and no case is known in which a nurse's right to practice was taken away because of participation in Nazi crimes.[204]

"Whatever proportions [National Socialist] crimes finally assumed, it became evident to all who investigated them that they had started from small beginnings. The beginnings at first were merely a subtle shift in emphasis in the basic attitude of the physicians.

"It started with the acceptance of the attitude, basic in the euthanasia movement, that there is such a thing as life not worthy to be lived. This attitude in its early stages concerned itself merely with the severely and chronically sick. Gradually the sphere of those to be included in this category was enlarged to encompass the socially unproductive, the ideologically unwanted, the racially unwanted and finally all non-Germans.

"But it is important to realize that the infinitely small wedged-in lever from which this entire trend of mind received its impetus was the attitude toward the nonrehabilitable sick."[205]

On the first day of World War II, 1 September 1939, Adolph Hitler charged Karl Brandt, official head of the medical profession, with this duty:

Reichsleiter Bouhler and Dr. Brandt, M.D., are charged with the responsibility of enlarging the authority of certain physicians to be designated by me in such a manner that persons who, according to human judgment, are incurably sick may, upon the most careful diagnosis of their medical condition, be accorded a mercy death.[206]

Two National Socialist propaganda movies—"Existence Without Life" and "Mentally Ill"—portray the killing of "life unworthy of life" as an act of mercy. Nazi documents discovered in Stasi files (East German secret police) after the fall of Communism confirm that the objects of the "euthanasia program" included anyone considered lazy or a drunk, and women who "kept a disorderly household" or had children by different men. Some 200,000 people were killed in the euthanasia program.

> Advocating that "incurables" be put to death by the state, the film said: "Every reasonable person would prefer death to such an existence," and that the mentally ill had a "right to die."[207]

The "patients" selected for such treatment included children and adults, with conditions such as blindness, deafness and epilepsy; mental disabilities such as Down's syndrome, and others "morally or socially feeble-minded." Michael Burleigh, a lecturer at the London School of Economics, discovered in a cellar of the Stasi archives both the National Socialist films and files on at least 70,000 people who were killed in the euthanasia program. (The Stasi had been using the records to blackmail doctors or professionals working in the West who had been involved in the euthanasia program.[208]) Might this be a future scenario for nurses who are now participating in dehydrating patients?

This is not 1939, and in the United States are many kinds of people. Citizens are not generally afflicted with aspirations to an ideal state inhabited by a pure race. But as nurses struggle to make ethical decisions about dying people, should they keep in mind any possible analogy to that time and its aspirations?

Some people of the United States also saw euthanasia as a solution even at that time. The wish for euthanasia seems an undercurrent in society, being discussed openly when social conditions encourage it.

A 1939 Gallup Poll on euthanasia in the United States found that 46 percent of the people interviewed were in favor of legalizing euthanasia for "suffering incurables." In England, 69 percent of the people in the survey were in favor. An even larger percentage favored putting deformed infants to death in cases of highly defective children (a Down's baby was so considered at that time). A respected nursing ethics textbook of that era defined involuntary euthanasia as follows:

"Involuntary euthanasia refers to the practice of destroying deformed and mentally defective children or putting to death hopelessly insane or diseased adults who are incapable of exercising judgment."[209]

And, the textbook quoted an article in *Collier's Magazine* of 20 May 1939, titled "To be or not to be," in which the writer said:

To these unfortunates we surely might be allowed legally to grant a dreamless and unending sleep . . . [as an example an] idiot girl of four, unable to sit up or speak. She would follow a light and look toward a sound—and that was all.[210]

—Foster Kennedy

The nurse ethicist:

> "It is not clear at present just what the prevailing view of physicians will be regarding this difficult question."[211]

The euthanasia program of the Germans revealed the ease with which the concept of euthanasia slipped into wholesale killing of anyone who presented difficulty. "Controversial questions" for nursing ethics of that time were as outlined in Densford: Capital punishment, warfare, martyrdom, euthanasia, contraception, and abortion. What will the young nurse reading this book in the 1990s remember as nursing's present "controversial questions" fifty years hence?

Killing: Assisted Suicide

> *Assisted suicide* is ill-defined; in Holland it is defined "prescribing drugs for patients to poison themselves" (illegal there; but in the United States, legalized by a referendum in Oregon in 1994).
>
> Doing more than providing the poison or gun is actually doing the killing; the patient may volunteer or not.
>
> The distinctions of "voluntariness" are voluntary (patient requests), involuntary (patient does not request), and nonvoluntary (patient cannot request, so surrogate does) (euthanasia).
>
> Nurses face as much ethical (and legal) pain for assisted suicide or euthanasia as do doctors; such technical work is invariably delegated.
>
> Distinctions are made regarding whether the patient volunteers, whether the act is direct or indirect, and whether the killing is active or passive.
>
> Euthanasia by dehydration is confusing since it seems to "allow the patient to die naturally"—but allowing animals or convicted felons to "die naturally" by withholding water from them is considered cruel.

Increasingly, nurses and doctors are being asked to assist suicide (some experts *suggest* that they do so). This topic involves practitioner and patient autonomy; the freedom to kill (oneself or one's patient) and the freedom not to kill (oneself or one's patient). These freedoms are either expressions or violations of the value, Freedom. The topic is discussed here in this chapter on dying because such actions and law also dramatically express the value that society puts on living and dying.

Assisting suicide is not the act done when a nurse kills a patient with a drug (yet many proposals for "assisting suicide" incorporate this action). Providing the gun or the prescription is assisting suicide, but administering a drug or firing a gun is killing. It may not be murder if it is not forbidden by the law, and it may be called euthanasia instead of killing, if that word is preferred.

The difference between ventilators and feeding tubes is more than the emotional reaction to withholding food (emotions can be a valuable indicator of the rightness of an action, however). The real difference is: Removing a ventilator *may* result in death; while removing a feeding tube *will* certainly cause death (the action kills the patient).

Withdrawing the ventilator won't kill the patient (the underlying lung disease may cause death—not everyone removed from a ventilator dies). But *everyone* who does not get food and water, dies.

The issue for nurses: Doctors don't assist suicide for these patients; doctors don't nurse the patients for the 11 or 12 days it takes them to die. The doctor doesn't give a quick lethal injection and personally kill a person who's more burden than benefit. The *nurse* is asked to take responsibility.

Other-killing: Euthanasia

Euthanasia comes from the Greek for "well" (happy, good) and *thanatos* for "dying" (death)—a well or good death.

Some authorities say that as many as six concepts of death are possible (note that many theories are constructs of three conditions, each with two opposites). On this subject, the conditions are *active or passive* death, *direct or indirect* death, and *voluntary or involuntary* death. Suicide and assisted suicide are integral to the discussion of euthanasia; it is impossible to talk about suicide, assisted suicide, and euthanasia without mentioning all three.

In active death, the practitioner does something actively to cause the death of the patient. Passive death is withdrawing or withholding treatment that preserves life. As discussed earlier, these are not very helpful distinctions except in the most obvious cases, such as actively administering a lethal injection.

Direct death is a result of an act intended to cause death, while indirect death is the result of an act not intended to cause death in the first instance (but which has that result). An example of indirect death is that last injection of morphine for the pain, which also then causes respiratory depression and results in death.

Voluntary death is obvious—the patient wants/wishes the death. Involuntary is the opposite: Death is caused without the request or wish of the patient. Some assert that a middle level of voluntariness should apply to incompetent persons who are killed involuntarily: *Nonvoluntary*. That is, the person didn't volunteer (couldn't), nor did they object (so they weren't killed *in*voluntarily); therefore their death is "nonvoluntary."

In suicide, the patient kills him- or herself. Assisted suicide is prescribing poison or furnishing a gun. If the practitioner administers the poison, it is not assisting suicide, but directly killing the patient.

The main disagreement: whether voluntary, direct, active death should be permitted, and even authorized in law. If unassisted, that act is suicide. The issue for nurses is whether doctors and/or nurses should be permitted or sanctioned to *assist* people to suicide, or even to *kill* them if they are unable to kill themselves.

Euthanasia by Dehydration. Dehydration as a method of terminating life is discussed above, as is the condition of PVS. The topic of euthanasia by dehydration touches again on both of those subjects; the cross-fertilization of PVS, euthanasia, and dehydration will not be put into neat categories. The "messiness" of the topic makes it "messy" to discuss.

**A RESPECTED ETHICIST
ON EUTHANASIA BY DEHYDRATION:**

"[D]enial of nutrition may in the long run become the only effective way to make certain that a large number of biologically tenacious patients actually die. Given the increasingly large pool of superannuated, chronically ill, physically marginal elderly, it could well become the nontreatment of choice."[212]

In several cases earlier in this chapter, dehydration was used to cause involuntary, direct, passive death (*killing* the patient *without request*, but *not actively*). In the *Cruzan* and *Busalacchi* cases, it may be argued the deaths were *voluntary* in that the patients would have wished it (not that they actually did). Or it may be argued that the death was caused indirectly, since no lethal injection was administered. The indirect-direct distinction is as unhelpful here as the withholding-withdrawing distinction earlier.

The unwillingness to admit that the intent is to cause death (and the failure to take responsibility for causing it) is asserted to result in cruelty in letting these patients die "naturally." But some assert these patients don't feel pain; if so, then perhaps there's no ethical problem.

> *The animal analogy:* Animals are not killed at the pound by dehydration and starvation, but are quickly killed. Some assert that no less should be done for people (some assert, however, that people in PVS are not "people"—perhaps are not human).

The interests here: The individual, in life. That interest may be secondary to relief of pain, in which case the patient's interest really may be in dying. The family's interest is in helping the loved one (doing good/beneficence), which may translate into having the loved one dead. The family's interest is also in being free of grief and pain over this family member they believe is already dead. In that case the family is loyal to itself—the value is being true/fidelity.

The family's interest may also be peripherally in money—if the family is projected to get money from an insurance policy or trust on the death of their daughter—as in the *Cruzan* and *Busalacchi* cases.

The practitioner's interest is in helping (doing good/beneficence), in not harming (non-maleficence). Some assert the safety, lack of pain, and even euphoria of dying by dehydration. However, none of the authors cites evidence that a patient undergoing such death actually enjoys it (and none of the authors volunteers to undergo a period of such beneficial treatment). It is important to note that people do not commit suicide by dehydration if any other means is available, nor is dehydration suggested as a humane way to execute condemned felons.

Dehydration is advised as a compassionate treatment for patients who are actually dying (and it may be). Unfortunately, the logic immediately slides into the proposal that dehydration to cause death is also good for people who are *not* dying (people in nursing homes who are merely senile). When it is pointed out to one author that she has advocated termination of nondying senile patients by dehydration, the author responds that she has advocated dehydration for "dying patients only."[213]

The Laws

Analysis by Degree of Intent

Actions that cause death can be separated into those that are intended to cause death (suicide, murder, assisted suicide, euthanasia) and those that are not so intended (reckless act, negligence, increase in pain medication).

Suicide has been variously considered as good or bad in societies; to change the assistance of practitioners in suicide will have other consequences.

In criminal law, *intent* is crucial to determining culpability. Intent to cause death (as opposed to allowing death which is inevitable) may be in some situations considered a crime. In the area of euthanasia and assisted suicide intent is also crucial; the important distinction is between actions intended to cause death, and actions which are not intended to cause death.

Action Not Intended to Cause Death (Death is Not a Certain Result). If the intent is not to cause death (meaning that death is not a certain result of the action), no ethical or legal guilt should result. Example: Giving the appropriate dosage of morphine for pain in the patient's situation, even though the patient's respirations are further depressed and the patient dies, is usually ethical and so, legal.

The exception to that intent criterion is an action that is *not* intended to cause death, but which does so negligently. An unintended negligent action that causes death can give rise to a malpractice suit. Example: Giving 100 mg of morphine, though there was no intent to kill, can be punished in a civil lawsuit.

If the negligence rises to the level of *conscious disregard* of whether death will result, the crime of manslaughter could be charged. An example is realizing that 100 mg of morphine was given, and not reporting it, resulting in the death of the patient.

Action Intended to Cause Death (Death Was Certain to Occur from the Action). It may be determined legally whether the action that caused the death was *intended* to cause death (although the inside of the mind of the person who did the action can never be seen). A lengthy history of law using intent, infers the intent from the *knowledge of the result of the action.* The intent to cause death is inferred if the actor has certain knowledge that the action will cause death.

Voluntariness of the Person to Death. The next step in analysis is whether the patient wants the death done. If the patient wants to die, is she or he prepared to kill herself personally?

If YES = SUICIDE

If NO = SOMEONE KILLS THE PATIENT (some wrongly call this assisted suicide)

In voluntary death the patient commits suicide, either independent or assisted.

Involuntariness of the Person to Death. Involuntary death is either caused by disease (or accident) or is caused by a person. As noted above, some writers dislike the similarity to murder that results when an incompetent patient is involuntarily killed, so a third category is established: *"nonvoluntary"*—that is, the patient did not ask to be killed (voluntary), nor did the patient object to dying (if she had, that *involuntary* killing would be murder).

The patient was incapable of volunteering, so the *agent* volunteers (the patient is considered nonvoluntary). This reasoning allows the thinker to escape the moral difficulty of involuntary killing (which in any other situation would be murder). Is this new construction of intent an unnecessary escape? If people in a society believe that incompetent patients may be killed without their volunteering to die, can they face that fact without constructing an ethical (and resulting legal) fiction?

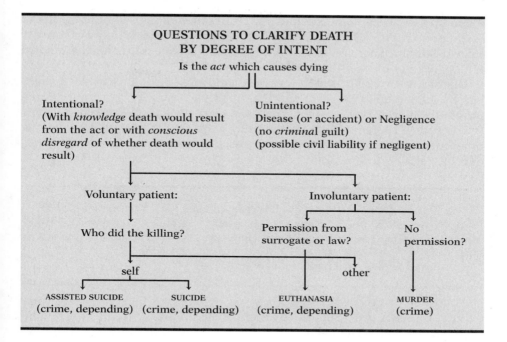

QUESTIONS TO CLARIFY DEATH
BY DEGREE OF INTENT

What distinguishes murder from involuntary killing (euthanasia) is an arbitrary line drawn by lawmakers, depending on motive for the killing and the status of the victim. And the arbitrary line moves; if the law permitting doctors and nurses to assist suicide in Oregon prevails, the law line will have moved further to the left.

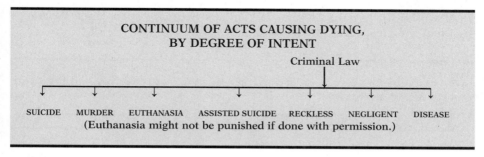

CONTINUUM OF ACTS CAUSING DYING,
BY DEGREE OF INTENT

Self-killing

In order to think clearly and ethically about assisted suicide, people must know their attitude toward suicide itself. The issue: Is it acceptable for people to kill themselves? Is it the ultimate in autonomy, or are they mentally ill, or depressed? Should such people be helped to live, or to die?

The issue of suicide expresses the value, Freedom (Autonomy). Self-killing (and assisting people to do self-killing, by giving them a prescription or a gun or a rope) can be distinguished from other-killing (all other forms of ending one person's life by another). Examples of other-killing are murder (illegal killing), abortion (legal killing), and euthanasia (technically illegal killing, but not often prosecuted).

One study showed that increases in suicide among people who used methods of suicide described in Derek Humphrey's *Final Exit* were not among terminally ill, but in the population of the mentally ill.[214] Virtually all people (studies say 95 percent) who kill themselves are depressed and/or have some other mental illness. Treatment for depression and some other mental disorders has become dramatically more effective in the last decades.[215]

> "We believe the line between [euthanasia and suicide] is becoming blurred in the eyes of the public. Efforts to destigmatize euthanasia or even encourage it for some groups may have the untoward effect of promoting suicide in other groups—for example, people with chronic, nonfatal medical illnesses and people with mental disorders."[216]

Suicide in History. Suicide is an old issue, as are so many ethical conflicts in this book. The behavior of aboriginal people is an indication that peoples in pre-history also dealt with the dying and their care (or non-care). The Greeks wrote about good death and suicide. The concept of suicide is inextricable from assisted suicide—in this context, killing the patients. Plato in his ideal society would have permitted voluntary, direct medical killing of the incurably ill or disabled. But Plato suggested that physicians who attempt to poison patients must be punished by death, and lay persons who did so should be fined. Aristotle thought that suicide and mercy killing violated the social contract that individuals had with each other. Worse, in his view, the acts were not virtuous.

> "I will neither give a deadly drug to anybody if asked for it, nor will I make a suggestion to this effect."
>
> —Hippocrates

From the attempt of this oath to discourage suicide, it can be assumed that doctors did perform such deadly care. Or perhaps that promise in the oath is an attempt to discourage doctors from giving poison to people who would use it on their enemies.

Sts. Augustine and Thomas Aquinas opposed suicide on religious grounds. They thought life (and suffering if a part of it) to be given by God. Utopians, as characterized in the writing of Sir Thomas More, thought suicide a be part of the "good life." Christians generally are against the practice.

The desire for suicide and the related wish to end lives not worth living are recurrent themes in human history. In 1994 a version of assisted suicide passed in Oregon in a public referendum; court challenges ensued. Legislatures and courts in several other states are considering the issue.

The state or society (all citizens together) have some interest in protecting people who are unable to protect themselves (doing good/beneficence). Is suicide in the best interest of people who don't want to live, whatever their reason? Can the state prohibit suicide, or prohibit nurses from helping people kill themselves? They may be in unknown psychic pain. Do nurses have a responsibility to help heal the pain, or help end it with death?

Societies prohibit suicide because it is assumed to be an irrational act. Life is assumed to be better than death; someone choosing death, who doesn't have physical pain, is deemed irrational. That is the reason for making assisted suicide illegal where it is; suicide itself may or may not be illegal in various states (but a successful suicide is unpunishable).

Many offer the rationale that allowing assisted suicide would allay the fear people have of dying a lingering death while attached to machines, among strangers, in pain, without dignity.

Official Positions on Suicide, Assisted Suicide, and Euthanasia

The Medical Society in Britain and the American and World Medical Associations condemn euthanasia/assisted suicide, but the Dutch Medical Association accepts it as part of medical practice. This is similar to the position of professional groups on abortion in the United States. The Dutch document states that physicians should not be required to administer euthanasia (kill patients) but should not impose their moral beliefs on the patient; they should refer the patient to another doctor who will kill her.

What do nurses say? The American Nurses Association opposes assisted suicide as proposed in Oregon, but does accept that nurses may dehydrate to death patients not dying if their surrogate wants. If a terminally or chronically ill patient chooses death, a line must be drawn between allowing suicide, encouraging suicide, assisting with suicide, or directly killing. The nurse must differentiate between injecting a consenting patient with a lethal injection for the purpose of causing death, inserting the needle so that the patient may inject the lethal dose personally; and prescribing the lethal dose. There are differences between action, facilitation, encouragement, and mere information,[217] and, in the cases of dehydration, inaction.

Organized nursing in the United States has several position statements on the nurse's role in "end-of-life" decisions.[218] Many of those statements as they pertain to euthanasia by dehydration are set out in Dehydration, above.

Australian Euthanasia

Some research on Australian nurse attitudes toward euthanasia reveals that 55 percent felt that they had been asked by a patient to hasten death. Almost all those nurses felt that such a request can sometimes be rational. Two-thirds of those nurses had been asked by a patient to forego life-sustaining treatments (what the authors called passive euthanasia). Ten percent of those nurses said they had done so on the patient's request. Two-thirds of the nurses who'd been asked to hasten death said the patient requested active death. Three-fourths of those nurses said they thought it was wrong to actively end a patient's life. Three-fourths of the nurses thought that the criteria said to operate in Holland would be a good idea to have in their country. (The criteria that are supposed to be followed are set out below.) The authors of the study concluded that if the Dutch euthanasia practice were permitted in their country, "there would be no shortage of nurses willing to assist in the provision of active euthanasia. . . ."[219]

Another study, done for an Australian criminal justice body, found similarly: The researcher found that 18 percent of doctors and nurses ignore the law and take active steps to hasten the death of their patients.[220] Other Australians worry that doctors and nurses should not follow the Dutch example (in which unauthorized, unasked-for killing is done).[221]

RESOURCES

Fisher, A., "The road to euthanasia," *Tablet*, 20 February 1993; pp. 235–237.

Robinson, J., "Euthanasia: The collision of theory and practice," *Law, Medicine & Health Care*, 1990; 18(1–2):105–7.

Jack Kevorkian is a retired Michigan pathologist who (depending on what one believes) has killed several people or helped them commit suicide in Michigan. (Assisted suicide was not, but is now, against the law of Michigan as it is in other states.) Kevorkian uses the same method of death as the Germans under National Socialism; Hitler's medical advisor, Werner Heyde, concluded that carbon monoxide gassing was the most humane way to kill people. National Socialist doctors stressed that only doctors should carry out the gassing. Carbon monoxide has no medical use but to kill (Pathologist Kevorkian had great difficulty in starting IV lines to use on early suicides, so he abandoned IV lethal injections as a method of death).[222]

As discussed regarding futility in Chapter Four, practitioners who have acquiesced to other patient demands will find it hard to take a high moral ground on this particular patient demand.

Only quadraplegics would need help to commit suicide if they really wanted to. If people don't want to make the effort to kill themselves, it might be questioned whether they really want to die. Should nurses help them to die even when the patient won't act personally?

Do patients ask for death on demand, to be relieved of the responsibility and to be approved in their choice? Are practitioners who take that responsibility giving approval to die by performing the task?

"Pro"—The patient needs relief of suffering. Causing death relieves and prevents loss of control at the end of life, ends fear of dying among strangers, on machines, without dignity. The individual has a right to his own body, his autonomy, his freedom; he can forego treatment, so he should be able to ask the practitioner to kill instead of having to suffer longer. If the person has no religion that says death comes when it is fated, then why shouldn't he die whenever he wishes?

"Con"—Assisted suicide is the slippery slope to killing. It is secret killing, because voluntary death will first be tolerated, then encouraged, and then pressure will be brought to bear to end life. The old will feel not-so-subtle pressure to request death, to leave their assets to others. Women, upholding their image of "giving" to the end, would be especially susceptible to pressure.

Immediately pressure would increase on surrogates to decide on death for patients who can't voluntarily request it, or who don't have good families who request it for them (like Nancy Cruzan's). If competent people are allowed to get out of terrible lives, discrimination against the incompetent, the helpless, could not be allowed. Subtle but real discrimination would occur when surrogates decide who would "want" involuntary good death. The poor, old, disabled, black, handicapped (mental and physical), alcoholic, drug-addicted, AIDS-infected, all might be seen as more miserable than others. Many people declared incompetent are poor, old, without family; they have a real stranger as a guardian (a public administrator who is guardian for perhaps thousands of other incompetent indigent people in her county). That person also may have a responsibility (an interest) in saving tax money.[223]

The U.S. government's position:

> Policies prohibiting direct killing may also conflict with the important value of patient self-determination . . . The Commission finds this limitation on individual self determination to be an acceptable cost of securing the general protection of human life afforded by the prohibition of direct killing.[224]

The Holland Experience

Doctors in Holland may kill patients (but not prescribe poisons) if several criteria are met; there is evidence that patients are killed without the criteria satisfied and without the deaths being reported as euthanasia.

Pain control is a related issue in that some patients are said to request euthanasia or assisted suicide because pain relief is inadequate; nurses continue to seek ways to meet patient needs short of killing them.

Holland has legalized killing by doctors. The law against killing patients will not be prosecuted (enforced) if certain conditions are met:

1. Patient must be competent (not Quinlan, Cruzan, newborns, handicapped, Alzheimer's, or senile dementia).
2. Patient must request voluntarily, consistently, repeatedly over a reasonable time and document (not an impulsive act).
3. Patient must suffer intolerably, with no prospect of relief (there's no need for the patient be terminal).
4. Physician performs, with analysis by another doctor not involved in the original care.

Usually a barbiturate is used to put the patient to sleep, then killing is done with curare to paralyze the muscles of breathing.

Estimates vary widely as to how many such deaths take place in Holland yearly, between 2,300 and 20,000. It is believed a minimum two percent of all deaths are caused by physicians; the actual number is not known because, despite the law's requirement, Dutch doctors don't put the required "unnatural causes" on the death certificate. If that is listed, a formal inquiry must be held. The doctors avoid reporting, although they have no liability if they comply with the list above.

Some 54 percent of Dutch doctors say they killed patients as above, or have assisted suicide. In Holland, *assisted suicide* is different from killing patients; in Holland, assisting suicide is prescribing drugs that patients later administer *themselves*. Prescribing is illegal in Holland, but it is the act approved by voters in Oregon in 1994.

Only 186 deaths by euthanasia were reported in Holland in 1988.[225] In an anonymous study, physicians admit to assisting 386 suicides by prescribing lethal drugs, to causing 2,318 deaths after request (with barbiturates and curare usually), and to causing 1,030 deaths *without request* (involuntary intentional death) (definition: murder).[226] Almost half of all lethal injections given to incompetent patients are given in cases in which the patient has never expressed a wish for death.[227]

Psychiatrists worry that many of the Dutch requesting death are depressed, and that they could be helped with therapy if they were treated by other than general practitioners.

The Dutch have no problem with directly causing death, but in the main are opposed to passive nonvoluntary euthanasia—in other words, dehydrating the nondying patient to death. The Dutch think that *Americans* are on the slippery slope regarding "allowing the patient to die" in ways that are not voluntary on the part of the patient.

Pain Control

Hospice nurses have said they have never had a patient who was free of pain and who felt wanted, express a wish to die—with or without help. Both of those are conditions nurses can affect.

25. Abortion data sources: The Alan Guttmacher Institute, New York, NY.
"Researchers Amass Abortion Data," *Journal of the American Medical Association*, 1989; 262:1431–1432.
And: "Abortion in context," *Family Planning Perspectives*, 1988; 20:273–275.
26. *Webster v. Reproductive Health Services*, 492 U.S. 490 (1989).
27. Harrison, M.R., "Unborn: Historical perspective of the fetus as a patient," *Pharos*, Winter, 1982; pp. 19–24.
28. *McNeil/Lehrer News Hour*, 29 December 1993.
29. *Washington Post*, 22 December 1993: A1. Also, *New York Times*, Editorial, 27 December 1993.
30. Post, S.G., "History, Infanticide, and Imperiled Newborns," *Hastings Center Report*, 1988; 18(4): 14–17.
31. English common law resource: Coke's Institutes, Blackstone, discussed in Stein, P., *Legal Institutions: The Development of Dispute Settlement*, London: Butterworths, 1984.
32. *Roe v. Wade*, 40 U.S. 113 (1973).
33. Resource: Carmen Werner, M.D., Denver Children's Hospital.
34. Beller, F.K., "The beginning of human life: Medical observations and ethical reflections," *Clinical Obstetrics and Gynecology*, 1992; 35(4):720–727.
35. deBlois, J., "Anencephaly and the management of pregnancy," *Health Care Ethics USA*, Fall 1993; pp. 2, 3.
36. *Planned Parenthood of Southeastern Pennsylvania v. Casey*, 505 U.S. 833 (1992).
37. *Barnes v. Mississippi*, 114 S.Ct. 468 (1993).
38. "Ginsburg on *Roe v. Wade*," in a speech to the New York University Law School, March 1993, reported in *Wall Street Journal*, 16 June 1993.
39. See discussion in: Annas, G.J., "The Supreme Court, liberty, and abortion," *New England Journal of Medicine*, 1992; 327(9):651–654.
40. Berlin, Germany: Associated Press, "Court: Abortion Law Is Unconstitutional," *Amarillo Globe-Times*, 28 May 1993, 25A.
41. Warsaw, Poland, Associated Press, "Senate Passes Strict Abortion Limits but Rejects Ban," *Amarillo Sunday News-Globe*, 31 January 1993, 21A.
42. Frates, M.C., *et al.*, "Pregnancy outcome after a first trimester sonogram demonstrating fetal cardiac activity," *Journal of Ultrasound in Medicine*, 1993; 12(7):383.
43. Evans, H., "Womb with a View: Unborn Babies Star in Fetal Film Fests," *Wall Street Journal*, 30 November 1993, A1, A5.
44. Wertz, D.C., and Fletcher, J.C., "Ethics and Genetics: An International Survey," *Hastings Center Report*, July/August 1989; pp. 20–24.
45. Vincent, V.A., *et al.*, "Pregnancy termination because of chromosomal abnormalities: A study of 26,950 amniocenteses in the Southeast," *Southern Medical Journal*, 1991; 84:1210–1212.
46. "Biomedical Ethics and the Shadow of Nazism: A Conference on the Proper Use of the Nazi Analogy in Ethical Debate," *Hastings Center Report*, August, 1976; Special Supplement, p. 20.
47. Toon, P.D., "Daughters, doctors and death," *Lancet*, October 1993; reporting on BBC 2 *Assignment*: "Let Her Die," aired 28 September 1993.
48. Wertz, *op. cit.*
49. Tanouye, E., "Abortion Procedure Is Found to Be 99% Effective," *Wall Street Journal*, 27 May 1993, B6.
Peyron R., *et al.*, "Early termination of pregnancy with Mifepristone (RU486) and the orally active prostaglandin Misoprostol," *New England Journal of Medicine*, 1993; 328 (21):1509–1513.
Tanouye, E., "Legal Import of Abortion Pill Appears Near," *Wall Street Journal*, January, 1994, B1, B3.
50. Weinstein, B.D., "Do pharmacists have a right to refuse to fill prescriptions for abortifacient drugs?" *Law, Medicine & Health Care*, 1992; 20(3):220.
51. *Rust v. Sullivan*, 500 U.S. 173 (1991).
52. Murphy, E., "Celebrating the Bill of Rights in the year of Rust v. Sullivan," *Nursing Outlook*, 1991; 39(5):238–239.
53. Data from The Guttmacher Institute (note 25, above).
54. *Michael H. v. Gerald D.*, 491 U.S. 110 (1989).
55. Densford and Everett, *op. cit.*

56. Reilly, P., *The Surgical Solution: A History of Involuntary Sterilization in the United States*, Baltimore: Johns Hopkins Press, 1991.

57. LA Times–Washington Post News Service, "Court Allows Woman to Reject Caesarean," Washington: *Amarillo Sunday News-Globe*, 19 December 1993, 3B.

58. "Brain-dead woman maintained on life support to carry fetus to term," *NURSEweek*, 2 November 1992, p. 4. (Berlin).

59. *International Union v. Johnson Controls*, 111 S.Ct. 1196 (1991).

60. Curtin, L.L., "Abortion: A tangle of rights," *Nursing Management*, 1993; 24(2):26, 28, 30–31.

61. "Mother Charged with 'Assault' in Birth of Intoxicated Baby," *Missouri Lawyers Weekly*, 9 December 1991, p. 1.

62. Hansen, M., "Courts side with moms in drug cases: Florida woman's conviction overturned for delivering cocaine via umbilical cord," *American Bar Association Journal*, November 1992, p. 18.

63. Section 1.205 RSMo (1994). A Missouri case has held that a parent can sue for wrongful death of a child killed *prior* to viability, based on this statute. *Connor v. Monkem Company Inc.*, No 77313 (Mo. banc April 25, 1995).

64. "Drunk Driver Gets Manslaughter for Viable Fetus' Death," and "'Viability' the New Battleground for Civil Suits, Too," *Missouri Lawyers Weekly*, 9 December 1991, pp. 1, 16–17.

65. *Lough v. Rolla Women's Clinic, Inc., et al.*, 866 S.W. 2d 851 (Mo. 1993).

66. Denniston, L., "Viable Fetuses Legally Protected from Killing, Okla. Appeals Court Rules," *The Baltimore Sun*, 26 January 1994, 7A.

67. Murray, J., and Bernfield, M., "The differential effect of prenatal care on the incidence of low birth weight among Blacks and Whites in a prepaid health care plan," *New England Journal of Medicine*, 1988; 319:1385–1391.
Oechsli, F.W., "Prenatal care and low birth weight among Blacks and Whites," *New England Journal of Medicine*, 1989; 320(15):1010.

68. Wilson, A.L., *et al.*, "Does prenatal care decrease the incidence and cost of neonatal intensive care admissions?" *American Journal of Perinatology*, 1992; 9(4):281–284.

69. Stahlman, M., "Ethical issues in the nursery: Priorities versus limits," *Journal of Pediatrics* 1990; 116(2):167–170.

70. Kempe, A., *et al.*, "Clinical determinants of the racial disparity in very low birth weight," *New England Journal of Medicine*, 1992; 327:1021–1024.

71. Interview with Ronald David, in March-April 1993 issue of *Harvard Magazine*; reprinted in *Wall Street Journal*, 15 March 1993, A10.

72. Tanouye, E., "Study Shows Even the Well-insured Fail to Meet Immunization-rate Goals," *Wall Street Journal*, 16 January 1994, B10.
Only 46% of children on AFDC got imminizations, though they were free. Dr. Demetria Montgomery, Texas Department of Health, 15 November 1995.

73. Lantos, J., "Survival after cardiopulmonary resuscitation in babies of very low birth weight: Is CPR futile therapy?" *New England Journal of Medicine*, 1988; 318(2):91–96; and Letters, *New England Journal of Medicine*, 1988; 319(3):176–178.

74. Sood, S., and Giacoia, G., "Cardiopulmonary resuscitation in very low birthweight infants," *American Journal of Perinatology*, 1992; 9(2):130–133.

75. Caron, E., and Mitchell, C., "Her only chance," *American Journal of Nursing*, 1991; 91(9):19–20.

76. Horbar, J., *et al.*, "Predicting mortality risk for infants weighing 501 to 1500 grams at birth: A National Institutes of Health Neonatal Research Network report," *Critical Care Medicine*, 1993; 21(1):12–18.

77. *Ibid.*

78. Costarino, A., "Can we predict mortality for low birth weight infants?" *Critical Care Medicine*, 1993; 21(1):2–3.

79. Storch, T., "Editorial board speaks: The unkindest cut," *American Journal of Diseases of Children*, 1990; 144:533.

80. Infant Health and Development Program, "Enhancing the outcomes of low birth weight, premature infants," *Journal of the American Medical Association*, 1990; 263:3035–3042.

81. *Ibid.*

82. Stevenson, D.K., *et al.*, "The 'Baby Doe' Rule," *Journal of the American Medical Association*, 1986; 255(14):1909–1912.

83. Burt, R., *Taking Care of Strangers: The Rule of Law in Doctor-Patient Relations*, New York: The Free Press, 1979.
84. 42 U.S.C. 5101, 45 C.F.R. 1340.14 *et seq.*
85. *Idem.*
86. 45 C.F.R. 1340.15.
87. *In re. T.A.C.P.*, 609 So.2d 588 (Fla. 1992).
88. Van Cleve, L., "Nurses' experience caring for anencephalic infants who are potential organ donors," *Journal of Pediatric Nursing*, 1993; 8(2):79–84.
89. Wilkinson, J.M., "Moral distress: A labor and delivery nurse's experience," *Journal of Obstetric, Gynecologic, & Neonatal Nursing*, 1989; 18(6):513–519.
    Mahon, M.M., "The nurse's role in treatment decisionmaking for the child with disabilities," *Issues in Law & Medicine*, 1990; 6(3):247–268.
90. Gero, E., and Giordano, J., "Ethical considerations in fetal tissue transplantation," *Journal of Neuroscience Nursing*, 1990; 22(1):9–12.
91. Martin, D.K., "Abortion and fetal tissue transplantation," *IRB: A Review of Human Subjects Research*, 1993; 15(3):1–3.
92. London, Associated Press, "Board to Probe Technology Ethics," *Amarillo Daily News*, 8 January 1994, 2A.
    See generally, Robertson, J.A., "Rights, symbolism, and public policy in fetal tissue transplants," pp. 5–7; and Nolan, K., "*Genug ist Genug*: A fetus is not a kidney," pp. 13–19, *Medical Ethics Advisor*, January 1992.
93. Williams, T.F., "Aging or disease," *Clinical Pharmacological Therapy*, December 1987: pp. 663–4.
94. Comfort, A., *A Good Age*, New York: Simon & Schuster, 1976.
95. Maturity News Service, "Study Uncovers Few Seniors on TV," *Amarillo News-Globe*, 31 October 1993; researchers James Robinson and Thomas Skill.
96. Excerpt from Friedan, B., *My Quest for the Fountain of Age* (New York: Simon & Schuster, 1993), in *Time Magazine*, 6 September 1993.
97. "Facts You Should Know," *American Nurse*, July/August, 1993, p. 13.
98. Litvak, J.A., "Challenge beyond the year 2000," *Bulletin of the Pan American Health Organization*, 1990; 24(3):330–334.
99. Solomon, M., *et al.*, "Decisions near the end of life: Professional views on life-sustaining treatments," *American Journal of Public Health*, 1993; 83:14–22.
100. Walford, R.L., *Maximum Life Span*, New York: Avon, 1984.
101. Yin, P., and Shine, M., "Misinterpretations of increases in life expectancy in gerontology textbooks," *Gerontologist* 1985; 25:78–82.
102. Dalton, R.H., "The limit of human life, and how to live long," *Journal of the American Medical Association*, 1893; 20:599–699.
103. "Facts you should know," *op. cit.*
104. Zedlewski, S.R., and McBride, T.D., "The changing profile of the elderly: Effects on future long-term care needs and financing," *Milbank Quarterly*, 1992; 70:247–275.
105. Clymer, A., "Hillary Clinton raises tough question of life, death and medicine," *New York Times*, 1 October 1993.
106. Olshan, A.F., *et al.*, "Paternal occupation and congenital anomalies in offspring," *American Journal of Industrial Medicine*, 1991; 20(4):447–475.
107. *Ibid.*
108. Rundle, R., "Study Suggests Electric Razor Link to Cancer," *Wall Street Journal*, 13 November 1992, B1, B14.
109. Bishop, J.E., "Statisticians Occupy Front Lines in Battle over Passive Smoking," *Wall Street Journal*, 28 July 1993, B1, B6.
110. Emanuel, E.J., and Emanuel, L.L., "The economics of dying: The illusion of cost savings at the end of life," *New England Journal of Medicine*, 1994; 330(8):540–544.
111. *Ibid.*
112. Kidder, D., "The effects of hospice coverage on Medicare expenditures," *Health Services Resource*, 1992; 27:195–217.
113. Hentoff, N., *et al.*, "Contested Terrain: The Nazi Analogy in Bioethics," *Hastings Center Report*, August/September: 1988; pp. 29–33.
114. Stoutman, K., Falk, I.S., "Health Indexes: A Study of Objectives Indexes of Health in Relation to Environment and Sanitation," *Bulletin of Health Organizations*, League of Nations, 1936; 5:901–996.

Cubbon, J., "The principle of QUALY maximisation as the basis for allocating health care resources," *Journal of Medical Ethics*, 1991; 17:181–184.

Harris, J., "Unprincipled QUALYs: A response to Cubbon," *Journal of Medical Ethics*, 1991; 17:185–188.

Editorial, "Which medical condition shall we treat first," *Lancet*, 29 November 1988; 2: 1175–1176.

115. Guyatt, G.H., *et al.*, "Measuring health-related quality of life," *Annals of Internal Medicine*, 1993; 118(8):622–629.

Jachuck, S.J., *et al.*, "The effect of hypotensive drugs on the quality of life," *Journal of the Royal College of General Practice*, 1982; 32:103–105.

116. Knaus, S.A., et. al., "APACHE II, A severity of disease classification system," *Critical Care Medicine*, 1985; 13:818–829.

117. Pearlman, R., and Jonsen, A., "The use of quality-of-life considerations in medical decision making," *Journal of the American Geriatrics Society*, 1985; 33(5):344–352.

118. Caron, E., and Mitchell, C., *op. cit.*

119. Jachuck, *op. cit.*

120. Fowler, M.D., "Slow code, partial code, limited code," *Heart & Lung*, 1989; 18(5):533–534.

121. Swidler, R.N., "The presumption of consent in New York State's do-not-resuscitate law," *New York State Journal of Medicine*, 1989; 89:69–72.

122. Taffet, G.E., *et al.*, "In-hospital cardio-pulmonary resuscitation," *Journal of American Medical Association*, 1988; 260(14):2069–2072.

Murphy, D.J., et. al., "Outcomes of CPR in the elderly," *Archives of Internal Medicine*, 1989; 111:199–205.

123. Landry, F.J., *et al.*, "Outcome of CPR in the intensive care setting," *Archives of Internal Medicine*, 1992; 152:2305–2308.

124. *Hospital Ethics*, November/December 1991, p. 7.

125. Sachs, G., Miles, S., and Levin, R., "Limiting resuscitation: Emergency policy in the EMS," *Archives of Internal Medicine*, 1991; 114:151–154.

126. Wachter, R.M., *et al.*, "Decisions about resuscitation: Inequities among patients with different diseases but similar prognoses," *Archives of Internal Medicine*, 1989; 111:525.

127. See, for example, Nicholson, L.G., "The ethics of limiting treatment: DNR decisions," *Nursing Management*, 1991; 22(2):64H, 64J, 64L, 64P.

Clarke, D.E., and Raffin, T.A., "Do-not-resuscitate orders in the ICU: Why are there so few?" *Chest*, 1993; 104(5):1322–1323.

128. AMA Council on Ethical and Judicial Affairs, "Guidelines for the appropriate use of DNR orders," *Journal of the American Medical Association*, 1991; 265:1868–1871.

129. Hackler, J.C., "Family consent to orders not to resuscitate: Reconsidering hospital policy," *Journal of the American Medical Association*, 1990; 264:1282–1283.

130. Scofield, G.R., "Is Consent Useful When Resuscitation Isn't?" *Hastings Center Report*, 1991; 21(6): 28–36.

Tomlinson, T., and Brody, H., "Futility and the ethics of resuscitation," *Journal of the American Medical Association*, 1990; 264:1276–1280.

131. Snider, G., "The do-not-resuscitate order: Ethical and legal imperative or medical decision," *American Review of Respiratory Diseases*, 1991; 143:665–674.

132. References for DNR in the OR:

Igoe, S., *et al.*, "Ethics in the OR: DNR and patient autonomy," *Nursing Management*, 1993; 24(9):112A, 112D, 112H.

Reeder, J.M., "Do-not-resuscitate orders in the operating room," *Association of Operating Room Nurses Journal*, 1993; 57:(4)947–951.

Murphy, E., "DNR in the OR," *Association of Operating Room Nurses Journal*, 1993; 58(2):399–401.

Walker, R., "DNR in the OR," *Journal of the American Medical Association*, 1991; 266:(17)2407–2411.

133. Hall, J.K., "Call the code: CPR should require consent," *Aspec Review*, 1989; 2:15.

134. Hippocrates, from *The Art*, Jones, W.H., Ed., vol. 2, Cambridge: Harvard University Press, 1923: pp. 193,203.

Hippocrates, from Chadwick J., and Mann, W.N., Eds., *The Medical Works of Hippocrates*, Boston: Blackwell Scientific Publications, 1950.

135. Knox, L.S., "Ethical issues in nutritional support nursing: Withholding and withdrawing nutritional support," *Nursing Clinics of North America*, 1989; 24(2):427–436.
136. Barnie, D.C., "Percutaneous endoscopic gastrostomy tubes: the nurse's role in a moral, ethical, and legal dilemma," *Gastroenterology Nursing*, 1990; 12(4):250–4.
137. Leff, B., Cheuvront, N., and Russell, W., "Discontinuing feeding tubes in a community nursing home," *Gerontologist* 1994; 34(1):130–133.
138. *Ibid.*
139. *Ibid.*
140. *Cruzan v. Harmon*, No. CV 384-9P, Circuit Court of Missouri (Mo. Cir. Ct. Jasper County Dec. 14, 1990) (Teel J.).
141. *In re: The Matter of Christine Busalacchi, incapacitated and disabled*, Department of Health and Missouri Rehabilitation Center v. Peter J. Busalacchi, father and guardian of Christine Busalacchi, Missouri Supreme Court No. 73677.
142. House of Lords, *Airedale NHS Trust (Respondents) V Bland (Acting by his guardian "ad litem") (Appellant)*, London: House of Lords, 1993.
    Wright, S., "What makes a person," *Nursing Times*, 1993; 89(21):42–45.
143. Wright, *Ibid*.
    Hall, J.K., "Death by dehydration issue needs heads-on discussion," *Nursing Times*, 1993; 89(30):12.
144. Brahams, D., "Persistent vegetative state," *Lancet*, 1992; 340:1534–1535.
145. Allen, A., "Right to die, freedom of choice, and assisted death: Implications for nurses," *Journal of Post Anesthesia Nursing*, 1991; 6(2):150–151.
146. Further discussions: Hart, C.A., "The role of psychiatric consultation liaison nurses in ethical decisions to remove life-sustaining treatments," *Archives of Psychiatric Nursing*, 1990; 4(6):370–378.
    Wilson, D.M., "Ethical Concerns in a long-term tube feeding study," *Image—Journal of Nursing Scholarship*, 1992; 24(3):195–198.
    Marsden, C., "Technology assessment in critical care," *Heart & Lung*, 1991; 20(1): 93–94.
    Marsden, C., "Ethical issues in critical care: Real presence," *Heart & Lung*, 1990; 19:(5Pt1):540–541.
147. Hager, P., "Fighting for His Death," *California Lawyer*, July 1993, p. 27.
    Crabtree, P., "Patient's Condition Was Key Question," *Rutland Herald*, 19 November 1993; pp. 1, 16.
    In re: Guardianship of Ronald Comeau, Bennington Superior Court, Docket No. S0325-93, 12 November 1993.
148. Johnstone, M-J., *Bioethics: A Nursing Perspective*, Sydney: W.B. Saunders, 1991; pp. 249–250.
149. About Busalacchi generally: Tighe, T., "Busalacchi's Death Offers Few Answers," *St. Louis Post-Dispatch*, 9 March 1993, p. 1.
    Editorial, "Body and Mind, Family and Faith," *St. Louis Post-Dispatch*, 10 March 1993.
150. Exodus 20:13, Old Testament.
151. *Superintendent of Belchertown v. Saikewicz*, 370 N.E.2d 417, 425 (Mass. 1977).
    Satz v. Perlmutter, 326 So.2d 160,162 (Fla. 1980).
152. Position Statement on Capital Punishment, American Nurses Association, Kansas City, Mo. 1988. A similar but more specific statement was adopted by the Missouri Nurses Association in 1993.
153. Code for Nurses with Interpretive Statements, American Nurses Association, Kansas City, Mo. 1986.
154. *Ibid.*
155. Hall, J., quoted in "Providers balk at withdrawal of nutrition, hydration," *Medical Ethics Advisor*, 1992; 8(8):85–89.
156. American Nurses Association Committee on Ethics, *Guidelines on Withdrawing or Withholding Food and Fluid*, Washington, DC: American Nurses' Association, 1992.
157. American Nurses Association Position Statement on Promotion of Comfort and Relief of Pain in Dying Patients, *American Nurse*, February 1992; p. 7.
158. Position Statement on Foregoing Artificial Nutrition and Hydration, American Nurses Association, Washington, DC: 1992.
159. RSMo. §404.872 (1994).
160. RSMo. §459.040 (1994).

161. *In re. Jobes*, 529 A.2d 434 (N.J., 1987). Justice O'Hern, Dissenting.
162. House of Lords, Lord Mistill, *op. cit.*
163. *In re. Quinlan*, 70 N.J. 20, 355 A 2d 647 (NJ 1976).
164. Fiesta, J., "Refusal of treatment," *Nursing Management*, 1992; 23(11):14–18.
165. Kjervik, D.K., "Legal and ethical issues. The choice to die," *Journal of Professional Nursing*, 1991; 7(3):151.
166. *Cruzan v. Director, Missouri Department of Health*, 497 U.S. 261 (1990).
167. Lippman, H., "After *Cruzan*: The right to die," *RN*, January 1991; 65–73.
168. Justice Cardozo in *Schloendorff v. Society of New York Hospital*, 105 N.E. 92, 93 (N.Y. 1914).
169. Hall, J.K., "Cruzan II," *Journal of American Medicine*, 1993; 94:115.
    Also, on *Cruzan*, see: Fairman, R.P., "Commentary: Withdrawing life-sustaining treatment—lessons from Nancy Cruzan," *Archives of Internal Medicine*, January 1992; 152:25–27.
170. Wolfe, J.F., "Nurses' groups join court debate in right-to-die case," *Joplin Globe*, 25 August 1992.
171. St. Louis, Associated Press, "Missouri's 2d Right-to-Die Case Ends with Death of Christine Busalacchi," *West Plains Daily Quill*, 18 March 1993, p. 9.
172. *In re. O'Connor*, 53 NE 2d 607 (NY 1988).
173. For example: "Comatose Woman's Wakening a 'Miracle,' " *St. Louis Post-Dispatch*, 22 December 1991.
174. *Bouvia v. Superior Court for Los Angeles County*, 225 Cal. Rptr. 297, 307 (Ct. App. 1986).
175. *Rojas v. District Attorney Erkenbrack*, Civil Action No. 973V142. Filed January 20, 1987, District Court, Mesa County.
176. Fish, A., and Singer, P.A., "Nancy B: The criminal code and decisions to forgo life-sustaining treatment," *Canadian Medical Association Journal*, 1992; 147(5):637–642.
177. *In re. Guardianship of Browning*, (State v. Herbert) 568 So. 2d 4 (Fla., 1990).
178. *In re. matter of Claire C. Conroy*, 486 A 2d 1209 (N.J. 1985).
179. Lo, B., "The death of Clarence Herbert: Withdrawing care is not murder," *Archives of Internal Medicine*, 1984; 101:248–251.
180. Jennett, B., and Plum, F., "Persistent vegetative state after brain damage, a syndrome in search of a name," *Lancet*, 1972; 1:734.
181. Celesia, G.G., "Persistent vegetative state," *Neurology*, 1993; 43:1457–1458.
182. American Neurological Association Committee on Ethical Affairs, "Persistent vegetative state: report of the ANA CEA," *Annals of Neurology*, 1993; 33:386–390.
    Institute of Medical Ethics Working Party on the Ethics of Prolonging Life and Assisting Death, "Withdrawal of life support from patients in a persistent vegetative state," *Lancet* 1991; 337:96–98.
    Brown, J., "The PVS: Time for caution?" *Postgraduate Medical Journal*, 1990; 66:697–698.
    Wikler, D., "Not Dead, Not Dying? Ethical Categories and Persistent Vegetative State," *Hastings Center Report*, 1988; 18:41–47.
    Brody, B.A., "Ethical Questions Raised by the Persistent Vegetative Patient," *Hastings Center Report*, 1988; 18:33–37.
    Ashwal, S., *et al.*, "The persistent vegetative state in children: Report of the Child Neurology Ethics Committee," *Annals of Neurology*, 1992; 32:570–576.
    Weiner, J.D., "Legal issues regarding patients in coma or in persistent vegetative state," *Physical Medicine and Rehabilitation*, 1990; 4:569–578.
183. Tresch, D.D., et al., "Clinical characteristics of patients in the persistent vegetative state," *Annals of Internal Medicine*, 1991; 151:930–932.
184. Levin, P., *et al.*, "Vegetative state after closed-head injury," *Archives of Neurology*, 1991; 48:580.
185. Childs, N., *et al.*, "Accuracy of diagnosis of persistent vegetative state," *Neurology*, 1993; 43:1457–1458.
186. Penticuff, J.H., "Ethical issues in redefining death," *Journal of Neuroscience Nursing*, 1990; 22(1):48–49.
187. Baron, C., "Why withdrawal of life support of PVS patients is not a family decision," *Law, Medicine & Health Care*, 1991; 19:1–2, 73–75.
188. Goodwin, J., "Mercy killing: Mercy for whom?" *Journal of the American Medical Association*, 1991; 265:326.

189. Riesman, D., *The Story of Medicine in the Middle Ages*, New York: Hoeber, 1935; pp. 233–240.
190. Keatings, M., "The biology of the persistent vegetative state, legal and ethical implications for transplantation: Viewpoints from nursing," *Transplantation Proceedings*, 1990; 22(3):997–9.
191. Veatch, R.M. "The Impending Collapse of the Whole-Brain Definition of Death," *Hastings Center Report*, 1993; 23(4):18–24.
192. Wikler, D., and Weisbard, A., "Appropriate confusion over brain death," *Journal of the American Medical Association*, 1989; 261:2246.
193. For examples of nurses who did: Steppe, H., "Nursing in Nazi Germany," *Western Journal of Nursing Research*, 1992; 14(6), 744–753.
194. Wikler, D., and Weisbard, A., *op. cit.*
   For the nurse's view: Foy, J.M., "Duty to respect the dead body: A nursing perspective," *Transplantation Proceedings*, 1990; 22(3):1023–1024.
195. "Brain-dead woman maintained on life support to carry fetus to term," *op. cit.*
196. Harris, M.D., "Death pronouncement by registered nurses," *Home Healthcare Nurse*, 1992; 10(2):57–59.
197. Pallis, C., "ABC of brain stem death," *British Medical Journal*, 1983; 280:209, and 1982; 285:1720–1723.
   Setzer, N., "Brain death: Physiologic definitions," *Critical Care Clinics*, 1985; 1(2):375–423.
198. Wolf, Z.R., "Nurses' experiences giving post-mortem care to patients who have donated organs: A phenomenological study," *Transplantation Proceedings*, 1990; 22(3):1019–1020.
199. Veatch, R. *op. cit.*
200. Botkin, J.R., and Post, S.G., "Confusion in the determination of death: Distinguishing philosophy from physiology," *Perspectives in Biology and Medicine*, 1992; 36(1):129–138.
201. Burt, R., *Taking Care of Strangers, op. cit.*
202. Summerfield, D.A., "Doctors and torture," *Lancet*, 1990; 336(8715):634.
203. Steppe, H., *op. cit.*
204. Steppe, H., "Nursing under Totalitarian Regimes: The Case of National Socialism," paper presented at the Congress: Nursing, Women's History and the Politics of Welfare, Nottingham, England, 23 July 1993.
   Also see: Brink, P.J., "When patientology is ignored: The case of Nazi Germany," *Western Journal of Nursing Research*, 1991; 13(2):162–163.
205. Alexander, L., "Medical science under dictatorship," *New England Journal of Medicine*, 1949; 241(2):39–47.
206. "Biomedical Ethics and the Shadow of Nazism: A Conference on the Proper Use of the Nazi Analogy in Ethical Debate," *Hastings Center Report*, op. cit.
207. "Selling Murder: The Killing Films of the Third Reich," The Discovery Channel, aired September 18, 1995.
208. Horner, R., London Observer news service, "Opened Files Detail Nazi Program to Kill 'Defectives'," *St. Louis Post-Dispatch*, 26 September 1991, C1.
209. Densford and Everett, *op. cit.*, pp. 181–182.
210. *Ibid.*
211. *Ibid.*
212. Callahan, D., "On Feeding the Dying," *Hastings Center Report*, 1983; 13(5):22.
213. Printz, L., "Terminal dehydration, a compassionate treatment," *Archives of Internal Medicine*, 1992; 152:697–700.
   Hall, J.K., "Dehydrating to terminate is different from dehydrating the terminal," *Archives Internal Medicine*, 1993; 153:399.
214. Marzuk, P., *et al.*, "Increase in suicide by asphyxiation in New York City after the publication of *Final Exit*," *New England Journal of Medicine*, 1993; 329(20):1508–1510.
215. Rich, C.L., *et al.*, "The San Diego suicide study. 1. Young vs. old subjects," *Archives of General Psychiatry*, 1986; 43:577–582.
216. Marzuk, *op. cit.*
217. Kowalski, S., "Assisted suicide: Where do nurses draw the line?" *Nursing & Health Care*, 1993; 14(2):70–76.
218. American Nurses Association, Center for Ethics and Human Rights, Task Force on

the Nurse's Role in End-of-life Decisions, Washington, DC: American Nurses Association Publications, 1993.

219. Kuhse, H., and Singer, P., "Euthanasia: A survey of nurses' attitudes and practices," *Australian Nurses Journal*, 1992; 21(8):21–22.

220. Stevens, C.A., and Hassan, R., *Management of Death, Dying and Euthanasia: Attitudes and Practices of Medical Practitioners and Nurses in South Australia*, Adelaide: Flinders University, 1992.

221. Winton, R., and Pollard, B., "Why doctors and nurses must not kill patients," *Medical Journal of Australia*, 1993; 158:426–429.

222. Annas, G.J., "Physician-assisted suicide—Michigan's temporary solution," *Legal Issues in Medicine*, 1993; 328(21):1573–1576.

223. Singer, P., and Siegler, M., "Euthanasia: A critique," *New England Journal of Medicine*, 1990; 322:1881–1883.

224. President's Commission on the Study of Ethical Problems in Medicine and Biomedical and Behavioral Research. *Decisions to Forego Life-Sustaining Treatment*, 1983; Washington, D.C.: U.S. Government Printing Office, p. 236.

225. van der Maas, P.J., *et al.*, "Euthanasia and other medical decisions concerning the end of life," *Lancet*, 1991; 338:669–74.

226. Fleming, J.I., "Euthanasia, the Netherlands, and Slippery Slopes," *Bioethics Research Notes Occasional Paper No. 1*, June 1992; 4(2):1–4.

227. Smith, M.L., *et al.*, "A good death: Is euthanasia the answer?" *Cleveland Clinic Journal of Medicine*, 1992; 59:99–109.
Battin, M.P., "Seven caveats concerning the discussion of euthanasia in Holland," *Perspectives in Biology and Medicine*, 1990; 34(1):73–77.

228. Jacox, A., *et al.*, "New clinical practice guidelines for the management of pain in patients with cancer," *New England Journal of Medicine*, 1994; 330(9):651–655.

229. Cleeland, C.S., "Pain and its treatment in outpatients with metastatic cancer," *New England Journal of Medicine*, 1994; 330(9):592–596.

230. Austin, TX, Associated Press, "Doctors Support Cancer Pain Control," *Amarillo Sunday News-Globe*, 1 November 1992, 7A.

231. American Nurses Association Position Statement on Promotion of Comfort and Relief of Pain in Dying Patients, *op. cit.*

INDEX

A

Abortion, 10, 383–399
    and conscience clauses, 397
    and prenatal testing, 393–395
    and right of privacy, 76
    and sex of child, 388, 395–396
    cross-cultural view of, 392–393, 395–396
    data related to, 385
    ethics issues in, 384
    father's interest in, 399
    federal power over law and, 78
    historical view of, 387–388
    late abortions, 397–398
    legal developments in, 388–391
    legal versus ethical issue of, 4
    methods of, 396, 397
    mother's interest in, 399–400
    nurse participation in, 6, 384–385, 397, 398
    pre-abortion counseling issue and, 398–399
    reasons for, 393–396
    state laws and, variations in, 393
    terms related to, 386
    viability of fetus and, concepts of, 389–391
Abuse, child, 179–180
    drug, discipline for, 201
    intentionally injured adults and, 181
    of dependent persons, 180–181
Accidents, Good Samaritan statutes, 138–139
Accreditation, and documentation, 153
Acts/actions, legal/ethical/practical, 4
    unintended consequences of, 11
Acute Physical Assessment and Chronic
    Health Evaluation (APACHE), 406, 428
Administrative Hearing Commission, 91
Administrative law, 69, 88, 91–93. See also
    Regulations.
Administrative procedure act, and due proc-
    ess, 91
    nature of, 90
Adoption, ethical issues in, 378
    surrogate motherhood and, 376–379
Advance directives, 240–244
    and competence of person, 242–243
    and Danforth amendment, 253–255
    cautions about, 255–256
    durable power of attorney and, 9, 249–260
    elderly fear of, 259
    ethical problems of, 261
    historical view of, 241–242
    living wills as, 9, 244–249
    purposes of, 241
    wills as, 240, 243–244
Advanced practical nurses (APNs), roles of,
    280
Adverse drug reactions, reporting of, 362
African-Americans, and advance directives,
    259
    and low birth weight infants, 403, 404
    and organ donation, 259
Age discrimination, 327
Age Discrimination in Employment Act,
    327
Ageism, meaning of, 413, 414
AIDS. See HIV/AIDS.
Alcohol intoxication, of newborn, 401
Alternative dispute resolution (ADR), 145–146
    arbitration in, 145–146
    mediation in, 145
Altruism, and professionals, 22
Alzheimer's disease, 251
American Association for Respiratory Care
    Code of Ethics, Preamble to, 29
    role model statement in, 37
    values reflected in, 31, 33, 34–37, 340, 352
American Law Reports (ALR), 286
American Medical Association Principles of
    Medical Ethics, Preamble to, 30
    values reflected in, 32–37, 341, 353
American Nurses Association (ANA), Center
    for Ethics and Human Rights and, 19–
    20, 66
    and standards of care, 114, 115
    member characteristics of, 20
    membership size of, 19
    on nurse education, 208–209
    role of, in ethics/law in nursing, 19–20
    union movement by, 20

American Nurses Association Code of Ethics, ethics test based on, 55
  lack of Preamble to, 29
  values reflected in, 31–36, 340, 352
Americans with Disabilities Act (ADA) (1992), 201, 322–324
  and illness care, 324
  and license law, 324
  and protection of HIV-positive practitioners, 274–275
  provisions of, 322–323
Amniocentesis, 394–395
Anencephalic infants, as organ donors, 409–410
Animals, dangerous, 130
  in research, 191–192
  transplants from, 269
Anti-dumping, 182–184
  meaning of, 182–183
Anti-trust law, 309
  Clayton Act (1915) in, 331
  medical practitioner use of, 331, 332
  necessity of, 331
  Sherman Act in, 330, 331
APACHE, 406, 428
A posteriori thinking, 44
A priori thinking, 44, 49
Appeal, case law process of, 97–98
Arbitration, process of, 145–146
Aristotle, 46, 109, 387
Artificial insemination, 10, 371–373
  donor screening for, 371
  ethical issues in, 373
  health insurance coverage for, 372–373
  procedure in, 371
  sperm bank for, 372
Assault, 9, 167
  in medical context, 167
  meaning of, 167
Assignment (payment), Medicare, 84
Assisted suicide, 467, 472–473. See also Suicide.
  and Kevorkian, 480
  nurse participation in, 6, 293, 472–473
  pros/cons of, 481
Assumption of risk, 130–131, 229
Attorney in fact, 251
Attorney-client privilege, meaning of, 156
"At will" doctrine. See Employment "at will."
Autonomy, 3, 26. See also Nurse autonomy.
  advance directives and, 240–244
  autopsies and, 269–270
  consent and, 222–240
  durable power of attorney and, 249–260
  for nurse. See Nurse autonomy.
  for patient/nurse, 221
  freedom versus justice concept of, 221–222
  HIV/AIDS and, 270–278
  in codes of ethics, 30, 35–36

living wills, 244–249
  meaning of, 9
  relative nature of, 220–221
  suicide and, 279
  transplants and, 263–269
  versus individualism, 41
Autopsies, 269–270
  elective, 270
  reasons for, 270

B

Baby Doe case, 179, 408
Battery, 9, 166
  defense for, 166, 223
  in medical context, 166
  meaning of, 166
Behavior, and law, 49, 50
  limits on, 11
  versus beliefs, 55–56
Beliefs, versus behavior, 55–56
Belmont Report, 186
Beneficence, 3, 26
  and malpractice, 108–123
  and nursing profession, 107
  and paternalism, 107–108
  in codes of ethics, 30
  meaning of, 8, 106
  other values related to, 106–107
Benefit-burden analysis, 429
Bennett, William, 8
Bentham, Jeremy, 48
Bills, lawmaking process, 83
Bioethics, meaning of, 14
BIOETHICS database, 12
Birth, cesarean section in, 400
  crack-addicted babies at, 401–402
  neonates and, issues related to, 405–410
  rights of unborn and, 402–403
  very low birth weight infants at, 404
Blood products, as service, 131
Blood transfusions, as transplants, 269
Board of Healing Arts, 73–74
Boards of nursing, and licensure, 200
Bouvia, Elizabeth, case, 59, 460
Brain death, 461
  and transplants, 264
  criteria for, 466
  versus higher brain death, 465, 467
Brazen rule (Sagan's), 41
Breach of standard of care, evidence of, 113–114
  in malpractice, 112–116
  meaning of breach, for nurses, 113
  meaning of, 112–113
  no breach as defense in, 121
Burke, Edmund, 42
Busalacchi case, 446, 458–459

C

Cadaver, use of term, 266
Camus, Albert, 47
Captain of the Ship doctrine, 133
Cardiopulmonary resuscitation (CPR), 435–436
  and lawsuits, 436
  for very low birth weight infants, 405–406
  proposed policy for, 438
  uses of, 435
Care continuum, 21
Caring ethic, in feminist thought, 56–57
Case law, 69, 93–99
  basis of, 93–94
  changes to, 73–74
  elements of, 72
  sources for locating of, 98–99
Case law process, 94–98
  appeal in, 97–98
  discovery in, 95
  initial conflict in, 94–95
  opinion in, 97
  trial in, 95–96
Case review, by ethics committees, 59
Casuistry, 48
Causation, establishment of, 118
  in malpractice, 118–119
  loss of chance in, 118
  no causation as defense in, 121
  res ipsa loquitur in, 118, 119
  substantial factor in, 118
Center for Ethics and Human Rights, 19–20, 66
Cesarean section, historical view, 400
  white women and, 400
Charaka, 17
Charitable immunity, 70, 133
Chemical codes, 435
Child abuse, 179–180
  medical context of, 179–180
  neglect as, 180
Child Abuse Amendments of 1984, 179, 408
Child Abuse Prevention and Treatment Act (1974), 179
Children, consent and, 230–231
  malpractice suits by, 402
  research on, consent to, 187–188
  suits against parents by, 402
Civil law, 69
  compared to criminal law, 81
  "wrong" in, 301
Civil rights, 324–328
Civil Rights Act (1964), 326
Civil Rights Act (1991), 325
Claims-made policies, malpractice insurance, 123, 124, 125
Clayton Act (1915), 331
Cloning, zygotes, 376
Code of Federal Regulations, 85, 92

Codefendants, and contribution, 136
Code of Hammurabi, 69–70
Codes of ethics, 26–37
  and values, 26–27
  compared to codes of conduct, 26
  competence reflected by, 30–32
  major concerns of, 28
  nursing, historical view of, 28
  Preambles to, selected codes, 29–30
  professional versus nonprofessional ethics and, 26
  purpose of, 26–27
  use of "should" in, 29
  values reflected in, 30–37, 340–341
  versus law, 27, 29, 30
  violations of, 27–28
  writers of, 27
Collective bargaining, in units, 329
  legal aspects of, 328–329
  nurses and, 329–330
Collectivism, as philosophy, 44–45
Colloquium, 174
Commission on Graduates of Foreign Nursing School (CGFNS) exam, 199
Commitment, 236
Common law, statutes and, 82. *See also* Case law.
Communism, as philosophy, 44
Comparative negligence, 120
  meaning of, 122–123
Competence, 30, 212–214. *See also* Incompetent patients.
  and advance directives, 242–243
  and freedom, 431
  and living wills, 245–246
  assessment of, 213
  compared to performance, 213
  meaning of, 212
  referred to in codes of ethics, 30–32
Computer documentation, 154
Confidentiality, 3, 27, 351–358
  and employee assistance professionals, 356
  and HIV/AIDS, 355–356
  and medical records, 353–354
  and National Practitioner Data Bank, 354
  as value, 339–340
  doctor-patient privilege and, 156
  importance of, 352
  in codes of ethics, 34–35, 352–353
  legal aspects of, 355–357
  privileged communication and, 357–358
Conflict, ethical, 37–40
  professional, sources of, 24
Conscience clauses, abortion procedures and, 397
  problems of, 450
Consent, 222–240
  and autonomy, 223
  and do not resuscitate (DNR) orders, 437
  and incompetent patients, 232–234

Consent *(continued)*
  and minors, 230–231
  as defense, 119–120, 166, 170, 172, 176, 223
  basic rule in, 223
  for organ donation, 265–267
  incompetent refusal in, 237
  informed consent in, 229–230
  leaving against medical advice as, 235–236
  nurse responsibility for, 224–225
  proxy decision makers in, 237–241
  refusal of treatment as, 234–235
  state statutes of, 232–234
  versus express, 225, 226–227
  versus implied, 227–229
Consent to research, 187–189
  and children, 187–188
  and incompetent patients, 188–189
Constitution (U.S.), rights enumerated in, 75–76
Constitutions, as law, 72
Construct, word *ethics* as, 14
Continuing Education (CE), mandatory, 90–91, 209–212
Continuity of care, and documentation, 153
Contraception, 379–383
  Norplant as, 381–382
  overpopulation problem and, 380–382
Contracts, 341–350
  as covenants not to compete, 345–346
  as guidelines for nurses, 349–350
  components of, 343
  employment "at will" and, 346–349
  essence of, 342
  for nurse/patient, 342–343
  requirements for enforcement of, 344
  spoken and written, 343, 344
Contribution, meaning of, 136
Contributory negligence, 120
  and strict liability, 130
  meaning of, 122
Conversion, as intentional torts, 172
Convoy, Clair, 460
Cost, in illness care market, 314–316
Courage, as Platonic ideal, 43
Court of appeals, 97–98
Covenants not to compete, 345–346
  enforceability of, 346
  rationale for, 345–346
CPR. *See* Cardiopulmonary resuscitation (CPR).
Crack-addicted babies, 401–402
Credentialing, as nonlegal credentialing, 196. *See also* Licensure.
  nurse autonomy and, 285
Crime, reporting injuries from, 182
Criminal law, 69, 79–80
  and nurses, 80
  basis of, 79, 80
  compared to civil law, 81

procedure in, 80–81
  "wrong" in, 301
Cruzan case, 44, 74, 235, 240, 245, 246, 455–458, 460
  and Danforth amendment, 254
  and right to refuse treatment, 457–458
  details of, 455–458
  nurse actions in, 240
Customs, as ethics, 40
Cystic fibrosis, 375

D

Damages, as "non-compensatory," 117–118
  as punitive, 125–126
  in malpractice cases, 117–118
  mitigation by plaintiff, 117
Danforth amendment. *See* Patient Self-Determination Act.
Database, BIOETHICS as, 12
  of law library, 99
Death. *See also* Dying.
  brain, 461, 466
  by assisted suicide, 472–473
  by euthanasia, 473–475, 479–482
  by suicide, 477–479
  causation of intent in, 475–477
  changes in definition of, 16, 461, 464–466
  definition of persistent vegetative state, 462 464
  higher brain, 465, 467
  intentionally caused, 467
  lawsuits after, 132
  legal aspects of, 475–477
  pain control and, 482–484
Deceit, misrepresentation, 177–178
Decision making, ethical, 61–66
Declaration of Independence (U.S.), 46
Deduction, in idealist thought, 43
Defamation, 9, 173–175
  as libel, written, 174
  as slander, 174
  defense to, 175
  examples of, 174–175
  meaning of, 174
Defective technology, 148
Defense of property, as defense, 173
Defensive medicine, 142
Defining Issues Test (DIT), 55
Dehydrating to death, 443–460, 474–475
  and competent patients, 459–460
  and living will statutes, 246–247
  and nondying patients, 444–451
  and retraining to oral feeding first, 443–444
  Bland case as, 445
  Busalacchi case as, 446, 458–459
  Cruzan case as, 240, 246, 455–458, 460
  decision making in, 452–455, 460

nurse participation in, 6, 445–451
O'Connor case as, 459
untreatable infants and, 179–180
Demand, in illness care market, 314–316
Deontology, ethical system of, 45
Dependent persons, abuse of, 180–181
Depositions, 95
Depression, and suicide, 478
Descartes, René, 44, 47
Determinism, philosophy of, 48
Dialysis, 16
   and advance directives, 257
   in Great Britain, 6
   universal access to, 311–312
Dignity, losses to, 9
Discovery, case law process, 95
Discrimination, 302–303
   age-based, 327
   in employment, 321, 323–327
   pregnancy-based, 326–327
   punishment for, 302
   race/national origin-based, 325
   religion-based, 325
   sex-based, 325
DNR. *See* Do not resuscitate (DNR).
Doctor-patient privilege, meaning of, 156
Doctors, education of, 20–21
Documentation, 151–157
   and continuity of care, 153
   and licensure law, 151–152
   and malpractice law, 152–153
   and reimbursement/accreditation, 153
   by computer, 154
   guidelines for, 153–156
   incident reports as, 156
   nurse notes as, 157
   standard for, 151
Do no harm. *See* Non-maleficence.
Do not resuscitate (DNR), 241, 436–439
   and type of condition, 437
   as futility issue, 437–438
   compared to living will, 258–259
   during surgery, 437
   family consent and, 437
   nurse reaction to, 437
   proposed policy for, 438–439
Dörfel, Emmy, 469
Down's syndrome, 394
   and abortion, 16
Drug abuse, discipline for, 201
Drug Enforcement Administration (DEA),
   numbers for mid-level practitioners, 287
Drug reactions, adverse, reporting of, 362
Drug testing, 321–322
   ethical issues in, 322
   situations for, 322
Due process, 81, 89–91
   and investigation by licensing board, 204
   as substantive process, 90–91
   as procedural process, 89–90

meaning of, 81
nurses' right to, 81
source of, 89
Dumping of patients, 140–141. *See also* Anti-
   dumping.
   motive for, 183
   remedies for, 184
Durable power of attorney (DPA), 9, 245,
   249–260
   and incompetent patient, 251–252
   nurse questions about, 262
   sample form for, 252–253
   springing, 260, 267
Duty, as deontological view, 45
   for nurses, 113
   in malpractice, 111–112
   meaning of, 111
   no duty, as defense, 121
Duty to inform, and whistle-blowing, 362–363
Dying, and cost of care, 423–425
   and incompetence, 431–434
   and old people, 413–415
   and quality of life, 426–431
   as term for end of life, 416
   CPR and, 435–436
   dehydration to death in, 443–460
   do not resuscitate (DNR) and, 436–439
   risk probability and, 420–422
   withholding treatment and, 439–443

E

Economics of illness care. *See* Illness care
   market.
Education, of professionals, 20–21. *See also*
   Nurse education.
Efficiency, of ethical behavior, 4–5
Egalitarians, 303
Elderly, views of, 415
Emergencies, and anti-dumping, 183–184
   Good Samaritan statutes and, 138–139
   implied consent in, 228–229, 233
Emergency Medical Transfer and Active La-
   bor Act (EMTALA), 183
Emotion, and decision making, 39
   and ethical conflict, 38–40
Emotional distress, and negligent infliction,
   171
   and transferred intent, 171
   in medical context, 170–171
   infliction of, 9, 170–171
   meaning of, 171
Emotivism, philosophy of, 38, 39, 49
Employer policies, and professionals, 24–25
Employer/employee conflicts, 22–23
Employment "at will," 346–349
   ethical factors in, 347–348
   exceptions to, 348–349, 363
   nature of, 346–347

Employment discrimination, 321,
323–327
and disabled, 323–324
Employment relationship, "at will,"
346–349
Employment status, independent contractors versus employees, 318–320
Encyclopedia of Bioethics, 17
End-Stage Renal Disease (ESRD) program,
311–312
Enlightenment, as cultural concept, 46, 47
Enterprise liability, 141–143
and HMOs, 142–143
meaning of, 141–142
Entitlements, economic consequences of,
311
effects of, 310–312
ethical issues in, 311–312
meaning of, 74, 75
Environment, threats to and research on,
192
Epicureans, 46–47
Equality in Retirement Income Security Act
(ERISA), 327–328
and health insurance reform, 327–328
Equipment instruction books, and standards of care, 114
Ethical behavior, and codes of ethics, 73
and compliance with law, 4
and instincts, 15
as practical, 5–6
efficiency of, 4–5
in statutes, 73
Ethical conflict, 37–40
and emotion, 38–40
and self-interest, 38
Ethical decision making, and fear of courts,
65–66
and values assessment for nurses, 64
ethical problem in, 61–62
medical aspects in, 62
outside information approach, 62
stop/look/listen process in, 63–65
Ethical duty, and relationship to legal duty, 6
to care as, 5
Ethicists, and decision making. *See* Ethical
decision making.
role of, 60–61
Ethics. *See also* Codes of ethics; Nursing
ethics.
and origin of word, 40
and public opinion, 74
and religion, 41
and use of term, 52
as basis of law, 3, 8
as construct, 14
codes of, 26–37
compared to law, 3–4, 5, 68, 71
contextual, 56
customs and, 40

feminist moral philosophy in, 56–57
historical view of, 15–16
major publications on, 12, 66–67
narrative, 56
professional versus nonprofessional, 26
teaching of, 60–61
to law, a continuum, 50–51
Ethics committees, 58–60
activities of, 58–59
as ethics courts, 59
criticisms of, 59
historical view of, 18
in research, 60
institutional review boards as, 60
lawsuit against, 59
members of, 58
Ethics information, centers of ethics study,
12, 66
major publications on ethics, 12, 66–67
Ethics for Modern Nurses (Densford and
Millard), 18
Ethics test(s), Defining Issues Test (DIT) as,
55
Judgments About Nursing Decisions
(JAND) as, 55
Eugenics, 372, 375–376
and cloning, 376
as pre-pregnancy procedure, 375–376
Euthanasia, 473–475, 479–482
active/passive, 473
Australian nurse attitudes on, 480
by dehydration, 474–475
direct/indirect, 473
impact of, for nurses, 76
in Holland, 479, 481–482
in 1930s Germany, 468–472
nurse participation in, 6, 16
opinion poll on, 16
voluntary/involuntary, 473
Euthanasia Society of America, 241–242, 257
Evidence in court cases, 95–96
beyond a reasonable doubt, 456, 457
clear and convincing, 456
preponderance of, 456
Execution, in prison system, 6
Executive branch, laws of, 72
Existentialism, philosophy of, 47
Expert witness, nurse as, guidelines for,
96
Express consent, 225, 226–227
spoken, 227
written, 226–227

F

Fair Labor Standards Act (1938), 320–321
Fairness. *See* Justice.
False imprisonment, 9, 167–170
defense to, 170

in medical context, 168, 169
  meaning of, 167–168
Family and Medical Leave Act (1993), 332–333
Father, and his interests in abortion, 399
Federal law, sources for locating laws, 85, 86
Federal Register (U.S.), 85, 92
Federal Tort Claims Act, 133–134
Feeding tubes, as means of retraining to oral feeding, 443–444. *See also* Dehydrating to death.
  reimbursement factors and, 444
Feminist ethics, 38
Feminist moral philosophy, 56–57
  caring ethic as, 56–57
  definition of, 56
  highest values in, 56
Feminist views, of moral development, 53–54
  of reproductive technology, 383
Fetal tissue research, 410–411
Fetal-protection policies, 326–327
Fetus, in abortion discussion, 386, 389–391
Fidelity, 3
  and managed care patient, 350–351
  as truth telling, 358–360
  as whistle-blowing, 360–364
  confidentiality and, 339–340, 351–358
  in codes of ethics, 32–33, 35–36, 340–341
  in contracts, 341–350
  in employment law, 341
  loyalty as, 339
  meaning of, 338–340
Fifth Amendment (U.S. Constitution), 305, 345
  and due process, 89, 90, 204
  rights of, 75, 81
Final Exit (Humphrey), 478
Finders' fees, for research subjects, 191
Food and Drug Administration (FDA), medical devices regulation and, 184
Foreign nursing schools, graduates of, examination for, 199
Fourteenth Amendment (U.S. Constitution), 305, 345, 399
  and due process, 89, 90, 204
  and right to refuse treatment, 457
  rights under, 75, 76
Fraud, and nurse autonomy, 284
  misrepresentation as, 177–178
Fraudulent concealment, 137
Freedom. *See* Autonomy.
Free speech, and truth telling, 359–360
Freudian theory, philosophical basis of, 46
Futile treatment, 9, 289–293
  and competent patient, 292
  and DNR, 437–438
  and incompetent patient, 292–293
  example of, 291
  meaning of, 289–290

G

General intent, meaning of, 164
Genetic defects, and abortion, 393–395
Germany (1993), 392
Germany (c. 1935–1945), 468–470
  euthanasia program in, 468–472
  forced sterilization in, 395, 400
  killing of defectives in, 427, 471
  nurses' participation in, 18, 28, 51, 164
  research experiments of, 186
Gilligan, C., on moral development and justice, 53–54
Golden Rule, 44
Golden rule (Sagan's), 41
Good Samaritan statutes, 111, 138–139
  and nurses' liability, 138–139
  meaning of, 138
Governmental immunity, 134
Guidelines, and tort reform, 140–141

H

Health maintenance organizations (HMOs), lawsuits against, 142–143
Health-Related Quality of Life, 428
Hedonism, 46–47
Helga Wanglie, In re., case, 291
HIV/AIDS, 270–278
  and protection under Americans with Disabilities Act, 274–275
  and tuberculosis, 276–278
  as autonomy issue, 270
  confidentiality in, 355–356
  nurses' fear of, 271–272
  patients' fear of, from nurse, 273–274
  prevention of, education for, 276
  reporting of, 182
  statistics related to, 275–276
Hobbes, Thomas, 43
Holland, euthanasia in, 479, 481–482
Honesty, in codes of ethics, 33–34
"Hospice Six," case, 203
Humanism, philosophy of, 47
Hume, David, 49
Humphrey, Derek, 478
Huntington's disease, 251
Hysterectomy, 140

I

Idealism, 43–46
  philosophical concepts related to, 43–46
Illness care market, 307–317
  cost controls in, 310
  cost in, 314–316
  demand in, 314–316
  historical view of, 307–308

Illness care market *(continued)*
  legal entitlements in, effects of, 310–312
  monopsony in, 309
  myths about, 316–317
  nurse attitudes toward, 312–313
  nursing economics of, 313–317
  supply in, 314–316
Immunity, charitable, 133
  intrafamily, 132–133
  qualified, 181
  sovereign, 133–134
Implied consent, 227–229
  by patient action, 227–228
  in emergency, 228–229, 233
  patient, information waived by, 228
Inception statutes, 94
Incident reports, 156
  privilege for, 156
  purpose of, 156
Incompetent patients, 431–434
  and consent, 232–234
  and consent to research, 188–189
  and decisional capacity, 433
  and durable power of attorney, 251–252
  and loss of rights, 251
  determination of competency guidelines
    for, 234
  futile treatment of, 292–293
  incapacitated, use of terms, 432
  legal actions related to, 434
  stigma attached to, 432
  treatment for, refusal of, 235, 237, 248
Indemnity, 136
  meaning of, 136
Independent contractors, 318–320
  Internal Revenue Service (IRS) determi-
    nants of, 320
  nurse/agency relationship and, 319
Indexes, legal, 87
Indictment, process of, 80
Individualism, factors related to, 41
  philosophy of, 47
Induction, as reasoning method, 48–49
Infant Care Review committees, 180
Infanticide, 16, 387, 388
  examples of, 388
  of females, 388, 395
Infections, 148
Information, ethics, centers of, 12, 66
Informative model, of practitioner-patient re-
  lationships, 108
Informed consent, 10, 229–230
  and truth telling, 359
  for noncompliant patients, 137
  standards for, 229–230
Injury, damages in, 117–118
  in malpractice, 116–118
  no injury as defense in, 121
Innuendo, 174
Instinctive values, 15

Institutional licensure, 214–215
  benefits of, 215
Institutional Review Boards (IRBs), 60
  and research, 186–190
  review of quality assurance projects by,
    190
Insurance, malpractice, under employer,
  123–124
Intent, as general, 164
  as specific, 164–165
  as transferred, 165
  compared to motive, 165
  to cause death, 475
Intentional torts, 110, 120, 164–173
  compared to negligent torts, 165
  conversion in, 172
  defenses to, 172–173
  emotional distress in, infliction of, 170–
    171
  for assault, 167
  for battery, 166
  for false imprisonment, 167–170
  for trespass to chattels, 171
  for trespass to land, 171
Intentionally injured adults, 181
Interests, 399–411
  child's, 401–405
  father's, 399
  mother's, 399–401
International Council of Nurses (ICN), 18
Interrogatories, 95
Intrafamily immunity, 132–133
Intrauterine device (IUD), 396
Intuitionism, philosophy of, 39–40, 49
Invasion of privacy, 9, 175–177
  defense to, 176
  in medical context, 176
  statutes on, 177
In vitro fertilization, 10, 373–375
  as ova frozen for later use, 374
  legal aspects of, 374–375
  procedure in, 373–374
Iron rule (Sagan's), 41

J

John, King of England, 70
Joint Commission on the Accreditation of
  Health Organizations (JCAHO)
  and standards of care, 114, 115
  mandate for ethics mechanism of, 58
Joint and several liability, 134–126
  concept of, 134–135
  contribution and indemnity in, 136
Journals, and standards of care, 116
Judeo-Christian religion, 40–41
Judgments About Nursing Decisions
  (JAND), 55
Judicial branch, laws of, 72

Jury, selection of, 95
Jus talionis, 80
Justice, 3, and illness care market, 307–317
  as nursing value, 54–55
  as Platonic ideal, 43
  civil rights as, 324–328
  compared to justice, 301
  distributive, 303, 304–305
  drug testing as, 321–322
  Gilligan's theory of, 53–54
  Knowledgeable Position (Rawls's) on, 306
  Kohlberg's concept of, 52
  labor law under, 317–321, 328–334. *See also* Americans with Disabilities Act (ADA).
  meaning of, 9–10, 300–302
  Original Position (Rawls's) on, 305–306
  social, 9–10, 304–305, 306
  theories of, 303–306

K

Kafka, Helene, 469
Kaiserwerth, 17, 41
Kant, Immanuel, 44, 78, 80, 220, 221
Kevorkian, Jack, 480
Kohlberg's moral development theory, 52–53
  and ethics of nurse-women, 54–56
  criticism of, 53–54
  stages of, 53
Kutner, Luis, 242

L

Labor law(s), 317–321, 328–334
  anti-discrimination, 322–328
  anti-trust, 330–332
  Fair Labor Standards Act (1938) as, 320–321
  Family and Medical Leave Act (1993) as, 332–333
  for nurses as independent contractors, 318–320
  information on, sources of, 334
  National Labor Relations Act (1935) as, 328–330
  necessity of, 318
  Occupational Safety and Health Act (OSHA) (1970) as, 333
  work-related offenses in, contacts for, 317–318
  worker compensation, 333–334
Laissez-faire philosophy, 41
Law(s), 49–51
  administrative, 69, 91–93
  and behavior, 49, 50
  and constitutions, 72

and due process, 81, 89–91
and power, of lawmaking, 78
and religion, 40, 70
and rights, 74–78
basis of, ethics as, 3, 8
case, 69, 72, 93–99
civil, 69
compared to ethics, 3–4, 68, 71
criminal, 69, 79–80
enforcement of, 50–51
ethics/law continuum and, 50–51
historical view of, 69
lawmaking process and, 83
lobbying for, effects of, 73–74, 84
negative, 71
nursing, 70–71
philosophies of, 68–69
procedural, 69
regulations, 72, 88–89
rules of, 88–89
statute, 69, 72, 82–88
subject of, divisions in, 69
substantive, 69
written, 72
Lawsuits, and documentation, 151–157. *See also* Malpractice defenses; Tort law.
  and steps to take when sued, 149
  common reasons for, 148
  immunities from, 132–134
  law resulting from, 72
  nurse actions leading to, 147
  prevention of, 147–148
  statistical information about, 144–145
  statutes of limitation on, 136–137
  survival of, 131–132
  versus alternative dispute resolution (ADR), 145–146
  witness to, guidelines for, 149–151
Lawyers, attorney fee reform and, 140
  contingency fee for, 117
  number of in U.S., 99
League of Women Voters, as information source, 83, 85
Leaving against medical advice, 235–236
  nurse actions in, 236
  release in, 236
Legal duty, relationship to ethical duty, 6
  to care as, 6
Legal Research: How to Find and Understand the Law (Elias), 93
Legislative branch, laws of, 72
Leprosy, 464
Libel, meaning of, 174
Libertarians, 303
Library, locating laws in, 85, 86, 92
Licensure, 192–215
  alternatives to, 214
  and boards of nursing, 200
  and competence, 212–213
  and nurse autonomy, 284–285

Licensure *(continued)*
    as discipline to a license, 200–201
    as due process in investigations, 204
    as legal credentialing, 197–198
    as mandatory and permissive, 197
    board decisions in, contestng, 202–204
    common provisions of, 198–201
    compared to certification, 197
    contacting state authority for, 193
    effects of, 194–196
    examinations for, 199
    exemptions from, 199
    institutional, 214–215
    liabilities of, 204–205
    mandatory CE rule in, 90–91, 209–212
    minimum qualifications for, 198
    nurse education for, entry level, 208–209
    purposes of, 192–194
    reciprocity in, 199
    record of, 205–206
Licensure law, 9, 15
    and Americans with Disabilities Act
      (ADA), 324
    and documentation, 151–152
Life, abortion and, 383–399
    artificial insemination and, 371–373
    birth issues in, 400–410
    contraception and, 379–383
    eugenics and, 375–376
    in vitro fertilization and, 373–375
    interests in, 399–411
    surrogate motherhood and, 376–379
    value of, 3, 10, 27, 368–369
Life expectancy, meaning of, 417–418
Life span, average, 419
    meaning of, 418–419
    myths about, 419–420
Life support termination, decision making
    in, 452–455
    dehydration to death as, 443–460
    meaning of, 441
    myths about, 442–443
    Quinlan case on, 453
Limiting treatment, decision makers about,
    290–291
    meaning of, 248
Living will statutes, 76, 242, 245, 246
Living wills, 9, 244–249
    and competency, 245–246
    and noncompliance by practitioners, 256–
      257
    as refusal of treatment for incompetent, 248
    compared to DNR orders, 258–259
    economic factors in, 259–260
    information sources on, 249
    nurse questions about, 262
    specificity of, 248–249
    specific provisions of, 244–247
    spoken directives as, 247–248
    withdrawal of food/water under, 246–247

    written directives as, 247
Lobbying, 83–84
    and changes in law, 73–74, 84
Locked-in syndrome, 462
Loss of chance, 119
Low birth weight infants, 404, 407–408
    among African-Americans, 403, 404
    and disabilities, 407–408
    as mortality risk predictor, 406
    as *very* low, CPR for, 405–406
    cross-cultural view of, 403–404
Loyalty, conflicts in, 339
    in codes of ethics, 33–34

M

Magna Carta, 70, 93
Malicious prosecution, 177
    proof in, 177
Malpractice, 9, 108–123
    and documentation, 152–153
    causation in, 118–119
    coverage under employer, 123–124
    for breach of standard of care, 112–116
    duty in, 111–112
    historical view of, 109
    injury in, 116–118
    problems with system of, 145
Malpractice defense, 120–122
    arguing in the alternative as, 120
    comparative negligence as, 122–123
    contributory negligence as, 122
    no breach of standard of care as, 121
    no causation as, 121
    no duty as, 121
    no injury as, 121
Malpractice hearing officers, 146
Malpractice insurance, 123–126
    claims-made policies as, 123, 124, 125
    coverage under employer as, 123–124
    noncoverage for criminal acts in, 126
    noncoverage of punitive damage in, 125–
      126
    occurrence policies as, 123, 124
    tail coverage in, 125
    umbrella policy as, 125
Maltreatment prohibitions, 178–182
    abuse of dependent person in, 180–181
    child abuse in, 179–180
    intentionally injured adults in, 181
    reporting statutes of, 182
Managed care, and nurse duty to patient,
    350–351
    and use of term, 316
    as limits on care, 350
Mandatory Continuing Education (MCE),
    90–91, 209–212
    challenges to law of, 211
    purpose of, 209, 210

Maryland Health Care Decisions Act (1993), 246, 247
Materialism, philosophy of, 48
Mediation, process of, 145
Medicaid, beginning of, 308
  minimum fee for, doctor acceptance of, 204–205
Medical devices, legal aspects of, 184
Medical neglect, definition of, 408
Medical records, and confidentiality, 353–354
Medicare, anti-kickback provision in, 284
  assignmnet (payment) of, 84
  average market price of, 309–310
  beginning of, 308
  fraud in, 80
  Relative Value Rating Base System (RVRBS) for, 310
Medication, errors in, 148
Medications, administration of recording of, 5
Medwatch, 362
Mentally ill, consent from, 228. *See also* Incompetent patients.
Metaphysics, meaning of, 40
Mexican-Americans, pregnant, treatment of, 404
Michael H. v. Gerald D., case, 399
Mill, John Stuart, 8, 48, 220, 221, 304
Minors, and consent, 230–231
  consent of, to research, 187–188
  mature/emancipated, 231
Misrepresentation, 177–178
  in medical context, 177–178
Monetary interests, in codes of ethics, 35
Monopoly, meaning of, 309
Monopsony, and Medicare/Medicaid, 308
  meaning of, 308, 309
Moore, John, 190
Moral development, 6, 52–54
  Gilligan's theory of, 53–54
  Kohlberg's theory of, 52–53
Moral imperatives, 11, 51
Moral principles, types of, 3
Moral reasoning, justice-based, 54–55
  meaning of, 52
Morals, 51–52
Motive, compared to intent, 165

N

Narrative ethics, 56
National Institutes of Health (NIH) Revitalization Act (1993), 189
National Labor Relations Act (1935), 328–330
  nurse bargaining under, 329–330
  provisions of, 328–329
National Organ Transplant Act (1984), 268

National Practitioner Data Bank, 206–207
  and confidentiality, 354
Natural law, 11
  and founding fathers, 46
  as philosophical view, 46
  elements of, 10
  nature of, 68
NCLEX (licensure test), 197, 199
Necessity, as defense, 173
Neglect, as child abuse, 180
  medical, definition of, 408
Negligence, comparative, 122–123
  contributory, 122
  compared to intentional torts, 165
  in patient fall lawsuit, 94–97
  in tort law, 110
  per se, 115–116
Negligence law, components of, 110
Neonates, 10, 405–410
  CPR for, 405–406
  low birth weight, 404, 407–408
  survival probability of, 406–407
  withholding treatment for, 408–410
Nightingale, Florence, 17, 21, 41, 280
Ninth Amendment (U.S. Constitution), 75
Noble Savage, 45
Non-maleficence, 3, 27
  and licensure, 192–215
  and medical devices, 184
  anti-dumping and, 182–184
  in codes of ethics, 30
  in intentional torts, 164–173
  in maltreatment prohibitions, 178–182
  in quasi-intentional torts, 173–178
  in research, 185–192
  meaning of, 9, 162–163
Noncompensatory damages, 117–118
Norplant, 381–382, 402
"Notes for Nurses" (Nightingale), 21, 280
Nurse autonomy, 279–293
  and credentialing, 285
  and fraud, 284
  and licensure, 284–285
  and negligence liability, 286–287
  and participation in assisted suicide, 293
  and prescriptions, 287–288
  and relationship to patient autonomy, 288–289
  economic factors in, 281–283
  historical view of, 280–283
  to withhold futile treatment, 289–293
Nurse education, as standard for practicing, 207–208
  entry level, for licensure, 208–209
  levels of, 209
  Mandatory Continuing Education (MCE) in, 209–212
  standardization of, 208
  with master's degree, 285
Nurse notes, as documentation, 157

Nurse organizations, lobbying of, 73–74
Nurse practitioners (NPs), 279
Nursing, compared to medicine, 440–441
Nursing ethics, as basic professional values, 3, 8–10, 14
  as moral reasoning of nurses, 54–56
  caring ethic in, 56–57
  historical view of, 16–18
  in younger versus older nurses, 55
  JAND ethics test, 55
  reasons for study of, 13–14
  Nursing Ethics for Hospital and Private Use (Robb), 18
Nursing law, development of, 70–71
  relationship to nursing ethics, 71
Nutrition, withholding, living will statute on, 246–247. *See also* Dehydrating to death.

O

Oaths, and ethical principles, 28
Occupational health nurses, and confidentiality, 356
Occupational Safety and Health Act (OSHA) (1970), 333
  on universal precautions, 275
  purposes of, 333
Occurrence policies, malpractice insurance, 123, 124
Oligopoly, meaning of, 309
Opening statements, at trial, 95
Opinion, case law process, 97
Organization, of professions/professionals, 19–20
Organ transplantation. *See* Transplants.
Outside information approach, ethical decision making in, 62

P

Pain control, 482–484
  insufficient medication in, reasons for, 483
  nurse goals in, 483–484
Partial codes, 435
Paternalism, 107–108
  meaning of, 107–108
Patient Self-Determination Act (1990), 59, 242, 253–255
  compliance with, 255
  development of, reasons for, 254255
  intent of, 254
  requirements of, 253–254
Peer review, historical view of, 21
Pellegrino, Edmund, 13
Perceived Quality of Life (PQOL), 428
Performance, assessment of, 213
  compared to competence, 213

Persistent vegetative state (PVS), 416
  age and prognosis in, 462
  as definition of death, 462–464
  characteristics of, 462
  cost of care in, 463
  decisions about termination of treatment in, 464
  declaring dead in, implications of, 464, 465–465
  misdiagnosis of, 463
  patients in, as research subjects, 189
  recovery from, 463
Philosophy, ethics as subject of, 42
  idealism as, 43–46
  intuitionism as, 49
  meaning of word, 40
  realism as, 46–49
Physical restraint, as false imprisonment, 168–170
Physician assistants, 280, 282
Planned Parenthood, 380
Planned Parenthood v. Casey, 391
Plato, 16, 43, 109, 387, 388, 478
Poland, abortion laws in, 392
Policies, employer, 24–25
Population control, and contraception, 380–382
Positivism, philosophy of, 49
Positivist law, nature of, 68
Postconventional reasoning, 53
Power of attorney, durable, 9, 245, 249–260
  springing, 260
Practicality, of ethical behavior, 5–6
Preconventional reasoning, 53
Pregnancy Discrimination Act (1978), 326–327, 401
Pregnant women, in research studies, 189–190
Prenatal testing, and abortion, 393–395
Prescription writing, and nurse autonomy, 287–288
Prison system, execution and, legal power of, 6
Privileged communication, 357–358
  exceptions to, 358
  meaning of, 357
Procedural due process, 89–90
Procedural law, 69
Products liability, 131
  illness care products/services in, 131
  satisfaction and release in, 131
Professional misconduct, 200–201
  examples of, 201
Professions/professionals, altruism of, 22
  and employer policies, 24–25
  codes of ethics of, 26–37
  conflicts among, sources of, 24
  education/training of, 20–21
  elements of, 19
  employed, conflicts of, 22–23

image of, 19
organization of, 19–20
review of, 21
self-interests and work interests of, 25–26
Promissory estoppel, 347–348
Property rights, 75
Protocols, and standards of care, 114
Proxy decision makers, accuracy of decisions of, 239–240
  consent by, 237–241
  if lack of guardian, nurse actions, 238–239
  proxy decisions versus practitioner decisions under, 239–240
Psychological General Well Being (PGWB), 428
Public opinion, and ethics, 74

Q

Quadriplegics, dehydrating to death, 460
Qualified immunity from liability, 181
Quality Adjusted Life Years (QUALYs), 427–428
Quality assurance projects, review issue, 190
Quality improvement programs, and standards of care, 114
Quality of life, 369, 426–431
  and futile treatment, 292–293
  and Nazi Germany, 426–427
  assessment of, 62
  definitions of, 429
  ethical issues related to, 429–431
Quality of Life Improvement Scale (QLIS), 429
Quality of life measures, by Acute Physical Assessment and Chronic Health Evaluation (APACHE), 428
  by Health-Related Quality of Life, 428
  by Perceived Quality of Life (PQOL), 428
  by Psychological General Well Being (PGWB), 428
  by Quality Adjusted Life Years (QUALYs), 427–428
  by Quality of Life Improvement Scale (QLIS), 429
  by Sickness Impact Profile (SIP), 428
  in benefit-burden analysis, 429
Quasi-intentional torts, 110, 173–178
  defamation in, 173–175
  invasion of privacy in, 175–177
  malicious prosecution in, 177
  misrepresentation in, 177–178
Quinlan case, 58, 74, 453, 456

R

Race, discrimination based on, 325
Rational basis test, 205
Rawls, John, 305–306

Realism, 46–49
  philosophical concepts related to, 46–49
Reasoning, conventional, 53
  deductive, 43
  inductive, 48–49
  moral, 52, 53
Reciprocity, licensure, 199
Records, of licensure, 205–206. *See also* Documentation.
Refusal of treatment, 234–235
  by incompetents, 235, 237
Registration laws, 197, 198
Regulations, 88–89
  as over-regulation, 91
  changes to, 73
  development of, 72, 88
  finding, sources of, 85, 92–93
  functions of, 88
Reimbursement, and documentation, 153
Relative Value Rating Base System, 310
Release, and leaving against medical advice, 236
Religion, 40–41
  and ethics, 41
  and idealism (Christian) of, 45
  and law, 40, 70
  and values (Christian) from, 41, 45
  as limit on behavior, 11
  discrimination based on, 325
Reporting of disease, 182
  caution related to, 182
  rule for, 182
Reproduction technology, artificial insemination, 371–373
  fear of, 382–383
  in vitro fertilization as, 374–375
Research, 185–192
  aborted fetuses in, 410
  animals in research, 191–192
  consent to, 187–189
  environmental risks in, 192
  ethics committees in, 60
  finders' fees for subjects of, 191
  issues related to, 185–186
  on pregnant women, 189–190
  on women, 189
  quality assurance projects as, 190
  tissue ownership issue in, 190–191
Res ipsa loquitur, 118, 119
  meaning of, 118, 119
Respondeat superior, 142
  meaning of, 127
Retirement plans, federal pension law, 327–328
Retribution, right of, 80
Right to die, 76–77
  and Constitution (U.S.), 76
  and *Cruzan* case, 76, 455–458
  and incompetent patients, 251–252
  and living wills, 244–249

Right of liberty, and court opinions, 76
and right to refuse treatment, 76–77
Right of privacy, and abortion, 76
Right to refuse treatment, 76
and right to liberty, 76–77
basis of, 457–458
Rights, 74–78
constitutional, 75–76
in decisions by courts versus legislatures, 77–78
legal definition of, 75
meaning of, 75
Risk probability, 420–422
Robb, Elizabeth Hampton, 18
Roe v. Wade, 385, 388, 389, 392
Rojas, Hector, 460
Role model statement, in codes of ethics, 37
Roman Catholic Church, on artificial insemination, 373
on in vitro fertilization, 374
on suicide, 478
Roman civil law, 70
Romanticism, 45
Rousseau, Jean-Jacques, 45
RU486, 397
Rules, 88–89
development of, 88
Sagan's, 41
Rust v. Sullivan, 398–399

S

Safe Medical Devices Act (1990), 184, 362
Sagan, Carl, 41
Salary, of nurses, 214
Sanger, Margaret, 380
Sartre, Jean-Paul, 47
Self-defense, as defense, 172
Self-employed, payor-practitioner relationship, 23
Self-insured plans, 328
Self-interest, and ethical conflict, 38
combined with work interests, 25–26
types of, 22
Sermchief v. Gonzales, 287
Services, in products liability, 131
Seventh Amendment (U.S. Constitution), 140
Sex discrimination, 325, 326
Sexual harassment, forms of, 325
Sherman Act, 330, 331
Sickness Impact Profile (SIP), 428
Silver rule (Sagan's), 41
Sisters of St. John's House, 17
Sixth Amendment (U.S Constitution), 363
Slander, meaning of, 174
Slow codes, 435
SOAPIE method, 154
Socialism, as philosophy, 44
Socialized medicine, 308

Social justice, 9–10, 304–305
application of, 306–307
meaning of, 9, 304
in moral development theories, 52, 53–54
Society, in codes of ethics, 36–37
Society for Right to Die, 242
Sonograms, 393–394
Sovereign immunity, 133–134
Specific intent, meaning of, 164–165
Sperm bank, 372
Staffing, unsafe, 128
Standards of care, breach of. *See* Breach of standard of care.
case examples of, 115
sources for, 113, 114–116
Standing orders, and standards of care, 114
State, use of term, 411
State nurse association, method for contacting, 19
States, lawmaking by, 78
rights in, and medical lawmaking by, 76–77
State statutes, analysis of, guidelines for 97–98
consent, 232–234
importance of, to nurses, 83
sources of, finding, 85–87
Statute law, 69
Statute of limitations, 136–139
time limit for suit and, 137
Statutes, 82–88
administrative procedure acts as, 90
annotated and non-annotated, 86–87
as standards of care, 115–116
changes to, 73
examples of, 82
federal or state, determination of, 85
formulation of, 72
pros/cons of, 82
sources of, finding, 85–87
state, importance to nurses, 83
Steppe, Hilde, 469, 470
Sterilization, forced, 395, 400
of mental defectives, 400
reversible, forced, 402
Stoicism, 44, 46–47
Stop/look/listen, in ethical decision making, 63–65
Strict liability, 129–132
assumption of risk in, 130–131
in ultrahazardous activity, categories of, 129–130
meaning of, 129
non-maleficence and, 163
products liability under, 131
Substance abuse, and addicted newborns, 401–402
reporting of, by colleagues, 357

Substantial factor, 118
Substantive due process, 90–91
Substituted judgment, 452, 454–455
Suicide, 467, 477–479. *See also* Assisted sui-
    cide.
  and autonomy, 279, 477
  and depression, 478
  historical view, 478–479
Supervision, and vicarious liability, 126–129
Supply, in illness care market, 314–316
Surgery, and DNR during, 438
  retained instruments in, 147
Surrogate. *See* Proxy decision makers.
Surrogate motherhood, 10, 376–379
  attitudes of participants in, 378
  court cases on, 377–378
  issues related to, 377, 378
Symmetry, test of life, 390, 467
Syphilis research, 186, 259

T

Tail coverage, malpractice insurance, 125
Teleology, philosophy of, 48
Ten Commandments, 40, 70
Tenth Amendment (U.S. Constitution), 194
Third-party payor (3PP), relationship to pa-
    tient/practitioner, 23–24
Thirteenth Amendment (U.S. Constitution),
    75, 288
Tissue ownership, case example of, 190–191
Todd, Robert Bentley, 17
Tolling the statute, 137
Tortfeasors, 134
Tort law, intentional torts in, 110, 120, 164–
    173
  joint and several liability in, 134–126
  negligence in, 110
  quasi-intentional torts in, 110, 173–178
  strict liability in, 129–132
  vicarious liability in, 126–129
Tort reform, 139–146
  attorney fee reform in, 140
  enterprise liability in, 141–143
  limits on, 140
  related to guidelines, 140–141
Transferred intent, and infliction of emo-
    tional distress, 171
  meaning of, 165
Transplants, 263–269
  agency protocols related to, 265–266
  categories of, 264
  consent to donation for, 265–267
  cost of, 267
  fair allocation of organs for, 268
  from animals, 269
  payment for donors for, 267
  rationing of organs for, 268
  transfusions as, 269

use of body parts for, without consent, 268
Trespass to chattels, 171
Trespass to land, 171
Trial, case law process, 95–96
Truth, as defense, 175
Truth telling, 358–360
  and informed consent, 359
  and law, 359, 360
  risk of, 360
Tuberculosis, HIV/AIDS patients and, 276–
    278
  reactivation of, 277
  reporting of, 182
  transmission of, 277
Tuma case, 202

U

Ultra vires, 88–89
Umbrella policy, malpractice insurance, 125
Unborn, rights of, 402–403
Unions, 328–329
United Nations Universal Declaration of Hu-
    man Rights, 380–381
United Network for Organ Sharing, 268
United States Code Service, 85
Unlicensed assistive personnel (UAPs), 214
Utilitarians, 303
  philosophy of, 47

V

Values, and codes of ethics, 26–27. *See also*
    Ethics.
  and natural law, 10
  assessment of, for nurses, 64
  basic, to teach to young, 8
  Christian, 41
  ethical conflict about, 37–40
  in feminist moral philosophy, 56–57
  in professional nursing, 3, 8–10, 14
  instinctive values, 15
  use of term, 51–52
Veracity, 3
Verdict, 97
Veto, of bill, 83
Viability of fetus, 389–391
Vicarious liability, 126–129
  meaning of, 127
  supervisor responsibility in, 127–129
Virtues, of Plato, 43
Voir dire, 95

W

Wanglie case, 291
Webster case, 389–390
Wellness programs, 324

Whistle-blowing, 10, 360–364
  and child abuse, 408
  as duty to inform, 362–363
  negative consequences of, 361, 363–364
Wills, 241, 243–244
  nurse advice on, 243–244
Withholding treatment, 439–443
  as life support termination, 441
  compared to withdrawing treatment, 439–
    440
  for disabled neonates, 408–410
  general rules for, 439
  myths related to, 442

Witness, guidelines for, 149–151
Women, in research studies, 189–190
Worker compensation, 333–334
  provisions of, 333–334
Written consent, 226–227
Written contracts, 343, 344
Wrongful death suits, 132

Z

Zero population growth, 380